Clinical Assessment Procedures in Physical Therapy

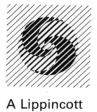

A Lippincott
Physical Therapy Title

Clinical Assessment Procedures in Physical Therapy

M. Lynn Palmer
PH.D., P.T.

Professor
Department of Physical Therapy
Graduate School for Health Studies
Simmons College
Boston, Massachusetts

Marcia E. Epler
M.ED., P.T., A.T.C.

Assistant Professor
Department of Physical Therapy
Temple University
Philadelphia, Pennsylvania

Illustrations by Michael Adams

J. B. Lippincott Company
Philadelphia

Grand Rapids   New York   St. Louis
San Francisco   London   Sydney   Tokyo

Acquisitions Editor: Patricia L. Cleary
Indexer: Barbara Farabaugh
Designer: Anne O'Donnell for Ruttle, Shaw & Wetherill, Inc.
Production: Ruttle, Shaw & Wetherill, Inc.
Compositor: Ruttle, Shaw & Wetherill, Inc.
Printer/Binder: Semline, Inc.

6   5   4   3   2

Library of Congress Cataloging-in-Publication Data

Palmer, M. Lynn.
    Clinical assessment procedures in physical therapy / M. Lynn
Palmer, Marcia E. Epler; illustrations by Michael Adams.
        p. cm.
    Includes bibliographical references.
    ISBN 0-397-54807-9
    1. Physical therapy. 2. Muscle strength—Testing. 3.
Joints—Range of motion—Measurement. I. Epler, Marcia
E. II. Title.
RM701.P35   1990   89-13150
615.8′2—dc20   CIP

The authors and publisher have exerted every effort to ensure
that drug selection and dosage set forth in this text are in
accord with current recommendations and practice at the time
of publication. However, in view of ongoing research, changes
in government regulations, and the constant flow of information relating to drug therapy and drug reactions, the reader is
urged to check the package insert for each drug for any change
in indications and dosage and for added warnings and precautions. This is particularly important when the recommended
agent is a new or infrequently employed drug.

Foreword

For years I have heard students and faculty colleagues grumble about the lack of a comprehensive text for musculoskeletal systems evaluation. To them all I say, here it is. No longer will you need to buy a goniometry text, a muscle testing text, and a clinical tests text. Palmer and Epler have provided a cohesive and readable text that brings together information about physical therapy diagnosis in the musculoskeletal systems into a single, well-organized volume.

Chapter 2 on examination techniques and orthopedic evaluation of synovial joints provides the framework for other kinds of physical therapy evaluation. The book's descriptions of measurement of joint motion (primary and accessory), muscle performance, and clinical tests, all clearly illustrated, are the answer to an instructor's prayers.

The physical therapy assessment as it is presented here—unencumbered by treatment approaches—removes bias from the process. The assessment stands alone as a means to clarify and quantify the patient's problems.

Lynn Snyder-Mackler, P.T., M.S.
Assistant Professor
Department of Physical Therapy
Sargent College
Boston University
Boston, Massachusetts

Preface

This clinical text has been designed to teach entry-level physical therapy students techniques for assessing persons who have neuromuscular or musculoskeletal disorders, according to standardized criteria. The book stresses that consistency of technique provides consistency of results. While intended for use by students, this book is also a well-illustrated reference for the practicing physical therapist.

The book begins by describing screening examinations and gross evaluations that enable students to determine the need for more definitive physical therapy examinations. Chapter 2 describes the principles of specific clinical assessments. Chapter 3 is devoted entirely to posture and muscle imbalance. Subsequent chapters focus on specific regions of the body, and their format follows the normal sequence of clinical assessment of those specific regions.

The appendices at the end of the book are in two parts. Appendix A contains recording forms that have been developed as guidelines for examiners as they assess their patients. The objective of an assessment procedure is to establish baseline data on the patient from which a treatment plan is developed. The examples of assessment forms included in Appendix A can be used for recording initial patient evaluations and for periodic reevaluation of patient progress.

Appendix B contains multiple-choice objective examination questions for readers to assess their knowledge of clinical assessment procedures. The questions are organized by chapter.

An outstanding feature of this book is the number of quality photographs and illustrations. They do not serve merely to support text, rather, they tell their own story and join with the text to form a total information package.

The material covering goniometry, functional muscle testing, and manual muscle testing was written by Dr. Palmer. Ms. Epler wrote the sections covering orthopedic examination, clinical tests, and joint play.

Acknowledgments

The authors would like to thank the following people for their contribution to the development and publication of this text:

Jan Bühler Callahan, M.Ed., P.T., E.M.T., for the researching and writing of the orthopedic clinical assessment portion of Chapter 7, Neck and Trunk.

Danny DiSabatino, P.T., for providing his time and expertise in composing the section on the "biomechanics of the ankle and foot" in Chapter 11.

J. Julian Washington and Gail Baker, whose expertise in photography is evident in the professional quality of the numerous photographs used throughout this textbook.

Michael Adams, whose illustrative talent is apparent in the accuracy and detailed complexity of his work.

Efrain Paz, Linda Miller, Janice Toms, Al Jette, Rauf Rashid, Jean Marchant, and Sandra Shirley for contributing their time to pose for the photographs contained within this book.

Lisa Biello, Sanford Robinson, Eileen Rosen, and the staff at the J.B. Lippincott Company for their inspiration, support, and expertise, which made this publication a reality.

Kathy Barrett and the staff at Ruttle, Shaw & Wetherill, Inc. for their expertise in the editing and composition of the book.

Finally, thank you to our colleagues, friends, and family, who in their own ways have helped us become the individuals and professionals that we are today.

Contents

Gross
Evaluations

Chapter 1

Cognitive and psychomotor skills are necessary to mastery of patient assessment. This process involves identifying the appropriate procedures, which are usually determined from the patient's chart, history, and other sources of information. Careful selection of assessment procedures is important and which procedures are appropriate depend on the patient's condition. Only assessments that contribute to developing treatment strategies should be performed. Unless accurate employment of technical skills during evaluation produces concrete information, the results will be meaningless and time will be wasted.[1]

Standardized criteria have been developed to establish a range of normal performance or functional mobility. Patients' results are compared with the established norms. The desirable level of function may depend on the patient's physical build, age, and previous activity level. The patient's performance is tested at intervals to monitor response to treatment. These assessments must also adhere to normative criteria and be conducted in a reliable manner.

Because the results of clinical assessment are used to develop a plan of care, to choose the appropriate treatment techniques, and to monitor the patient's functional and physiological changes, the consistency of technique cannot be overemphasized. When therapists evaluate the efficacy of a treatment they rely heavily on the quality of the measurements of the patients. Thorough and accurate patient assessment is necessary to prevent functional disability, to improve impaired function, and to maintain a given level of function.

Purpose

The purpose of assessment procedures is to gather data on the status of the patient at specific times. Assessments are performed to:

1. Develop a database to establish the patient's level of function, identify the patient's problem, and determine why the problem exists.
2. Plan a treatment program based on the results. The therapist analyzes the results, lists strengths and weaknesses, ranks the problems, develops treatment goals, and establishes the patient's outcomes. Prioritizing problems is important. For example, a patient needs to learn bed mobility activities before learning wheelchair transfers; joint range of motion is evaluated before muscle strength is determined.
3. Evaluate the results of the treatment program to know how treatments are affecting the patient.

4. Modify treatment to suit the patient or terminate the treatment.

Assessments are the basis of all physical therapy treatment. A complete and accurate evaluation allows therapists to establish a database against which to assess progress. It allows them to determine a level of function so that an appropriate treatment program can be developed and adapted to the changing status of the patient. At times it also allows therapists to identify the cause of the patient's problem.

For every type of assessment there is a set of criteria for performing the evaluation and a specific method of recording the results.

Reliability, Objectivity, and Validity

Assessments must be reliable and objective, and the results must be valid. Reliability is the extent to which comparable results are achieved every time a test is repeated. If a muscle test is repeated by one or more therapists who obtain the same grade every time, then the test is reliable. The key to reliability for manual muscle testing is to follow the standard procedure, performing the test in the same way each time and in the same way that other therapists perform it. Reliability is increased if the therapist gives clear instructions to the patient.

Evaluation procedures should exhibit interrater and intrarater reliability. Interrater reliability means that another person who performs the test should arrive at the same results. Intrarater reliability means that one person should come up with the same results on every repetition of the test. D.L. Riddle performed an intrarater-reliable test by examining the effects of goniometer size on the reliability of passive shoulder joint measurements. He concluded that goniometric passive measurement of the range of shoulder joint motion can be highly reliable when taken by a single therapist (intrarater reliability), regardless of the size of the goniometer. The degree of *interrater* reliability for those measurements appeared to be specific to the range of motion.[2]

Assessment procedure objectivity means that the findings are reported without distortion by personal opinion or feelings. Therapists should not let concern for the patient influence the results of an evaluation procedure. In manual muscle testing, the most difficult area in which to be objective is deciding whether the resistance the patient can tolerate is mimimal, moderate, or maximal. If the patient's weakness is unilateral, the therapist should test the opposite side and use the result as the baseline for normal. If the patient has bilateral involvement, the therapist must rely on experience in testing other patients to know what is normal for a particular muscle in a person of a given age, sex, size, and occupation.

Objectivity is of prime importance when third-party–payer systems are involved. These systems allow patients to receive many physical therapy services and require accurate and comprehensive documentation of treatments and patient outcomes.

Validity means that a test actually measures what it is supposed to measure. In muscle testing, therapists are testing the strength of a specific muscle. For a muscle test to be valid, the therapist must know the location and function of the muscle being tested and the location and function of surrounding muscles. Validity of assessments means that therapists evaluate exactly what they say they are going to and that the results are correct, or true.

Gross Muscle Screening

A quick screening evaluation of a patient is an important component of the entire evaluative process; it gives a picture of the patient's status and is a basis for planning effective treatments. Seeing a patient for the first time, the therapist performs subjective and objective assessments. The therapist takes a history and hears the patient's complaints. The therapist then performs a general evaluation to determine which specific evaluation procedures are indicated.

The purpose of a muscle screening test is to quickly determine a level of muscle strength. If the therapist finds weakness during the muscle screening test, a specific manual muscle test is then performed to focus on such factors as resistance, positions, grades, palpations, and substitutions. Muscle screening is not a detailed determination of strength; it simply classifies levels of strength as either normal or weak. The results of the evaluation provide physical therapy practitioners with sufficient information to devise a plan of care or to proceed with a definitive muscle test for areas found to be weak.

Following are some general considerations for the technique of a muscle screening test that will assist the therapist.

- Simple observation of the patient prior to the assessment may give a general idea of his or her strength.
- Explanation of the purpose and procedure of the test must be given in terms that the patient can understand.
- As many tests as possible should be performed

with the patient in one position to avoid unnecessary fatigue and discomfort.
- The assessment is based on movements usually performed in less than the full range of motion and tests groups of muscles performing a specific activity. Not all muscle groups need to be tested.
- A muscle screening test of the entire body should take no longer than 5 minutes.

The following are guidelines for a muscle screening test that may be altered to suit the patient and circumstances. The therapist should also keep these in mind when administering the test.

- The patient is directed to complete the test motion before the therapist provides resistance.
- The command, "Hold," to the patient precedes the application of resistance when using the "break test."
- Resistance is applied and released gradually, not quickly. Resistance is usually applied distally to the joint tested, unless otherwise indicated.
- The patient should perform most motions bilaterally simultaneously, except for motions of the hands. Bilateral motion provides the therapist the opportunity to compare one side with the other.
- Palpation is not usually done during a gross muscle test.
- Test positions may vary to allow for patient comfort: upper limb motions, for example, may be performed with the patient sitting in a wheelchair.
- Adequate stabilization is usually accomplished if the patient resists motions bilaterally. If testing is performed unilaterally, the patient must be stabilized.
- If a recording form does not exist, a summary of results should be entered in the patient's medical record, even if all muscles are found to be within normal limits.

Table 1–1 outlines the evaluation procedures for muscle screening tests.

Range of Motion Screening

The purpose of a screening evaluation for range of motion is to determine whether and where a specific goniometric assessment is necessary. The motions are performed actively. The patient should be comfortably positioned and stable; tight or binding clothing should be removed. General considerations for performing any assessment should be followed.

Table 1–1. Evaluation Procedures for Muscle Screening Tests

POSITION OF PATIENT	MUSCLE GROUP TESTED	INSTRUCTION TO PATIENT	THERAPIST'S ACTION
Supine	Neck and trunk flexors	1. Hold arms straight in front of body. Raise head and shoulders off table. Hold.	None
	Hip flexors	2. Keep legs straight. Raise both legs off table simultaneously. Hold.	None
	Hip abductors	3. Abduct legs to each side. Hold.	Attempt to bring legs together.
	Hip adductors	4. Keep legs together. Hold.	Attempt to separate legs.
	Hip extensors	5. Flex hips and knees, keeping soles of feet on table. Raise hips from table.	None
	Shoulder adductors	6. Bring hands together in front of chest, elbows straight. Hold.	Attempt to separate arms into horizontal abduction.
	a. Shoulder flexors and scapular upward rotators	7. Flex shoulder to 90 degrees, elbows straight. Hold.	a. Attempt to push arms into extension.
	b. Shoulder extensors and scapular downward rotators		b. Attempt to push arms into flexion.
	c. Shoulder horizontal abductors		c. Attempt to push arms together into horizontal adduction.
Supine or sitting	a. Shoulder abductors	8. Abduct shoulder to the side to shoulder level, elbows straight. Hold.	a. Attempt to push arms down to sides into shoulder adduction.
	b. Shoulder adductors		b. Attempt to push arms over head into shoulder abduction.
	a. Shoulder medial rotators	9. Hold arms at sides, elbows bent, forearms in neutral position. Hold.	a. Attempt to push arms outward into lateral rotation.
	b. Shoulder lateral rotators		b. Attempt to push arms in toward body into medial rotation.
	c. Elbow flexors		c. Attempt to push forearms toward table into elbow extension.
	d. Elbow extensors		d. Attempt to push forearms toward shoulders into elbow flexion.
	e. Supinators		e. Attempt to turn palms down into pronation.
	f. Pronators		f. Attempt to turn palms up into supination.
	g. Wrist extensors		g. Attempt to flex the wrists.
	h. Wrist flexors		h. Attempt to push palms away from body into wrist extension.

Table 1–1. *(continued)*

POSITION OF PATIENT	MUSCLE GROUP TESTED	INSTRUCTION TO PATIENT	THERAPIST'S ACTION
	Finger flexors	10. Squeeze my fingers. Hold.	Place index and middle fingers in patient's hands; attempt to pull fingers out.
	Finger extensors	11. Straighten fingers. Hold.	Attempt to push fingers into flexion.
	Palmar interossei	12. Adduct fingers. Hold.	Attempt to pull fingers into abduction.
	Dorsal interossei	13. Abduct fingers. Hold.	Attempt to push fingers into adduction.
	Opponens pollicis	14. Pinch my finger. Hold.	Place index finger between patient's thumb and each finger, one at a time.
Sitting	Latissimus dorsi and triceps	15. Place hands on treatment table next to hips, elbows straight, shoulders shrugged. Depress scapula by lifting buttocks off table.	None
	Upper trapezius and levator scapulae	16. Shrug shoulder toward ears. Hold.	Push shoulders down into depression.
	Medial rotators of the hips and everters of the feet	17. Evert feet. Hold.	Push on lateral borders of each foot, into inversion and lateral rotation.
	Lateral rotators of the hips and inverters of the feet	18. Invert feet. Hold.	Push on medial border of each foot into eversion and medial rotation.
Prone	Rhomboids, middle trapezius, and posterior deltoid	19. Bend elbows level with shoulders; pinch or adduct scapulae together, raising arms from table. Hold.	Attempt to push arms down.
	Elbow and shoulder extensors	20. Begin with arms at sides, elbows straight. Raise arms off table. Hold.	Attempt to push arms down.
	Extensors of the hips, back, neck, and shoulders	21. Begin with arms at sides. Arch back, raising head, shoulders, arms, and legs off table simultaneously. Hold.	None
Prone or sitting	a. Hamstrings	22. Flex knees. Hold.	a. Attempt to pull knees into extension.
	b. Quadriceps		b. Attempt to push knees into further flexion.
Standing	Gastrocnemius soleus	23. Stand on one leg. Rest fingers lightly on table. Rise up on tiptoes; repeat 10 times. Repeat with other leg.	None
	Dorsiflexors	24. Walk on heels for 10 steps.	None
	Hip and knee extensors	25. Do five partial deep knee bends.	None

Table 1–2. Range of Motion Screening Test

POSITION OF PATIENT	MOTION BEING TESTED	INSTRUCTIONS TO PATIENT
Sitting	Shoulder abduction and lateral rotation	1. Reach behind head and touch opposite scapula, or place hands behind neck and push elbows posteriorly.
	Shoulder adduction and medial rotation	2. Reach to opposite shoulder or touch the inferior angle or opposite scapula, or place both hands behind back as high as possible.
	Shoulder flexion and extension	3. Raise arms in front of body overhead and reverse to behind back.
	Elbow flexion and extension	4. Bend and straighten elbows.
	Radioulnar supination and pronation	5. With elbows flexed 90 degrees, supinate and pronate.
	Wrist flexion and extension	6. Flex and extend wrists.
	Radial and ulnar deviation	7. Move wrist laterally and medially.
	Finger abduction and adduction	8. Spread fingers apart and bring them together
	Finger flexion and extension	9. Make a tight fist and open fingers wide.
	Thumb flexion and extension	10. Bend thumb across the palm and out to the side.
	Neck flexion and extension	11. Place chin on chest, tilt head back.
	Neck rotation	12. Turn head to the right and left.
	Hip flexion and adduction	13. Sitting, cross one thigh over the other.
	Hip flexion, abduction, and lateral rotation	14. Uncross thighs and place the lateral side of foot on opposite knee.
	Ankle inversion	15. Turn foot in.
	Ankle eversion	16. Turn foot out.
Supine	Hip abduction and adduction	17. Spread legs apart and bring them together.
	Hip extension	18. a. Flex hips and knees; lift buttocks as in bridging.
Supine or sitting	Hip extension	b. Rise to standing from sitting position.
	Knee flexion and extension	19. Pull knees to chest, heels toward buttocks, and return.
Standing	Trunk flexion	20. Bend forward and reach for toes with knees straight.
	Trunk extension	21. Bend backward while I stand beside you.
	Trunk lateral bending	22. Lean to the left, then right while I stabilize your pelvis.
	Trunk rotation	23. Turn to the right and to the left while I stabilize your pelvis.
	Ankle plantar flexion and toe extension	24. Stand on tiptoes.
	Ankle dorsiflexion	25. Stand on heels.

The quick and easy evaluation of a patient's range of motion is also an important component of the entire evaluation process. It gives a quick picture of the patient's willingness to move.

If limitations in joint range of motion are identified, a specific goniometric test should be performed to obtain a detailed account of the restrictions in range of motion. A specific range of motion test is then performed to focus on such factors as position, stabilization, alignment of the goniometer, and recording of the limitations (Table 1–2).

References
1. Campbell SK: Measurement and technical skills: neglected aspect of research education. Phys Ther 61:523, 1981
2. Riddle DL, Rothstein JM, Lamb RL: The reliability of shoulder joint range of motion measurements in a clinical setting. Presented at the annual meeting of the American Physical Therapy Association, Chicago, 1986

Principles of Examination Techniques

Chapter 2

Clinical evaluation procedures have been developed to measure the function of joints, muscles, and soft tissues of persons who require the services of a physical therapist. The application of these techniques requires basic knowledge of the human body and well-developed practical skills. An understanding of the evaluation techniques and of the principles of application is required if reliable and valid results are to be obtained. The therapist assesses the results of the measurements and uses them to develop a plan of care.

This chapter is divided into sections dealing with goniometry, functional muscle testing, specific manual muscle testing, and peripheral joint assessment. Each section contains information on the purpose, techniques, and recording of measurements and on factors that influence the assessment.

Goniometry

Goniometry is the most commonly used evaluation technique in physical therapy practice.[15] Therapists have used it since the 1920s to assess joint range of motion. The range, or amount, of motion a joint is capable of is a function of joint morphology, shape, capsule, and ligaments, and of the muscles or tendons that cross the joint. The shape of the articular surfaces and the soft tissues surrounding the articular surfaces also influence the range of motion.

Joints are described as having degrees of freedom of movement. If the motion occurs in only one plane and around one axis, the joint is said to have one degree of freedom. Two degrees of freedom describes a joint that allows movement in two planes and around two axes. A joint that moves in three planes and around three axes has three degrees of freedom—the most that occur in any anatomical joint. Joints are physiologically "designed" to allow more motion at the end of the range as a protective mechanism.

Purposes of Joint Range of Motion Evaluation

1. To establish the existing range of motion available in a joint and to compare it to the normal range for that subject. The information will permit a therapist to establish a database for the patient. This information is used to develop goals and a treatment plan to increase or decrease the range of motion.
2. To aid in diagnosing and determining the patient's joint function. Goniometry reveals joint limitations in the arc of motion but does not identify the dysfunction. It does, however, provide information regarding limitations if joint disease is suspected.

Hypomobility or hypermobility of joints affects a patient's function in activities of daily living. Hypermobility—laxity in the joint or structures surrounding the joint—allows motion to exceed the normal range. Hypomobility is joint tightness or a less than normal range of motion. An example of joint hypomobility interfering with a person's daily living activities would be an inability to perform stair climbing because of a 70- to 80-degree restriction in knee flexion.

3. To reassess the patient's status after treatment and compare it to that at the time of the initial evaluation. Goniometric measurements are used to evaluate the effectiveness of treatment programs. If the range of motion is not increasing, the treatment program may need to be changed in order to obtain effective clinical results.
4. To develop the patient's interest in and motivation and enthusiasm for the treatment program. Most patients are aware of changes in joint motion and usually are motivated by these improvements to participate in the treatment.
5. To document results from treatment regimens for medicolegal reasons and to communicate with other medical personnel, third-party payers, and workmen's compensation companies.
6. To participate in vital research to improve function. Research has contributed, for example, to the design of chairs and desks and placement of pedals in cars that are ergonomically ideal for the average driver.

Several factors that influence range of motion must be considered to ensure that goniometry is an objective assessment.

Reliability. Although Moore and her associates showed that experienced therapists were reliable in taking goniometeric measurements,[16] there is still some concern about the clinical reliability of goniometry. Miller states, "Although the inferences that can be made from measuring joint motion are limited (validity), the measurement itself is invaluable as a basic indicator of patient status."[15]

When measuring, the therapist must try to rule out as many of the factors as possible that decrease reliability. Some of these factors that will improve reliability include removal of tight and restrictive clothing, duplications of positions used, and measuring at the same time of day.

Age. Generally, the younger the subject, the greater the range of motion. Bell and Hoshizak found that there was a decline in range of motion in most patients between age 20 and 30 years, followed by a plateau until the age of 60 years, after which a decline again occurred.[3]

Sex. Many studies have been performed to determine the difference in range of motion between men and women. Overall, it has been found that women tend to have greater ranges than men, but not all studies confirm that finding.[3]

Joint Structures. Some persons, because of genetics or posture, normally have hypermobile or hypomobile joints. Body type can influence joint mobility, as can flexibility of the tendons and ligaments crossing the joint.

Joints are structured so that motion is limited by the capsule, ligaments, and tendons, or by the bony configuration. Some motions are limited by soft tissue bulk of the segments and not by a limitation associated with the joint. For instance, elbow flexion is usually limited by the muscle bulk of the arm against the forearm.

Soft tissues such as ligaments, tendons, and capsules are dense, regular connective tissues with inherent elastic properties; they may become tight or loose and affect the motion available at joints. Muscles associated with the joints may become stretched or contracted thereby affecting the joint motion. The shape of the joint surfaces is designed to allow motion in particular directions. These surfaces may be altered by such factors as posture, disease, or trauma to allow more or less motion than normal at a joint.

Normally, each joint has a small amount of motion at the end of the range that is not under voluntary control. These accessory motions are not assessed during active range evaluation but are included under the realm of passive measurement. Accessory motions help protect the joint structures by absorbing extrinsic forces.

Examiners performing goniometric measurements should consider the "end feel" of each joint when determining passive range of motion. The structure or structures that limit the range of motion at a joint have a characteristic "feel" at the end of the motion. The feel is a subjective measurement of the resistance encountered at the end of the range of motion and is part of the range of motion evaluation.[17]

Dominance. Most researchers have found that there is essentially no difference for corresponding joints between the left and right sides of the body.[15] Comparative goniometry is done when a joint is involved unilaterally; the contralateral limb can then be used as the standard for normal range of motion for that subject.

Type of Motion. Active range of motion testing provides limited information regarding joint motion. Assuming that the subject has complete passive motion, an inability to actively move the segment completely through the motion must be attributed to muscle weakness. Active range grossly evaluates coordination of movement and functional ability.

Passive range of motion is usually evaluated in goniometry and is the amount of motion possible when the examiner moves a body part with no assistance from the subject. It is usually greater than active range of motion because the integrity of the soft tissue structures do not in themselves dictate the limits of movement. A passive range of motion test gives the examiner information about the integrity of the joint, but provides no information about the capabilities of contractile tissues.

Norkin and White state, "Comparisons between the passive and active ranges of motion provide information about the amount of motion permitted by the joint structure relative to the person's ability to produce motion at a joint."[17] A comparison may be an advantage in developing a patient's treatment plan or aiding in a diagnosis.

Instruments

The instruments practitioners use for measuring joint range of motion are called goniometers, or arthrometers. The tools, although varying in size, shape, and appearance, all possess the capabilities to provide specific information regarding joint motion. The widely used universal goniometer is durable, washable, and can be applied to almost all joints.

The goniometer is basically a protractor with two long arms. One arm is considered movable and the other stationary, and both are attached to the body of the protractor by a rivet or tension knob (Fig. 2–1).

A variety of goniometers have been developed to conform to specific joints. There are goniometers with short arms for short anatomical segments such as the digits. Such tools can be made easily by cutting down the arms of a plastic goniometer to about 1 inch (Fig. 2–2). The arms on finger goniometers are placed on the dorsal or ventral aspect of the joint being measured rather than on the lateral aspect of the joints (lateral placement is standard procedure).

Figure 2–1. A metal goniometer showing a moving arm (*A*), stationary arm (*B*), body, or protractor (*C*), and the axis (*D*).

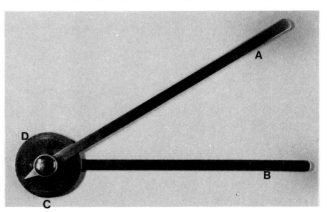

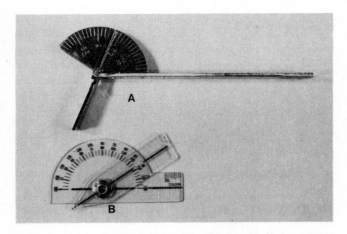

Figure 2–2. Two goniometers designed for measuring digits. (*A*) The first is constructed of metal and is placed on the dorsal or ventral surface for measurement at the joint. (*B*) The other is constructed of plastic, and the stationary and moving arms have been shortened to conform easily to the digits. They may be placed on the lateral, ventral, or dorsal side of the digits.

Another type of goniometer, which works like a carpenter's level, relies on the effects of gravity. The gravity-activated or fluid (bubble) goniometer has a 360-degree scale (Fig. 2–3).

Another type is designed with a needle or pointer instead of being fluid filled (Fig. 2–4). The device is strapped to or held firmly on the limb segment. This type of device is easy and quick to use because it is not aligned with bony landmarks; however reliability suffers as a result of a lack of landmark orientation.[15] In many instances, the armless goniometer is better than the universal (two-armed) goniometer because it does not have to conform to body segments. It is particularly useful for measuring joint rotation and axioskeletal motion.

In 1959, the electric goniometer was developed by Karpovich and Karpovich.[10] This device is attached to an electromyograph machine. The two arms of the goniometer are attached to a potentiometer and are strapped to the proximal and distal body segments. Movement from arms of the device causes resistance in the potentiometer, which measures dynamic joint motion. Aligning the arms of the electrogoniometer is difficult and time consuming.

Clinically, the most commonly used instrument is the universal goniometer, which has not changed in design in over 30 years. One type of instrument is the transparent plastic goniometer, which was developed by Wainerdi in 1952 to allow greater accuracy of alignment with the body segments.[20] A line on the goniometer along the stationary and moving arms facilitates alignment with body parts. Other universal goniometers are constructed of lightweight metals.

The goniometer's protractor has a full or a half circle. It is marked in increments of 1, 2, or 5 degrees. The degrees on the protractor are usually numbered in both directions from 0 to 180 degrees and 180 to 0 degrees. Full circle protractors indicate 360 degrees in both directions. The half circle goniometer has an advantage over the full circle type in that it can be applied easily to joints when the subject is supine or prone.

The stationary arm of the goniometer is aligned with the fixed body segment, and the moving arm, with the moving body segment. When a half circle goniometer is used, the two arms are interchangeable.

The rivet or fulcrum of the goniometer should be free to move without being too loose. Some metal goniometers are equipped with a knob to adjust the tension of the arms.

Figure 2–3. Fluid goniometer, which is activated by the effects of gravity.

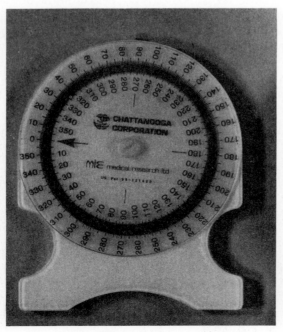

Figure 2–4. A goniometer without alignment arms has a level on the straight edge to indicate that the protractor is level.

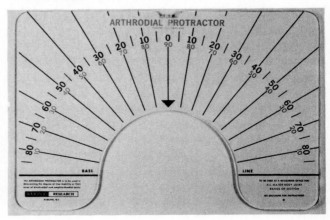

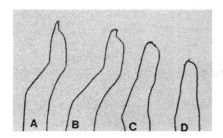

Figure 2–5. A starting position tracing for the (A) index, (B) middle, (C) ring, and (D) little fingers.

Large goniometers have 12- to 16-inch arms for use on the large joints of the body with long limb segments. Intermediate sizes developed primarily for the wrists and ankles have arms approximately 6 to 8 inches long. The intermediate-size goniometer is convenient because it fits easily into a pocket and can be used for most joint measurements. The fingers and toes are usually measured with a special goniometer or one whose arms have been shortened to ½ to 1 inch.[22]

Other devices, such as tape measures and rulers, may be used to assess trunk and scapular mobility. The tape should be made from a durable fabric that withstands washing and does not stretch.

X-rays may be made of joints, which then are measured with a ruler or goniometer. Tracings can be taken of motions to compare initial measurements with subsequent ones. Tracings are used most commonly with the fingers: the shape of each finger is drawn on a piece of paper (Fig. 2–5).

General Principles for Measuring Joint Range of Motion

Passive Range. Passive range of motion measurement is employed whenever possible to assess the extent of structural limitation to the available joint range of motion.

The therapist estimates available range of motion before actually placing the goniometer. Having a mental idea of the starting or ending range of motion helps the therapist minimize faulty readings from the instrument.

Starting Position. The anatomical position of 0 degrees is the starting position for all measurments except rotation at the shoulder and hip, and pronation/supination of the radioulnar joints. These exceptions are explained under the specific test motions (Chaps. 4, 5, and 9). In the starting position (preferred position) it is easy to isolate the movement, place the goniometer, stabilize the subject, and see the motions being performed. Tension in the muscles passing over adjacent joints and in the soft tissues surrounding the joint is lessened or

eliminated. For example, the measurement of knee flexion is performed with the hip flexed to eliminate tension in the rectus femoris muscle.

The end of the range is assisted by the weight of the limb, so the effects of movement against gravity are minimal. The subject usually lies supine on a firm, comfortable surface. The examiner should be comfortable and in a position to read the goniometer at eye level so as to avoid errors in visual perception (Fig. 2–6).

Alignment. For most measurements the goniometer is aligned on the lateral side of the test joint. This placement enables the examiner to see the protractor, and to properly align the goniometer arms with the bony landmarks of the body.

Axis. The axis of the goniometer is the intersection of the two arms and should coincide with the axis of the joint being tested. The axis of the joint will shift during the motion; therefore it is important to adjust the axes of the goniometer accordingly.

If the moving arm is placed parallel to the long axis of the moving body segment and the stationary arm is parallel to the long axis of the fixed segment of the joint, then the axis of motion will fall where the two intersect.

Moving Arm. The moving arm of the goniometer is aligned parallel and lateral to the long axis of the moving body segment. The therapist palpates the specific bony landmarks before aligning the moving arm of the goniometer. The moving segment of the body along which the moving arm is aligned is the segment distal to the test joint. The proximal portion of the movable arm near the fulcrum is either pointed, has a line through

Figure 2–6. The examiner reads the goniometer from the same horizontal level as the protractor. Hip extension is measured with the axis aligned with the greater trochanter, (A) the moving arm aligned with the midline of the femur in line with the lateral femoral epicondyle, and (B) the stationary arm aligned with the midline of the trunk.

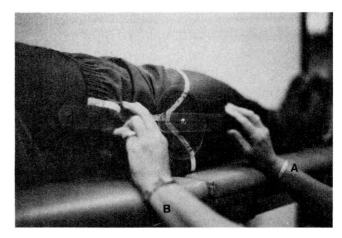

to the end, or is notched to enable the examiner to read the goniometer with ease.

Stationary Arm. The stationary arm of the goniometer is aligned parallel and lateral to the long axis of the fixed body segment. As with the moving arm, the therapist palpates the specific landmarks before aligning the stationary arm. The fixed segment is the proximal body segment and does not change position during the testing.

Numerical Expression of Joint Range of Motion

Most physical therapists use a system of measurement based on 0 to 180 degrees that was proposed in 1923 by Silver and is the method of the American Academy of Orthopedic Surgeons.[19] The subject is placed in the starting, or anatomical, position that represents the 0 position on the measuring device (rotation and forearm measurements are an exception). The arc of motion produced by the subject and the goniometer is based on 180 degrees. For instance, the starting position for measuring the elbow joint range of motion is 0 degrees of elbow extension. The elbow joint is then passively flexed through an arc of motion, followed by the goniometric arc of motion, through approximately a normal range of 145 degrees. As the joint increases in motion, the numbers on the goniometer scale increase and are positive.

Other methods of expressing range of motion have been developed, but they are not widely used as they are more difficult to interpret than the 0-to-180-degree method. Another method of measuring range of motion is based on a 360-degree arc to test motions of extension or adduction that go beyond the anatomical position. This method is also useful for measurements that are performed from a starting position of 180 degrees. The numerical values of abduction and flexion motions would decrease toward 0 degrees (Table 2–1).

Table 2–1. Hip Range of Motion Represented by Three Different Notation Systems

	0–180	180–0	360
Flexion	125	55	55
Extension	15	165	195
Abduction	45	45	135
Adduction	45	15	195
Internal rotation	45	135	45
External rotation	45	135	45

(Using "normal" values taken from Gerhardt JJ, Russe OA: International SFTR Method of Measuring and Recording Joint Motion. Bern, Huber, 1975. From Rothstein JM: Measurement in Physical Therapy, p. 118. New York, Churchill Livingstone, 1985)

Recording Measurements

Examples of recording forms appear in Appendix A.

The methods of recording range of motion have ranged from tables, charts, and graphs to tracings. The most common recording is based on a 0-to-180-degree scale. The starting and ending ranges of each motion are identified separately. The goniometer is aligned in the starting position or anatomical position at 0 degrees, except for rotation and ankle movements, in which cases the moving arm starts at 90 degrees.

A calculation must be done for motions in which the goniometer placement begins at 90 degrees to attain the starting and ending degrees in order to record the appropriate range of motion. For instance, to examine ankle dorsiflexion the goniometer is aligned at 90 degrees in the preferred position and recorded as 0 degrees. Following the dorsiflexion motion, the arc produced by the goniometer may show 100 degrees. It is recorded as 10 degrees of ankle dorsiflexion motion. If a subject lacks motion and is unable to assume the starting position, the goniometer is aligned as close to 0 degrees as possible.

For accuracy in measuring and recording limitation of joint motion, the therapist must be sure to use the preferred position or an alternate position and specific placement of the goniometer. Use of an alternate position is noted by an asterisk in the recording space and reasons for use of the alternate position are explained in the Remarks column. If neither the preferred nor an alternate position is used, the position and the reason for that choice of position are described in the Remarks column. Any deviation from the key, such as use of active range, presence of pain, or other limiting factors, should be also noted and explained in the Remarks column.

The goniometer is aligned and readings are made at the beginning and at the completion of each movement. The goniometer is removed from the subject during the motion and realigned at the completion of the motion. If the examiner is interested in the end of the range of motion, only that measurement need be taken. It would be assumed that the starting point was zero. The number of degrees of motion away from zero is recorded. If limited range prevents the patient from starting the motion at the preferred position, the amount of limitation is measured and recorded in degrees.

The range and date are recorded and the therapist initials the test form.

Whenever possible, the subject's normal range is determined by measuring the uninvolved limb.

Procedure for Measurement

Using the proper sequence and techniques for goniometry ensures reliability, validity, and objectivity:

1. Place the subject in correct body alignment, which should correspond as nearly as possible to the anatomical position. Rotations at the shoulder and hip joints and forearm motion are exceptions. The segment to be examined should be exposed and unrestricted, in the "preferred position."

2. Explain and demonstrate the desired motion to the subject.

3. Perform the motion passively two or three times to eliminate substitutions and tightness due to inactivity.

4. Stabilize the proximal body segment.

5. Locate the approximate center of motion (axis) actively or passively by palpating the appropriate bony landmark on the lateral aspect of the joint.

6. Place the stationary arm of the goniometer parallel to the longitudinal axis of the midline of the fixed segment in line with the designated bony landmark.

7. Place the movable arm parallel to the longitudinal axis of the moving segment, in line with the designated bony landmark.

8. Determine the axis of motion by the intersection of the midline of the two segments. Hold the goniometer between your fingers and thumb. Place it loosely against the subject so as not to compress soft tissues, possibly resulting in an erroneous reading or limitation of the range of motion. If you are unable to hold the goniometer steady, rest your forearms against the treatment table.

9. Align the goniometer and take readings at the beginning and at the completion of each movement. Remove the goniometer from the subject during the motion and realign it at the end of the motion. If you are interested only in the end range of motion, then the starting measurement need not be taken. It would be assumed that the starting point is 0 degrees (Fig. 2–7). Record the number of degrees of motion away from zero. If limitation in the range prevents the subject from starting the motion at the preferred position, measure the amount of limitation and record it in degrees.

Principles of Functional Muscle Testing

Manual muscle testing is an attempt to determine a subject's ability to voluntarily contract a specific muscle or group of muscles. This technique of muscle evaluation does not provide information on the ability to use the

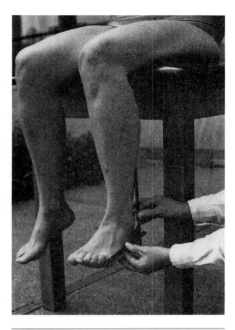

Figure 2–7. The arms of the goniometer are placed at a 90-degree angle indicating the starting position for ankle dorsiflexion measurements.

muscle in daily activities, nor does it provide information about the muscle's ability to interact with other muscles in a synergistic pattern. Functional muscle testing consists of activities to assess muscle group strength and the muscles' ability to function together as a unit in performance of an activity.

Jette states, "The restoration of the disabled to their highest level of physical, vocational, and social function is an important treatment objective for physical therapists."[8] This is the ultimate goal for all treatments and evaluations. Rather than traditionally testing specific muscle strength or range of motion or relieving pain, the clinician considers the subject's functional abilities, regardless of limitations in range of motion or weakness in specific muscles.

The activities and grading outlined in the following chapters have *not* been standardized. A functional muscle test can demonstrate reliability if, when the activities are used by therapists repeatedly, test results are identical or fall within a narrow specific range. Standardization is needed for functional muscle testing as well as other evaluation techniques that therapists use on a daily basis.

Muscles are tested as a group in relation to the joint axis and the plane of motion in which they contract to move a body segment. For instance, the hip flexors lie anterior to the hip joint axis and produce a motion in the sagittal plane. The muscles contract both eccentrically and concentrically during activities of daily living. Functionally, they are used to flex the hip joint in activities such as climbing stairs or during the swing phase of gait.

Therefore, a functional muscle test of the hip flexors would be aimed at evaluating the ability of the subject to ascend stairs or to walk a certain distance.

Testing specific muscle groups for function also includes coordination of the movement produced by the agonistic, synergistic, and antagonistic muscles. Time required to complete the activity and the ability to produce repetitions of the movements within a specific period are considerations in functional muscle testing. For instance, if the knee extensors have increased muscle tone and the knee is not able to "unlock" smoothly, knee flexion may be considered functionally poor or nonfunctional. Another example lies in the recognition that it requires 20 to 25 seconds to walk 30 feet. When a subject is uncoordinated or has altered muscle tone, this activity may require two to three times the average time, and the ambulatory distance would not be considered functional in a community environment.

Purpose

1. The purpose of functional muscle testing is to evaluate muscle contraction by having the patient perform activities or motions in positions in which muscles function in normal daily circumstances.
2. Functional muscle evaluation data can be used to indicate degree of impairment or disability to support decisions regarding eligibility for medical benefits or compensation resulting from an inability to return to work.[1]
3. An important use of functional assessment is in research. The data can play a role in studies of the incidence and prevalence of specific physical impairments and their associated disabilities.
4. Functional assessment data can be used to determine whether rehabilitation patients should be discharged from a hospital or sent to a long-term care facility.
5. Clinically, the results of a functional assessment are useful for selecting treatments, monitoring the course of patient responsiveness as a basis for possible treatment changes, and evaluating patient status at the end of treatment to determine whether treatment goals have been achieved.[1]

Factors That Influence Grading

Various factors influence the grading for functional muscle testing.

1. *Positions.* The evaluation has been developed to test the contraction and endurance of muscle groups with the subject in a position that is functional for that particular motion or activity. Lower limb tests are performed with the subject in the standing, or weight-bearing, position. The upper limbs are tested in a non–weight-bearing position in which most persons use their upper limb muscles (holding a newspaper, typing, eating, or doing resistive activities such as sawing wood or painting). The trunk musculature is assessed in either the supine or prone position, flexing forward or laterally, as in reaching for an object on a shelf.
2. *Activity.* The activity should be appropriate for the muscle groups being examined. This book suggests one activity for each muscle group, but many could be appropriate. The activity should be done in a weight-bearing position for the lower limb muscles, and a non–weight-bearing position for the upper limb muscles. The activities selected are based on the normal function of the muscle group being tested. A specific number of repetitions is identified for activities in which the muscles contracting are considered type II, or phasic, muscles. Some of the suggested activities are based on distance moved or number of times an activity can be completed within a specific period of time. The type I, or heavy-work, muscle groups are tested with one or two repetitions, and the subject may be asked to hold the position.
3. *Speed and Coordination.* The rate of muscle contraction during functional activities is determined by the voluntary control exhibited by the subject, and significantly influences how much tension a muscle can produce. When an activity requires an isometric muscle contraction, no movement occurs; therefore, no speed is required. But when a muscle contraction is either eccentric or concentric, the force developed by the muscles is directly related to the velocity of movement. Velocity and coordination necessary for a person to contract and relax muscles are based on factors such as muscle attachments and leverage, the ability of the bones to glide smoothly as joint angles change, the appropriateness of signals arriving at the myoneural junction, conduction of action potentials along the muscle fibers, and the willingness of the subject to cooperate in the testing. Changes in muscle contractibility caused by musculoskeletal or peripheral or central nervous system disorders could alter the rate of coordinated muscle contractions and result in ballistic muscle activity. Ballistic movements are a result of the inability to coordinate the speed of muscle contraction of the agonistic muscle group with relaxation of the antagonistic group.

The rate at which a subject is able to voluntarily contract and relax muscle groups influences the time that is required to complete an activity or task. The greater a person's muscle control, the greater are the person's chances of completing an activity within a reasonable time and of performing functionally.

4. *Endurance and Fatigue.* Endurance is the ability to perform an action a number of times in succession. Loss of endurance may be an early sign of a cardiopulmonary or a neurologic problem. Fatigue is defined as failure to maintain the required or expected force of muscle contraction.[13] The ability of a subject to complete the number of repetitions or to move a specific distance within a reasonable period of time without fatiguing defines endurance for functional muscle testing.

5. *Muscle Contraction.* Many activities performed on a daily basis are performed with muscles contracting eccentrically as well as concentrically. An eccentric contraction is a lengthening type of muscle contraction, resisting a stretching force. The movement usually occurs in a gravity-assisted position. Concentric contractions occur when the muscle shortens, the proximal and distal attachments come closer together, and tension develops to overcome resistance.

Isotonic contractions may be either concentric or eccentric and involve changes in muscle tension as well as muscle length. Many daily activities are performed isotonically by using concentric and eccentric types of muscle contractions.

The literature on evaluating or treating muscles during eccentric muscle contractions is sparse. In the 1940s, Signe Brunnstrom and Marjorie Dennen developed a system of grading movements rather than specific muscles. Their test used resistance and gravity and included fatigue as a factor in determining the strength of muscles.[5] In the chapters to follow, the functional muscle evaluations take into account the types of muscle contraction used to perform activities.

6. *Stability.* Many activities are performed in which proximal body segments are stabilized and the distal segments produce the motion. During some activities, the distal segment is stabilized while the proximal segment performs the motion. This type of movement can be seen in a closed kinematic chain or when a muscle contracts through reverse action. An example of reverse action of a muscle is walking with axillary crutches. The humerus is essentially fixed to the floor through the crutches and the latissimus dorsi muscle contracts to "swing" the trunk forward. Evaluation of the functional status of a muscle group for the lower limbs in the weight-bearing position requires that the proximal body segments be functional to provide sufficient stability

to accurately assess the distal segment motion. The converse is also true. If the test requires the subject to put weight on the foot to test hip musculature, then distal stability must be sufficient to obtain an accurate assessment of the proximal musculature.

The physical therapist should perform a gross muscle assessment to determine the stability around the joints before performing a functional muscle test.

7. *Sensation.* Sensation is important for normal performance of functional activities. Feedback to the muscles from the joints, ligaments, tendons, and the muscles themselves cannot be assessed in functional muscle testing, but should be evaluated with a detailed sensory examination. If the subject has a sensory deficit, movements may appear to be uncoordinated and lack adequate voluntary control. Because of commonly used movement patterns exhibited during functional activity, proprioceptive feedback may be enhanced through the use of functional muscle testing.

Criteria for Grading

Four grades are suggested to describe the levels of muscle function.

F (Functional).   The subject is able to complete the maximal number of repetitions or go a certain distance in a well-coordinated and timely manner.

FF (Functionally Fair).   The subject is able to complete more than half the desired number of repetitions or complete more than half the distance. The movement may be uncoordinated, the activity may require more time than normal, or the subject may complete the activity in a functional manner but have little endurance.

FP (Functionally Poor).   The subject is able to complete the activity 50 percent of the time or go half the distance but in an uncoordinated manner, or the subject requires an extended amount of time because of fatigue or a decrease in endurance.

NF (Nonfunctional).   The subject is unable to complete one repetition of the activity in a timely manner. Refer to the recording form in Appendix A.

Summary of Positions for Functional Muscle Testing

STANDING

UPPER LIMBS
Scapula abduction
Elbow extension

LOWER LIMBS

Hip
  Flexion
  Extension
  Abduction
  Medial rotation
  Lateral rotation
  Adduction
Knee
  Flexion
  Extension
Ankle
  Dorsiflexion
  Plantar flexion
Foot
  Inversion
  Eversion

SITTING

UPPER LIMBS

Shoulder
  Flexion
  Lateral rotation
  Extension
  Medial rotation
  Abduction
  Adduction
Scapula
  Elevation
  Depression
  Upward rotation
  Downward rotation
  Adduction
Elbow flexion
Wrist
  Flexion
  Extension
Hand in all positions
Trunk rotation

LOWER LIMB

Toes
  Flexion
  Extension

SUPINE

NECK AND TRUNK

Neck flexion
Trunk
  Flexion
  Rotation

PRONE

Neck extension

Principles of Manual Muscle Testing

Manual muscle testing (MMT) is one method by which muscle strength is defined and measured.[12] A manual muscle test is an attempt to determine the subject's ability to voluntarily contract a muscle or muscle group. Standard manual muscle tests as a measurement of strength are not suitable for persons who cannot actively or voluntarily control the tension developed in their muscles. As a result, subjects with disorders of the central nervous system who demonstrate spasticity are not appropriate candidates for muscle testing. Also, factors that activate the stretch reflex, such as gravity or manual resistance, will produce an inaccurate assessment of a subject's voluntary control of muscle activity. MMT is not as reliable, valid, and objective as other physical therapy testing procedures.

For MMT, *reliability* means that the test can be repeated by any therapist with results that vary by no more than one half of a grade. The measurement technique for determining strength of muscles is subjective, particularly in the area of manual resistance, and requires refinement. A half-grade interrater difference is acceptable. If the test is repeated by several therapists and the same grades are obtained, then the muscle test is said to be reliable. The key to reliable MMT is to follow the procedures that have been developed and used for the past 70 years. Reliability is increased by giving clear instructions to the subject. The therapist may help the subject understand the procedure by passively moving the joints through the motions, testing the opposite side, and demonstrating and explaining the movement.

Frese, Brown, and Norton tested interrater reliability by having 11 physical therapists test the middle trapezius and gluteus medius bilaterally on 100 patients.[6] They found that practitioners are reliable within one muscle testing grade of each other. They also found poor interrater reliability in grades below Fair, a finding that agrees with Beasley's findings of poor differentiation in grades below Fair.[2] Another study performed by Williams in the mid-1950s found that two examiners agreed on the muscle testing grade 60 to 75 percent of the time.[21]

A standardized method of MMT is needed so that comparable results can be obtained by different examiners. The resistance given for muscle testing grades of Fair Plus and above is subjective and needs standardization. The hand-held dynamometer developed by Smidt shows some potential for establishing reliability among therapists.[18]

Muscle strength testing should be a *valid* procedure—it must test the specific muscles that it purports to test. Validity can best be maintained by palpating each muscle, stabilizing the proximal segment, and preventing substitution of muscles or patterns.

Lamb states, "Manual muscle testing is hypothesized as a valuable tool for the clinical assessment of patients with neuromuscular problems. Information relevant to its reliability is sparse. More research must be done in today's clinical environment using appropriate research design. MMT appears to have content validity, however, there is no published evidence that gives credence to the degree to which an examiner can generalize the results of MMT to immediate and future behavior of patients."[12]

Objectivity means reporting the facts without distortion by personal opinion or bias. Following the standardized procedure and giving clear instructions help to make a muscle test objective. The most difficult variable to gauge objectively in muscle testing is the resistance the subject can take: is it minimal, moderate, or maximal?

The muscle test based on gravitational effects was developed by Dr. Robert Lovett, professor of orthopedic surgery at Harvard Medical School.[6] He developed this method of measuring specific muscle strength because of his involvement in the treatment of patients with poliomyelitis. In the 1940s and 1950s during the poliomyelitis epidemic in the United States, physical therapists developed skill in evaluating manual muscle strength. MMT continues to be useful for assessing muscle integrity for peripheral nerve lesions or musculoskeletal disorders. Even though the types of patients treated by physical therapists have changed over the past 30 years, the techniques developed continue to be useful for assessing strength of voluntary muscle contractions.

Manual muscle strength testing is usually performed by clinicians in a qualitative rather than a quantitative manner. The MMT method currently in use clinically is not sensitive enough to reveal and quantify subtle deficiencies in strength.

Uses of Manual Muscle Testing

1. To establish a basis for muscle reeducation and exercise. The therapist uses the data to develop a plan of care and to determine the patient's progress. Because it shows the effectiveness of the treatment, it evaluates the treatment program. MMT provides additional information before muscle transfer surgery. A muscle's strength should be rated Good or grade 4 before it is transferred because its strength will decrease one grade increment after the transfer.
2. To determine how functional a patient can be.
3. To determine a patient's needs for supportive apparatus, such as orthoses, splints, and assistive devices for ambulation.

4. To help determine a diagnosis. Some diseases affect only certain muscle groups. Peripheral nerve or nerve root lesions may affect all muscles served by that nerve or the cutaneous distribution. For example, muscular dystrophies and myopathies affect proximal muscle groups, and ulnar nerve lesions affect the intrinsic muscles of the hand.
5. To determine a patient's prognosis. A plateau in the progression of strength attained by the patient during treatment will be indicative of that patient's maximal level of function.

Factors That Contribute to the Effectiveness of Muscle Contraction

Muscle strength testing involves anatomical, physiological, and mechanical factors that influence muscle contractions.

The *length* of a muscle at the time of activation markedly affects the tension developed in that muscle. How much tension a muscle produces depends on its length in contraction. For some muscles the lengthened position is more favorable than the shortened position. Each muscle has its own optimal length to produce its optimal tension. As a one-joint muscle shortens or as the distal and proximal attachments of a two-joint muscle approach each other during a concentric contraction, the tension diminishes and the muscle may become actively insufficient. The patient may complain of pain and cramping in the tested muscle if it is in an actively insufficient position.

Physiologically, a muscle is capable of generating its greatest tension during an eccentric contraction. A muscle will generate less tension isometrically and even less when contracting concentrically.[2] Maximum isometric strength at any joint angle is always greater than the strength of a dynamic concentric contraction at the same angle. Maximum strength at a given joint angle is greatest when the muscle is lengthening eccentrically (as it attempts to overcome too great a load) than when it is contracting concentrically or isometrically.[2]

Skeletal muscles are composed of individual *muscle fiber types* that react differently to an action potential. Muscles classified as type I have a predominance of slow-twitch muscle fibers, which increase and decrease their tension slowly and are considered fatigue resistant. Muscles classified as type II have a predominance of fast-twitch muscle fibers, which increase and decrease their tension rapidly and fatigue quickly. All skeletal muscles have a mixture of both fiber types. Clinically, the speed of contraction and the resistance applied during the evaluation of strength must be considered. Much less resistance need be applied to muscles with a predominance of type II fibers to obtain a "normal" grade than to those that are predominantly type I fibers. An example that demonstrates a remarkable difference in natural strength is the amount of resistance applied to the sternocleidomastoid muscle, a type II muscle. The resistance used is much less than that applied to the soleus muscle (type I), yet the identical strength grade is obtained. The *speed* of muscle contraction is an important consideration when evaluating muscle strength. The rate and type of muscle contraction influence muscle strength and are determined by manual muscle testing. For the results of the test to be reliable, rate and speed of contraction must be consistent. If a concentric muscle contraction is the method of choice, a moderate speed is used. With an isometric muscle contraction, the muscle holds at the end of the test range and no motion occurs; the strength test result will be a whole grade higher than with the concentric muscle contraction.

If the test muscle is performing an eccentric contraction against resistance, the test results will be greater than with the isometric muscle contraction. The faster the eccentric contraction, the greater the tension that develops in the muscle. Isometric and concentric types of muscle contractions are used most commonly in specific manual muscle testing.

The rate of shortening substantially affects the force a muscle can develop. The faster a muscle produces a concentric contraction, the less ability the muscle has to generate tension. Therefore, as velocity increases, tension decreases. During an eccentric muscle contraction, the tension initially increases, then tapers off as velocity increases. This increase in tension associated with an increased velocity may help to provide protection from structural damage exceeding tissue limitations as muscle lengthening occurs. Isokinetic muscle contractions occur when the velocity of movement remains constant and the resistance accommodates to the external force with changing joint angle. The muscle can therefore maintain maximal output throughout the full range of motion.

Mechanical devices such as a dynamometer have been developed that control the velocity of movement (Fig. 2–8). Dynamometers are used extensively for evaluating and exercising muscles, but they do not replace MMT. Practitioners may apply manual resistance in an attempt to simulate the function of the mechanical dynamometer. With practice, the therapist can continuously adjust the amount of resistance being offered so that the motion produced is approximately constant throughout the range, thereby approaching an isokinetic condition.

Anatomically, many factors are involved in objectively assessing the strength of any given muscle. Factors that affect muscle strength include the number of motor units per muscle, functional excursion, cross-sectional area, line of pull of muscle fibers, number of joints crossed, sensory receptors, attachments and the relationship of the muscle to the joint axis, and the age and sex of the subject. These factors cannot be changed clinically; however, the literature has information on differences in strength for sex, age, and some occupations. In males, muscle strength tends to increase from 2 to 19 years of age, then it plateaus until age 30, after which it starts to decline. In females, muscle strength increases uniformly until age 20 and remains level for approximately 10 years, then begins to decrease. Criteria for grading are being developed on the basis of age, sex, and occupation of the population.

Lehmkuhl and Smith state that biomechanical leverage in a muscle is an important consideration for muscle contraction.[3] As muscles go through their range of motion, the torque generated varies with the length of the moment arm (the distance from the axis of rotation). For example, as the elbow moves from full extension in

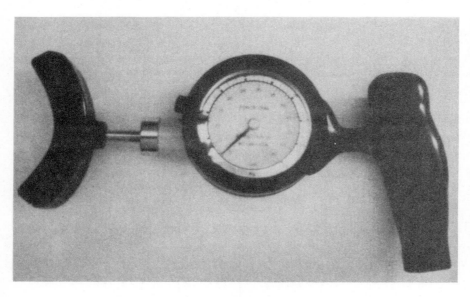

Figure 2–8. A hand-held dynamometer designed by G. Smidt (Spark Instruments and Academics Inc., P.O. Box 5123, Coraville, IA 52241) for measuring muscle strength.

flexion, the moment arm increases, reaching its maximum at 90 degrees of flexion, then decreases through the remainder of the range of motion.

Direct measurement of active voluntary tension developed in a muscle is not clinically practical. Muscle tension developed by a patient can be resolved into forces. One force is along the longitudinal axis of the segment on which the muscle attaches, and the other is at a right angle to the axis of motion. The component that is perpendicular to the body segment is called the rotary component; the component that is parallel to the body segment is the tension component when the direction of the force is away from the joint involved. It is called the compression component, or stabilizing force, when the direction of the force is toward the joint.[12] The rotatory force around an axis is the torque, which also can be expressed as muscle strength. Torque equals the product of the force and the perpendicular distance from the joint axis. The internal torque of muscle forces changes throughout the range of motion. Changes in the angle of attachment, which occur throughout the range of motion, produce changes in leverage and torque. The leverage of a muscle is greatest when the angle of insertion is 90 degrees.

Gravity (the weight of the body segment) also has a rotational component. It can be resolved in the same manner as muscle tension and acts in a direction opposite to that of muscle torque. The force of gravity has the greatest leverage and therefore is able to produce the greatest torque on a body segment when the segment is horizontal. External resistance applied to the moving segment must change as the body segment changes its position. Muscle torque must overcome applied external force and the weight of the limb in order to move or maintain a body segment in a specific position.

There are several mechanical methods of assessing muscle strength using instruments such as Kin Com, Lido, and Cybex dynamometers. The inherent properties of the instrument may dictate the mechanical factors relevant to the measurement, torque output. These factors include the capability of maintaining a constant moment arm, of assessing strength of different types of muscle contractions, and of maintaining a constant limb velocity. The segment to be tested can be positioned and the resistance applied where biomechanically and physiologically the muscle is at its best advantage to generate torque.

General Principles for Evaluating Skeletal Muscle Strength

In MMT the muscle grades express the examiner's objective evaluation of the functional strength of the muscle. Manual muscle tests are used to determine the degrees of muscle weakness resulting from disease, injury, or atrophy. The aim in muscle testing is to administer the test as accurately as possible. Knowledge of human anatomy and kinesiology is critical to success. The following factors are essential for therapists to make an accurate evaluation of muscle strength.

1. Anatomical, physiological, and biomechanical knowledge of skeletal muscle positions and stabilization.
2. Elimination of substitution motions.
3. Skill in palpation and application of resistance.
4. Careful direction for each movement that is easily understood by the patient.
5. Adherence to a standard method of grading muscle strength.
6. Experience testing many individuals with normal muscle strength and varying degrees of weakness.

Basic considerations in the technique of MMT are worthy of mention prior to an explanation of the procedure for evaluating muscle strength. MMT is preceded by a general review of the subject's medical history, interview, introduction to the subject and family, and a generalized or gross assessment of muscle strength. If the gross muscle evaluation shows specific muscle weakness, then those muscles are evaluated with specific MMT techniques. Seldom is an entire-body MMT performed; only muscles that have been identified previously warrant specific evaluation.

The examiner must explain the purpose of the test and give the directions in understandable terms. If the contralateral limb or segment is uninvolved, it is often useful to test that side first. Not only does it make the subject aware of the movement desired but it also provides a valuable standard for comparison.

The body area or segment to be evaluated is exposed, and the subject is properly draped. Each muscle to be tested must be palpated, and palpation through a hospital gown or clothing must be avoided as it will render the muscle test invalid. When possible the subject is evaluated in a quiet area free of distractions. The therapist requires the subject's cooperation and undivided attention in order to make an accurate determination of strength.

Results from the gross muscle evaluation will provide a general knowledge of total body muscle strength and enable the examiner to test all of the appropriate muscles in one position before having the subject change to another position, thus avoiding unnecessary fatigue and discomfort.

Grading

The examiner must be aware of variables that affect the grading of muscle strength. These variables are impor-

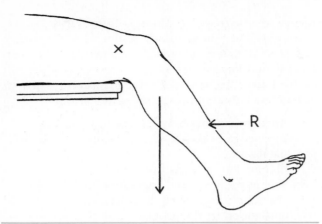

Figure 2–9. Illustration of resistance or rotational influence for knee extension. *X* is axis of knee joint, ↓ is gravitational force for leg and foot, *R* is external force applied to leg.

tant if MMT is to be clinically significant. The grading systems used in the practice of physical therapy are rather simple and easy to apply. Three basic factors are considered in MMT.

1. The weight of the limb or distal segment with a minimal effect of gravity on the moving segment. The muscle contracts in a plane horizontal to the effects of gravity. The test segment is supported on a smooth surface so that the frictional force is minimized during movement.
2. The weight of the limb plus the effects of gravity on the limb or segment. The motion occurs in a plane perpendicular to the effects of gravity.
3. The weight of the limb or segment plus the effects of gravity plus manual resistance. Practitioners must be consistent with respect to the point of application of resistance. Resistance is always applied at right angles to the long axis of the segment. The magnitude and direction of the resistance are opposite to that of the contracting muscle (Fig. 2–9).

The grading system for muscle strength is based on specific factors.

1. The amount of resistance given manually to a contracted muscle or muscle group determines strength. The force is applied by the tester in a direction opposite to the torque exerted by the muscle being tested.
2. The ability of a muscle or muscle group to move a part through a complete test range of motion is a measure of muscle strength.
3. Evidence of the presence or absence of a muscle contraction as determined by palpation and observation is critical to muscle strength evaluation.
4. Grades are obtained on the basis of the effects of gravity and manual resistance. Gravity affects movement depending on the position of the pa-

tient. When a muscle contracts perpendicular to the gravitational force, the position is referred to as *gravity-minimized (GM)*. When a muscle contracts against the downward gravitational force, the position is referred to as *against gravity (AG)*. The AG position may also involve the application of manual resistance.

The standard muscle testing grades are applicable to the adult population and may need to be adjusted for older or younger subjects. Grading criteria depend on the patient's body build, age, sex, and occupation. For example, a Good (4) grade for a professional football linebacker is not the same as the Good grade for a 75-year-old woman or a 3-year-old child. Some muscles within the body normally are not capable of exerting significant amounts of torque. The examiner must be aware of the variability of normal muscle function so as not to incorrectly assign a weak grade to a normal-functioning muscle.

Table 2–2 describes various grading systems that have been used in clinical practice over the past 60 years.

There are some basic differences between Lovett's (Daniels and Worthingham) and Kendall's method of grading.[13] Overall, because Daniels and Worthingham's method tests a motion that utilizes all agonists and synergists involved in the motion, it is a more functional approach. Kendall's approach tests a specific muscle rather than a motion, and requires selective muscle performance on the part of the patient. Specific muscle testing requires a greater knowledge of anatomy and kinesiology than testing voluntary motions. It gives accurate results of a muscle's function but is more time consuming for the examiner.

Kendall's method tests muscles isometrically in which the segment is aligned in the direction of the muscle fibers in a mid-range position and the patient is asked to hold against resistance. Kendall's technique maintains the patient in the same antigravity position and uses assistance to determine which grades the patient is unable to attain moving against gravity. In Lovett's technique the patient moves through the full test range, a concentric contraction, or holds at the end of the range while the muscle is in its shortened position. Although Lovett's is a more subjective test; it will identify where in the range weakness exists. Daniels and Worthingham place the patient in the GM position when the patient is unable to move against gravity. Both Lovett's and Daniels and Worthingham's techniques have an inherent subjectivity in the area of applied resistance.

Most physicians use the Medical Research Council scale, which is based on numbers that are easy to remember and to interpret.[6] The grades of 0, 1, and 2 are tested in the GM position. All others are tested against gravity. Resistance is applied as an isometric hold at the end of the test range to determine AG grades. Another infre-

Table 2–2. Comparison of Gravity-Resisted Muscle Grading Criteria

LOVETT AND DANIELS AND WORTHINGHAM[5]	KENDALL AND MCCREARY[11]	MEDICAL RESEARCH COUNCIL
N (Normal): Subject completes range of motion against gravity, against maximal resistance.	100%: Subject moves into and holds test position against gravity, against maximal resistance.	5
G+ (Good Plus): Subject completes range of motion against gravity, against nearly maximal resistance.		4+
G (Good): Subject completes range of motion against gravity, against moderate resistance.	80%: Subject moves into and holds test position against gravity, against less than maximal resistance.	4
G− (Good Minus): Subject completes range of motion against gravity, against minimal resistance.		4−
F+ (Fair Plus): Subject completes range of motion against gravity, against minimal resistance.		3+
F (Fair): Subject completes range of motion against gravity with no manual resistance.	50%: Subject moves into and holds a test position against gravity.	3
F− (Fair Minus): Subject does not complete range against gravity but does complete more than half the range.		3−
P+ (Poor Plus): Subject initiates range of motion against gravity or completes range with gravity minimized against slight resistance.		2+
P (Poor): Subject completes range of motion with gravity minimized.	20%: Subject moves through small motion with gravity minimized	2
P− (Poor Minus): Subject does not complete range of motion with gravity minimized.		2−
T (Trace): Subject's muscle can be palpated but there is no joint motion.	5%: Contraction is palpable with no joint motion.	1
0 (Zero): Subject exhibits no palpable contraction.	0%: No contraction is palpable.	0

quently used grading system is based on a numerical scale that ranges from 5 to 1, 5 indicating a trace of muscle strength and 1 indicating normal.

Body segments that have short lever arms are not significantly influenced by gravity. Their grades are determined by manual resistance or no resistance. The fingers and toes are short segments, and the effect of gravity on them is insignificant. Physical therapists in different areas of the country determine grades variously by means of palpation alone or by gravity assistance of the muscle. When a patient is unable to change testing positions or when the patient demonstrates weakness in the AG position and cannot be appropriately positioned in the GM position, other grading methods may be used.

When a patient is unable to assume standard test positions, grades may be determined by *palpation*. This type of grading is one for which considerable experience in palpating normal and weak muscle contractions is necessary.

GRADING BY PALPATION CRITERIA
N (Normal, 5): The muscle is well delineated and the contraction feels hard.
G (Good, 4): The muscle is well delineated and the contraction feels firm.
F (Fair, 3): The muscle outline is well delineated, but the contraction feels soft.
P (Poor, 2): The muscle is not well delineated, and a slight, mushy contraction is felt.
T (Trace, 1): A flicker or mere tension or relaxation after contraction is felt.
0 (Zero, 0): No muscle contraction is palpated.

Grades also may be determined by the *assistance* to the segment or body part when positions or other factors may prevent the subject from assuming the standard positions. The subject is positioned to allow the effects of gravity to assist the contraction of the muscle and a determination of strength is made by estimating the amount of assistance given to a weak muscle. The subject relaxes the part to be tested so the examiner can feel the weight of the test segment. As the patient moves through the range of motion, the examiner attempts to measure the decreased weight of the part. The examiner should guide the movement and give assistance but not precede the motion.

GRADING BY ASSISTANCE CRITERIA
0 (Zero): 100% of the weight of the segment is supported by the examiner throughout the test range.
T (Trace): 100% of the weight of the segment is supported by the examiner throughout the test range, but a contraction is felt or observed.
P− (Poor Minus): 75% of the maximal weight of the segment is supported by the examiner.

P (Poor): 50% or moderate assistance is required to move the part through the test range.
P+ (Poor Plus): 30% or minimal assistance is required to move the part through the test range of motion.
Higher muscle strength grades would be against the effects of gravity, as indicated above.

As stated earlier, grades obtained by experienced examiners should not vary more than a half grade when half grades are used (i.e., a grade difference of 3 versus 3+ [Fair and Fair Plus] is permissible, since MMT has not been professionally validated). If the examiner is undecided between two grades, it is best to record the lower one to establish a treatment plan that is appropriate for the patient. Recording the lower grade may also serve to motivate the patient by demonstrating gains in strength between sessions.

Factors Affecting Manual Muscle Testing Results

The examiner must be aware that some musculoskeletal disorders or weaknesses cause muscles to fatigue more easily and rapidly than normal. Fatigue is a reason to test various areas of the body during one evaluation session rather than several muscles around a single joint or limb. For example, test a few hand muscles, then move to the lower limb, then come back to the upper limb.

There are patients who are unable to complete the test range of motion because of joint limitation rather than muscle weakness. A patient with rheumatoid arthritis may have limited range in the wrist or knee joints. The test range of motion is determined by the amount of passive range of motion available in the joint. In such a situation, a *range grade–strength grade* is used to determine strength and record the measurements. The purpose is to assign a grade of strength to a muscle in which the passive test range is incomplete. Range grade–strength grade is used to evaluate muscles that are incapable of contracting through a complete test range because of joint limitations but that can complete the available range and can hold against resistance. For example, tightness of a muscle or lack of joint stability may give such a grade. The limited range should be measured before muscle strength is evaluated. Range grade–strength grade is recorded as a fraction whose numerator is the number of degrees completed through the available passive limited range of motion and whose denominator is the strength. If knee extension is lacking 20 degrees and the strength of the quadriceps muscle is Good (4), the range grade–strength grade is stated as −20 degrees / 4 Good.

The numerator of range–strength grades also may be stated as F− or P+. F− means that the test range is not complete but the motion is over one half the standard test range of motion. P+ means that the test range is less than one half the test range.

A question mark in MMT is used when the validity of the strength is in doubt. For instance, if the subject has a painful joint that limits the muscle's contractile force, one may use the question mark or write on the form "pain—unable to test."

Sliding grades have been recorded when muscle strength ranges between two grades. For instance, T to P− (Trace to Poor Minus) indicates the grade is better than a trace but does not demonstrate sufficient strength to be assigned a grade of Poor Minus. There can be only a half grade difference when using the sliding grade scale.

Subjectivity becomes a factor in determining muscle grades any time one uses manual resistance, assistance, or palpation to determine muscle strength.

Grades obtained during MMT do not represent the absolute amount of muscle tension developed during contraction. A muscle grade of 4 (Good, 75%) is not equivalent to 75% of the strength represented by a grade of 5 (Normal, 100%). It is a natural grade determined by the effect of gravity, manual resistance, patient's age, degree of disability, and so forth. Absolute muscle strength is determined by the physiological cross-sectional area of the muscle and is an indication of the muscle's functional capacity. The larger the cross-sectional area, the more tension can be produced. The cross-section alone, however, does not determine how much work the muscle is able to produce. To determine the muscle's work capacity, the distance a muscle can shorten must be known. Rudolph Fick computed work capacity of individual muscles by multiplying 3 to 4 kilograms (kg) of force per square centimeter (cm^2) by the cross-sectional area. Tables have been developed and published for individual muscles. It is obvious that absolute muscle strength is not a practical criterion for evaluating muscle strength in the clinical setting.

Positions

Positioning a patient for testing varies with the muscle tested, its strength, and the overall condition of the patient. The patient and the part to be tested should be positioned comfortably on a firm surface. The body part must be exposed and the individual properly draped. Not all patients can be examined using the standard test positions. Patients may be on frames or may be medically unable to tolerate certain positions. In these situations, grades may be determined by palpation or by allowing gravity to assist the motion.

Two test positions (GM and AG) are used as standard positions to determine the strength of muscles based on the effects of gravity.

GM (Gravity-Minimized). The test segment is positioned to minimize or diminish the effects of gravity

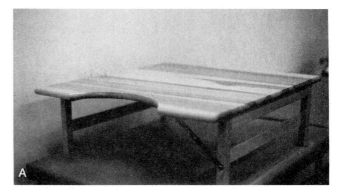

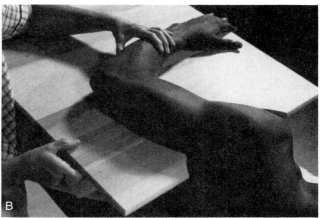

Figure 2–10. (*A*) A powder board, made of wood and treated to permit movement on a smooth, frictionless surface. The board is lightly covered with powder to reduce friction on the test segment during gravity-minimized muscle strength testing. (*B*) Placement of the powder board with the subject in a sidelying position. A pillow may be placed under the board if it rests on the subject.

for a specific muscle. The term "gravity-eliminated" is used by Daniels and Worthingham to describe this position,[4] although gravitational effects are eliminated only in a weightless environment. Movements are not assisted or resisted by gravity. The testing surface is free of friction. A powder board is often used to reduce friction from the patient's skin and the supporting surface. It is usually constructed of wood or lightweight plastic (Fig. 2–10*A* and *B*).

Muscles that flex and extend in the sagittal plane against gravity are tested in the transverse plane for GM testing. The subject lies on one side. There are no gravitational effects on the contracting muscle.

Muscles that produce motions against gravity in the coronal plane are tested in the transverse plane with the subject in a prone or supine position. To test in the GM position for abductor and adductor muscles, the patient is usually in the sitting position. The body segments for the rotator muscle groups tested in the GM position are positioned parallel to gravity.

AG (Against-Gravity). The subject is positioned so that the effects of gravity are working against the test segment. The patient is positioned so that the body segment contracts against the downward gravitational force.

The list Positions for Testing Against Gravity, later in this chapter, contains a summary of test positions. Positioning details for specific muscles are presented in subsequent chapters.

Test Range. The test range is the amount of motion a joint completes by contraction of the test muscle. The range of motion for specific muscle testing is not necessarily the complete range of motion that the muscle can produce at that joint. For instance, the muscles involved with shoulder flexion are able to contract through a range of motion of 180 degrees, but the manual muscle testing range is only 90 degrees.

Range of motion testing is initially performed passively to determine any limitation within the joint that the muscle to be evaluated is going to move. The practitioner assesses the test range before making a judgment on the strength of a muscle.

If the test range of motion is limited by a joint problem, manual muscle strength can still be tested and graded (see range grade–strength grade, above).

Palpation. Palpation should be done to assess the contraction of the muscle being tested. The number of fingers used depends on the size of the muscle or tendon being palpated. If the muscle is small, the middle finger is the most sensitive to tension in muscle contraction. Every muscle evaluated must be palpated to make MMT a valid assessment tool. Palpation is necessary to determine exactly which muscle is being contracted and to allow the examiner to detect substitutions by adjacent muscles.

Resistance. Resistance is the force applied at the end of the test range (break method) or throughout the test range (make method) in a direction opposite the muscle's rotatory component. Manual resistance is applied at right angles to the long axis of the segment. Resistance may be applied at the end of the test range, with the muscle providing an isometric hold as described by Daniels and Worthingham, or throughout the test range while the muscle is performing a concentric type of contraction.

The results in the assessment of muscle strength differ depending on the method used. The isometric hold, or the break test, shows the muscle to have a higher test grade than the resistance given throughout the range in the make test. In either method, manual resistance is applied gradually and released gradually, giving the pa-

tient time to contract the muscle and then to relax it before the resistance has been removed.

The skill and consistency with which the examiner applies the manual resistance to the segment are important. The force should be applied gradually in a direction opposite the muscle's rotatory component and at a consistent location—distally without crossing another joint—on the moving segment.

The effect of manual resistance on muscle torque is a function of the distance of its application from the joint axis. The tester who changes the point at which resistance is applied to the body segment will find that the muscle torque exerted will also change. This inconsistency in technique will prevent the examiner from developing an appreciation for what is "normal strength" relative to an individual's sex, age, body type, and lifestyle.

The proper location for the application of resistance is as far distal as possible from one joint axis of movement on the moving segment without crossing another joint. Resistance should never cross an intervening joint unless the integrity of the joint has been assessed and is considered normal.

The manual muscle testing developed for this book allows the examiner to apply resistance using either the isometric muscle contraction break test or the concentric muscle contraction make test. The important factor is consistency for each patient and among the coworkers who may be evaluating and treating the patient.

Stabilization

Extrinsic stabilization, or fixation, is counterpressure to resistance that provides support for the subject and helps prevent substitute motions. Manually or with an external support, the tester stabilizes the proximal segment while contraction of the muscle moves the distal segment. Stabilization adds validity to the muscle test. To evaluate the strength of the quadriceps, for example, the therapist would stabilize the thigh. If the proximal attachment of a muscle is unstable, the rotatory component of the contracting muscle will not have an adequate advantage.

Intrinsic methods of stabilization are achieved by structures or factors found inherently within the body. For example, the importance of the scapula in providing stability for shoulder and upper limb function is widely accepted.

Substitution

Substitute motions occur when muscles are weak or movement is uncoordinated. Synergistic muscles contract to produce the desired motion with or without the action of the agonist muscle.

Subjects typically use any muscle to produce a desired motion when the muscle being tested is too weak to perform the action. Substitution movements by synergist muscles are common in normal persons. When the therapist applies too much resistance, the subject is tempted to use substitute muscles to do the desired motion. In evaluating wrist flexion, for instance, if too much manual resistance is applied, the subject substitutes with the finger flexors.

Substitutions can be minimized by careful and appropriate positioning and stabilizing. Detection of substitutions is obvious when the examiner palpates the muscle being evaluated.

Recording Measurements

Refer to Appendix A for an example of the MMT recording form. Recording forms vary in format from clinical facility to clinical facility. Forms are designed to record muscle strength grades by peripheral nerve innervation, by specific muscle, or by muscle group actions. The grades that are recorded on the forms also vary by the method chosen.

At the bottom of the MMT form is an area in which to record any comments about the subject. For example, the subject may experience pain on motion, a variation from the standard position may have been used, or the subject may have appeared confused or disoriented during the evaluation. All are events that should be noted in the Comment section of the recording form. It is important to record muscle strength status as part of the patient's medical record, to develop a treatment plan, for documentation, and for reimbursement of medical services.

The form is designed for recording three to four measurements on subsequent evaluations. The records are dated and written on the designated side, right or left, with the muscle grade written on the inside column and subsequent recordings added to the outside columns. If all the muscles test Good to Normal in strength, it is not necessary to record the finding for each muscle on the form. It is necessary, however, to record the findings and include them in the patient's medical record.

General Procedure for Specific Manual Muscle Testing

Performing the test in the prescribed sequence benefits subject and examiner. When the sequence is followed, the test is performed without omissions, and the results should be valid and reliable.

1. Following the gross muscle test, the first step is to position the subject in the AG position, unless that is contraindicated. The subject should be positioned so that the muscle contracting and the motion being performed can be ob-

served easily. If muscle weakness is evident in more than one area, all muscles that can be tested in one position should be. Changing positions tires the subject and may yield an inaccurate evaluation of muscle strength. The subject should be stabilized and positioned comfortably. It also is important for the examiner to be comfortable while testing.

2. The body part or segment to be tested is exposed and the rest of the body is well draped.

3. After explaining the test and demonstrating it to the subject, the examiner determines the available range of motion associated with the test muscle. Usually the test range is evaluated passively unless the examiner knows that the muscle is functional and can move the part through the entire test range, in which case active motion may be performed. If the subject also requires goniometry of the joint, such measurement should precede the manual muscle evaluation.

4. The body part or segment to be evaluated is aligned according to the direction of the muscle fibers. This alignment allows optimal muscle function.

5. Before the subject contracts the muscle, the therapist provides adequate stabilization to the proximal segment.

6. During proximal segment stabilization the subject attempts to contract the muscle to move the distal segment throughout the test range of motion. The moving segment may also be placed at the end of the range of motion, in which case the subject is asked to hold the contraction. Speed of the contraction is moderate; accuracy is more important.

7. During the active contraction, the examiner observes the movement and the muscle and palpates the tendon or muscle belly. The therapist can help avoid substitutions by palpating the muscle that should perform the desired movement. As a rule, the joint is not graded on motion alone—the therapist should *always palpate*.

8. The examiner applies resistance to the muscle that is able to complete the test range against gravity. Application and release of resistance are firm and smooth. Resistance is applied at the distal end of the segment, without crossing an intervening joint, in a direction as nearly opposite the line of pull of the muscle fibers as possible. The subject is instructed to establish a maximum contraction before resistance is given. The therapist may apply resistance at the end of the test range, as in the break test, or throughout the range, as in the make test.

The movement is repeated until the muscle strength grade has been determined, but not so many times that the subject becomes fatigued. Muscle testing is designed to test strength, not endurance. The subject should be able to perform three consecutive repetitions at the same grade level. It is advisable to compare the strength with that of the uninvolved muscle, if possible. Fatigue of a muscle may be a diagnostic sign of a neuromuscular disorder. Also, fatigue with repetitions may be an early sign of nerve root compression.

9. The final step in the MMT evaluation is to record the grade and date and initial the test form.

10. The assessment of the patient's performance is derived from the recording form, and the patient's treatment plan is developed therefrom.

Preferred Positions for Against-Gravity Testing

SITTING

LOWER LIMBS

Hip
  Psoas major
  Iliacus
  Sartorius
Knee
  Quadriceps Femoris
    Vastus medialis
    Vastus lateralis
    Vastus intermedius
    Rectus femoris
Ankle/foot
  Anterior tibial
  Toes

UPPER LIMBS

Scapula
  Upper trapezius
  Levator scapulae
Shoulder
  Deltoid—middle, anterior
  Brachioradialis
  Coracobrachialis
  Pectoralis major—clavicular
  Supraspinatus
Elbow/radioulnar joint
  Biceps brachii
  Brachialis
  Brachioradialis
  Pronator teres
  Supinator
  Pronator quadratus
Wrist/hand
  Flexor carpi radialis

Flexor carpi ulnaris
Extensor carpi radialis longus and brevis
Extensor carpi ulnaris
All finger muscles
All thumb muscles
Neck and Trunk
  None

SUPINE

LOWER LIMBS

Knee
  None
Ankle/foot
  None

UPPER LIMBS

Scapula
  Serratus anterior
Shoulder
  Pectoralis major
  Anterior deltoid
Elbow/radioulnar joint
  Triceps brachii
Wrist/hand
  All, if not tested sitting

NECK AND TRUNK

Neck
  Sternocleidomastoid
  Scalene
Trunk
  Rectus abdominis
  Oblique internal abdominal
  Oblique external abdominal
Pelvis
  None

PRONE

LOWER LIMBS

Hip
  Gluteus maximus
Knee
  Hamstrings
    Biceps Femoris
    Semitendinosus
    Semimembranosus
Ankle/foot
  Gastrocnemius
  Soleus (NWB)

UPPER LIMBS

Scapula
  Middle and lower trapezius
  Major and minor rhomboids
Shoulder
  Latissimus dorsi
  Teres major
  Subscapularis
  Infraspinatus

Posterior deltoid
Elbow/radioulnar joint
 Triceps brachii
Wrist/hand
 None

NECK AND TRUNK
Neck
 Splenius capitis and cervicis
 Semispinalis capitis and cervicis
 Erector spinae capitis and cervicis
Trunk
 Thoracic and lumbar erector spinae
Pelvis
 None

SIDELYING

LOWER LIMBS
Hip
 Gluteus medius
 Gluteus minimus
 Adductors longus, brevis, magnus, gracilis, pectineus
 Tensor fasciae latae
Knee
 None
Ankle/foot
 Posterior tibialis
 Peroneus longus and brevis

STANDING

LOWER LIMBS
Hip
 None
Knee
 None
Ankle/foot
 Gastrocnemius
 Soleus

UPPER LIMBS, NECK, AND TRUNK
 Quadratus lumborum

Preferred Positions for Gravity-Minimized Testing

SITTING

LOWER LIMBS
None

UPPER LIMBS
Scapula
 Serratus anterior
 Major and minor rhomboids
 Middle trapezius
Shoulder
 Anterior and posterior deltoids
 Pectoralis major
Elbow/radioulnar joint

Biceps brachii
Brachialis
Brachioradialis
Supinator
Pronator teres
Triceps
Wrist/hand
 All

NECK AND TRUNK
Neck
 Sternocleidomastoid
Trunk
 Thoracic and lumbar erector spinae
Pelvis
 None

SUPINE

LOWER LIMBS
Hip
 Gluteus medius and minimus
 Tensor fasciae latae
 Adductor longus, brevis, magnus, gracilis, pectineus
 Lateral rotators
 Sartorius
Knee
 None
Ankle/foot
 Posterior tibialis
 Peroneus longus and brevis
 Toes
UPPER LIMBS
Scapula
 Upper trapezius
Shoulder
 Middle deltoid
Elbow/radioulnar joint
 None
Wrist/hand
 All
NECK AND TRUNK
Neck
 None
Trunk
 None
Pelvis
 Quadratus lumborum

PRONE

LOWER LIMBS
None
UPPER LIMBS
Scapula
 Upper and lower trapezius
Shoulder
 Latissimus dorsi

Teres major
Subscapularis
Pectoralis major
Supraspinatus
Teres minor
Infraspinatus
Elbow/radioulnar joint
  None
Wrist/hand
  None

NECK AND TRUNK
Neck
  None
Trunk
  None
Pelvis
  Quadratus lumborum

SIDELYING

LOWER LIMBS
Hip
  Psoas major
  Iliacus
  Gluteus maximus
Knee
  Quadriceps Femoris
    Vastus lateralis
    Vastus medialis
    Vastus intermedius
    Rectus femoris
  Hamstrings
    Biceps femoris
    Semitendinosus
    Semimembranosus
Ankle/foot
  Gastrocnemius
  Soleus
  Tibialis anterior

UPPER LIMBS
Scapula
  None
Shoulder
  Anterior and posterior deltoid
  Coracobrachialis
  Pectoralis major—clavicular
  Latissimus dorsi
Elbow/radioulnar joint
  None
Wrist/hand
  All

NECK AND TRUNK
Neck
  Sternocleidomastoid
Trunk
  None

Pelvis
  None
STANDING
None

Orthopedic Examination of Synovial Joints

It is important that orthopedic assessment of a joint be carried out systematically. Accurate evaluation and assessment depend on complete information regarding patient history, a thorough examination of clinical signs and symptoms, and a comprehensive medical workup.

Clinicians need to establish their own ways of performing a musculoskeletal assessment. When a systematic approach is followed repeatedly, it is unlikely that any information relative to the correct diagnosis will be overlooked.

This section deals with the components of synovial joint assessment and is divided into the following sections:

1. patient history,
2. gross observation and palpation,
3. examination of inert and contractile structures,
4. special tests, and
5. joint play movements.

Patient History

Before examining the patient, the clinician should thoroughly review the medical chart, paying specific attention to parts that are clinically relevant to the diagnosis. It is vitally important that the patient have a complete medical diagnostic workup. Information such as radiology reports, laboratory tests, and electrodiagnostic testing assist in definitively confirming or ruling out orthopedic and neurologic pathology.

The therapist next obtains information from the patient, and it is this portion of the examination process that may yield the most constructive information. An astute clinician many times is able to arrive at an accurate diagnosis on the basis of a very complete and thorough history related by the patient.

Questioning of the patient should be done in a systematic manner. It is important that the examiner not "lead" the patient in the course of questioning. Questions should be asked that require specific answers. For example, the clinician should not say, "Does this increase your pain?" but instead, "Tell me if this alters your symptoms in any way." The examiner should not accept vague responses that do not specifically answer the question and should persist with a question until a satisfactory response is obtained.

Answers to the following questions should be obtained as part of the subjective examination:

1. The first question should be, "What is the complaint that has brought you here today?" This question not only sets the tone for the rest of the interview, but also allows patients to describe the problem in their own words.
2. The next question should inquire into the occupation, athletic endeavors, and hobbies of the patient. Answers will provide the examiner with information regarding stresses and postures typical of the patient and may suggest the mechanism of injury.
3. "Was the onset of the problem sudden, or did the problem appear gradually over a period of hours, days, or weeks? Were you able to relate it to a specific activity or posture? Was the onset associated with direct trauma in a contact injury or with an indirect, noncontact situation?"
4. "Is this the first time that this particular problem has occurred? If not, how do the symptoms now compare to past experiences? How long did the problem persist in previous episodes? How were you treated for this problem in the past, and was that treatment regimen successful in relieving the symptoms?"
5. "How long have you had your present symptoms?" This information may help the examiner determine the acuteness or chronicity of the problem.
6. "How are your symptoms today as compared to the first day they became apparent?" Response to this question will yield information about the stage of healing or will indicate if the condition is getting worse.
7. "What is the nature of your symptoms?" If the patient expresses pain as the primary complaint, the examiner must delve thoroughly into the nature of the pain. It is important that the patient describe the type of pain. Is it sharp, dull, achy, or throbbing? "Is the pain constant or intermittent? If the pain is intermittent, do certain postures or activities exacerbate or relieve it? Do rest and activity make your pain worse or better, or do they have no effect?" For example, rest usually alleviates a mechanical problem in or around the joint. Pain felt in the morning that diminishes progressively as the day goes on is indicative of a chronic inflammatory process, such as arthritis. Pain and stiffness felt at the beginning of activity that subside as the activity continues may indicate a muscle problem. An increase in pain noted in the morning also may relate to sleeping postures, mattresses, or pillows.

"Can you pinpoint the pain, or is it diffuse or radiating?" Bone pain tends to be very deep and localized, whereas nerve root pain characteristically radiates following a dermatomal pattern. Muscle pain tends to be somewhat diffuse.

8. "Are you now experiencing or have you experienced sensations other than pain?" These may take the form of pins and needles, tingling, numbness, or anesthesia. These symptoms are usually associated with neurologic involvement.
9. "Do you experience any joint locking or 'giving way'?" Locking may be a result of internal derangement, as in a meniscal tear or the temporary lodging of a loose body between articular surfaces. Giving way is often related to ligamentous instability or reflex muscle inhibition.
10. "Have you experienced any dizziness or fainting spells?" These symptoms may be representative of a more serious underlying neurologic disorder.

Gross Observation and Palpation

Observation should begin as the patient is entering the department or examination area. The gait pattern may be observed and any gross deviations noted. An antalgic gait pattern may indicate to the examiner which joints are affected and may demonstrate the patient's willingness or reluctance to bear weight on the affected limb. Examination of the expression on the patient's face may provide information about the degree of pain.

The patient's freedom of movement should also be noted during removal of coats, pullover sweaters, and shoes and socks. The ease or difficulty with which the patient gets on the examining table and assumes various positions should be noted as it may suggest the necessity for more specific assessment.

Once the patient has exposed the body part to be examined and is properly draped, the examiner can make the following observations.

1. The examiner should look for any gross postural deformity or abnormality that may be associated with fractures, scoliosis, or traumatic incidents.
2. The examiner should compare the contours in the involved and the uninvolved sides.
3. The examiner should note any evidence of atrophy.
4. The examiner should note the color, texture, and temperature of the part being examined. Temperature elevation usually indicates an active inflammatory state, whereas a cooler temperature usually reflects vascular compromise. Trophic changes such as shiny skin, hair loss, and brittle nails may be evidence of diabetes, vascular problems, or peripheral nerve lesions.

5. The examiner should look for scars, indicating past trauma or surgery. Open or closed sinus tracts are typical of infections such as osteomyelitis.
6. The examiner should look for edema or effusion in or around the problem area.
7. The examiner should palpate for pulses and compare the findings to those for the uninvolved limb. The pulses that should be checked as part of this assessment include the brachial, radial, femoral, popliteal, and dorsalis pedis.
8. The examiner should palpate for any muscle spasm, indicating an attempt by the musculature to "splint," or immobilize, a traumatized or pathologic area.

Examination of Inert and Contractile Structures

In the assessment of a synovial joint, it must be remembered that all of the structures comprising the joint, as well as the musculature that moves the joint, are stressed when the patient moves actively. Therefore, specific examination techniques must be employed that isolate inert structures from contractile elements. A systematic approach to the identification of the structures responsible for the patient's complaints follows.

Active Movements

Little objective information is obtained from active movement, as both contractile and inert structures are moving and, therefore, stressed. Active motion, however, does provide information about the patient's willingness to move. As the patient moves, the examiner is able to generally assess whether other joint movements are substituting for the desired movement and where in the available range of motion pain is experienced, discern the quality and pattern of the movement, and get an idea of the restriction of the movement.

Passive Movements

The examiner passively moves the joint through the available range of motion in all directions of movement that the joint is capable of. Passive range of motion assesses the integrity of the inert structures of the joint by stressing them at various points in the range. These inert structures, which have no inherent ability to contract, include the capsule, ligament, bursa, cartilage, nerves and nerve sheaths, and dura mater. Objective information regarding the status of the joint may be gained through passive testing. The identification of the sequence of pain and resistance, end feel, and capsular patterns provide invaluable information about the pathologic state of the joint.

Sequence of Pain and Resistance. The sequence of pain and resistance provides the examiner with information about the acuteness or chronicity of joint pathology.

Stage 1. The patient experiences pain before the examiner feels any resistance to the passive range of motion. This stage is representative of an acute joint.
Stage 2. The patient feels pain at the same time the examiner feels resistance to the passive range of motion. Stage 2 indicates a subacute condition present in the joint. The clinician can be slightly more aggressive with this joint than at the previous stage.
Stage 3. The examiner feels resistance to the passive range of motion before the patient experiences pain. This joint has no active inflammatory process going on and therefore is considered chronic. With this stage, the clinician can treat aggressively.

End Feels. An end feel is the feeling imparted to the examiner's hands as the end point of passive range of motion is reached. It can provide information regarding the nature of the restriction responsible for terminating the range of movement. Each synovial joint in the human body has a normal end feel, which is how the resistance feels at the end point of the normal range of motion. It is during pathologic restrictions of range of motion that the clinician need be concerned with the assessment of end feel.

The types of end feel commonly found include:

1. Soft: The feeling of soft tissue compressing soft tissue; it is normally found in elbow flexion and knee flexion.
2. Bony: The feeling of bone impacting against bone, normally found in elbow extension; it is pathologic if found in other joints of the body or in restricted elbow extension.
3. Springy: The feeling of the joint stopping and then rebounding, normally not found in the body. It is associated with internal derangements, usually in joints with menisci or cartilaginous disks.
4. Capsular: A feeling of a firm but slightly yielding stop, as if two pieces of hard rubber were pressed together. Normally it is found with shoulder and hip joint rotations; it is pathologic if found in other joints or in restricted ranges of shoulder and hip joint rotation.

Table 2–3.   Capsular Patterns of Joints

JOINTS	CAPSULAR PATTERN
Glenohumeral	External rotation (ER)>abduction (abd)>internal rotation (IR)
Sternoclavicular	Pain at extremes of range of motion (ROM)
Acromioclavicular	Pain at extremes of ROM
Humeroulnar	Flexion (flex.)>extension (ext.)
Radiohumeral	Flex.>ext.
Proximal radioulnar	Pronation (pro.) = supination (sup.)
Distal radioulnar	Pro. = sup.
Radiocarpal	Equal restriction all motions
Midcarpal	Ext.>flex.
Carpometacarpal (2–5)	Equal restriction all motions
Carpometacarpal (1)	Abd. > ext.
Metacarpophalangeal (2–5)	Flex. >ext.
Interphalangeal (1–5)	Flex.> ext.
Hip	IR>abd.>flex.>ext.>adduction ER
Tibiofemoral	Flex.>ext.
Talocrural	Plantar flexion>dorsiflexion
Subtalar	
Metatarsophalangeal (2–5)	Flex.>ext.
Metatarsophalangeal (1)	Ext.>flex.
Interphalangeal	Flex.>ext.
Atlanto-occipital	Ext. equal to side flex.
Cervical spine	Side flex.=rotation (rot.); ext.
Thoracic spine	Side flex.=rot.; ext.
Lumbar spine	Side flex.=Rot.; ext.
Temporomandibular	Limited ability to open mouth

(Adapted from Kaltenborn FM: Mobilization of the Extremity Joints. Oslo, Olaf Norlis Bolchandel, 1980)

5. Empty: A feeling that there is nothing restricting the ability to perform passive motion except the patient's considerable pain. Normally not found in the body, it is associated with acute episodes or neoplasms.

Capsular Patterns.   When a synovial joint is traumatized, inflamed, or immobilized, the capsule of that joint undergoes a unique pattern of proportional limitation. Each synovial joint in the body has its own pattern of proportional limitation, or capsular pattern. The presence of a capsular pattern is determined through the comparison of passive range of motion measurements in a given joint. When a capsular pattern is identified, it is an indication that the capsule is involved in its entirety. It must be remembered, however, that a capsular pattern need not be present to have hypomobility in certain parts of the capsule.

Table 2–3 lists the common capsular patterns present in joints in the sequence of most to least restricted.

Contractile Testing

Contractile testing is performed to assess the integrity of the contractile structures about the joint. Stuctures iden-

tified as being contractile include muscles, tendons, and tendinous attachments to bone.

Contractile testing is performed *isometrically* at a neutral midposition within the range of motion to ensure that positioning alone does not stress these structures. It must be remembered that during isometric contraction, compressive forces are transmitted to the joint. These compressive forces may be minimized with proper technique and by applying slight traction before asking for a response.

The results of contractile testing will yield the following descriptions:

- Pain-free and strong (indicates normal muscle).
- Painful and strong (indicates a minor lesion in the contractile unit, e.g., tendinitis).
- Pain-free and weak (indicates a peripheral nerve lesion or muscle rupture).
- Painful and weak (indicates serious pathology, e.g., fracture, unstable joint, or metastatic lesion).
- All movements painful (usually represents fatigue or emotional problems).

Contractile findings may be positive during inert passive testing, a result of the muscle being stretched while performing passive range of motion in the antagonistic direction. Muscles that test weak should be specifically examined with MMT to determine the degree of weakness.

Special Tests

Ligament Instability

Ligament testing should be performed as part of the joint examination in the assessment of inert structures. Normal end feel or stability is based on and compared to that of the counterparts on the uninvolved side. Joint instability related to ligament laxity is graded on a scale of 0 to 3:

1. Zero instability indicates no difference in joint excursion between the ligament on the uninvolved side and the ligament on the involved side.
2. First-degree instability indicates an excursion of less than 0.5 cm of the involved ligament compared with the uninvolved ligament.
3. Second-degree instability represents an excursion of 0.5 to 1 cm of the involved ligament compared with the uninvolved ligament.
4. Third-degree instability indicates an excursion of more than 1 cm of the involved ligament compared with the uninvolved ligament.

Traction (Distraction)

Traction or distraction in this instance is defined as a movement performed passively (by the examiner) that results in separation of joint surfaces. The clinical significance of assessing joint distraction is that it may yield information about the integrity of the joint.

1. If traction relieves pain, joint surfaces may be involved. The relief is probably secondary to the removal of compressive forces.
2. If traction increases pain, a complete or partial tear of connective tissue may be present.
3. If traction reveals limited range, there may be contracture of connective tissue.
4. If traction indicates increased range, the joint may be hypermobile and supporting structures may be damaged.

Compression

Compression of the joint is accomplished by the examiner passively pushing the joint surfaces together. The clinical significance of assessing compression is to provide information about the state of the joint surfaces, as noted below:

1. An increase in pain associated with compression may be an indication of possible internal derangement or of a loose body.

Table 2–4. Upper Quarter Screening Examination

Cervical postural assessment
Active cervical range of motion
Passive overpressures, if no signs or symptoms are found actively
Contractile testing of cervical spine

Myotomal Testing

MOTION	MYOTOME
Cervical rotation	C1
Shoulder shrug	C2,3,4
Shoulder abduction	C5
Elbow flexion	C5,6
Wrist extension	C6
Wrist flexion	C7
Elbow extension	C7
Thumb extension	C8
Little finger abduction	T1
Finger adduction	T1

Dermatomal Testing

AREA OF SKIN INNERVATED	DERMATOME
No innervation to skin	C1
Posterior aspect of head	C2
Posterior aspect of neck	C3
Acromioclavicular joint	C4
Lateral arm	C5
Lateral forearm and palmar tip thumb	C6
Palmar distal phalanx middle finger	C7
Palmar distal phalanx little finger	C8
Medial forearm	T1
Medial arm	T2

Reflexes

TENDON	SPINAL CORD SEGMENT
Biceps	C5
Brachioradialis	C6
Triceps	C7

Pathologic Reflexes

Wrist clonus
Ankle clonus
Babinski

(Adapted from Cyriax J: Textbook of Orthopedic Medicine, 8th ed, Vol 1, Diagnosis of Soft Tissue Lesions. London, Balliere Tindall, 1982)

2. A decrease in pain noted during compression may be related to increased lubrication of the articular cartilage resulting from the compressive forces.

Screening Examinations

Screening examinations are extremely helpful to the clinician in assessing the location and nature of the patient's complaints. Often it is difficult to determine whether the source of pathology is localized in the periphery or referred from the spinal nerve roots, or whether the problem lies somewhere in the nervous system. An upper or lower quarter screen should be performed anytime there is a question of unclear involvement. The screening process is a combination of mobility and neurologic testing of the cervical spine and upper limbs, or lumbosacral spine and lower limbs.

Upper Quarter Screening Examination. The upper quarter screening examination begins with an examination of the cervical region. The examiner should do a postural assessment for any deviations, muscle spasm, or limited movement as the patient actively performs range of motion movements. If all active ranges appear normal and the patient does not complain of pain, the motions are repeated and the examiner applies gentle overpressure at the ends of the range. If there are no signs or symptoms during the active motion and overpressure, the cervical spine may be considered "clear" for involvement of the joints. Resisted motions of the cervical regions are assessed next. The patient's cervical spine is held in neutral position while cervical movements are tested isometrically. If no associated pain or weakness is found during contractile testing, the musculature is considered clear.

Next the upper limbs are assessed for sensation, myotomal integrity, and reflexes. Upper motor neuron testing is also performed to rule out central nervous system involvement. As in the cervical region, active motion is performed at each peripheral joint, with passive overpressure if the patient is symptom free. The results of the screen will indicate whether there is a pattern consistent with a specific nerve root level, or a specific localized problem. If there appears to be nerve root involvement, the examiner must then thoroughly evaluate the musculature and sensory distribution supplied by that nerve root. If the results indicate a localized joint problem, that particular joint should be examined as outlined previously in this chapter. Table 2–4 outlines the sequence of procedures in the upper quarter screen.

Lower Quarter Screening Examination. As with the previous screen, active motion of the lumbar spine is assessed. If movement is symptom free, passive overpressure is applied at the ends of the range. The patient is then asked to perform functional muscle tests of heel walking (L5) and toe walking (S1). The lumbar spine is cleared if the active motion with overpressure is symptom free. The lower limbs are examined in the manner stated in the previous screen.

Table 2–5 presents the format for the lower quarter screen.

Dermatomal Testing. A dermatome is defined as an area of skin innervated by a single segmental sensory nerve. Examination of the integrity of a dermatomal distribution should be performed in all apparent or suspected cases of peripheral nerve and nerve-root pathology and central nervous system involvement. In addition, thorough sensory testing should be done on those patients who demonstrate sensory abnormalities during an upper or lower quarter screening examination.

A chart illustrating the dermatomes of the body is shown in Figure 2–11.

Myotomal Testing. A myotome is defined as a distribution of musculature that is innervated by a given segmental motor nerve. Assessment of myotomes is performed in any pathologic condition of nerve or muscle

Table 2–5. Lower Quarter Screening Examination

Postural assessment of lumbar region
Active range of motion of lumbar spine
Passive overpressure if symptom free
Heel walking (L5)
Toe walking (S1)

Myotomal Testing

MOTION	MYOTOME
Hip flexion	L1,2
Knee extension	L3,4
Ankle dorsiflexion	L4,5
Great toe extension	L5
Ankle plantar flexion	S1
Bowel/bladder problems	S2,3,4

Dermatomal Testing

AREA OF SKIN INNERVATED	DERMATOME
Anterior thigh, 2–3 inches below anterior superior iliac spine	L2
Middle third of anterior thigh	L3
Patella and medial malleolus	L4
Fibular head and dorsum of foot	L5
Lateral side and plantar surface of foot	S1
Medial aspect of posterior thigh	S2
Perianal area	S3,4

Reflexes

TENDON	SPINAL CORD SEGMENT
Patellar	L4
Posterior tibial	L5
Achilles	S1

Pathologic Reflexes

Babinski
Ankle clonus

(Adapted from Cyriax J: Textbook of Orthopedic Medicine, 8th ed, Vol 1, Diagnosis of Soft Tissue Lesions. London, Balliere Tindall, 1982)

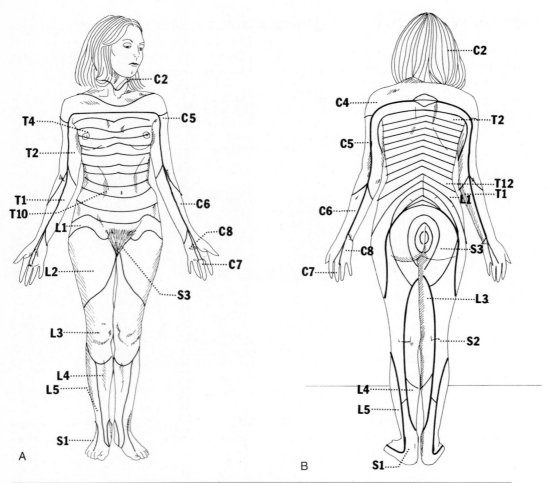

Figure 2–11. Dermatomal sensory pattern. (*A*) Anterior; (*B*) posterior. (Adapted from Haymaker and Woodhall: Peripheral Nerve Injuries, 2nd ed. Philadelphia, WB Saunders, 1953)

where muscle weakness is apparent or suspected. Also, a finding of weakness during the upper or lower quarter screening examinations should alert the examiner that thorough muscle testing needs to be carried out on all of the muscles innervated by that particular segmental nerve. Myotomal testing should not be performed in musculature where spasticity is evident.

Explanation and illustration of the myotomes of the body are found throughout this text under the headings of Manual Muscle Testing.

Joint Play Movements

Joint play testing is performed as part of the testing of inert structures; primarily it assesses the integrity of the capsule. Joint play or accessory movements are those movements that are not under voluntary control but are necessary for full and painless range of motion of the joint. The testing techniques presented later in this text may also be used as treatment techniques.

Joint play should always be assessed in the open-packed position where laxity of capsule and ligaments is greatest, and there is the least bone contact. The greatest amount of joint play is available in the open-packed position. Accessory movements should not be assessed or treated in the closed-packed position, where the ligaments and capsule are tautest and the most bone contact occurs between the articular surfaces. The least joint play is evident in the closed-packed position.

In determining the direction of glide to be performed in restoration of joint play, the type of surface of the moving segment must be considered. The articular surfaces of synovial joints are described as either concave or convex. Arthrokinematically, the direction of gliding that occurs in a joint where the moving partner is concave is the same as that of the bony movement. For example, in considering the radiohumeral joint to restore elbow extension, the concave superior surface of the radius normally glides dorsally on the convex capitulum of the humerus. This dorsal glide must be replicated if attempts

Table 2–6. Open- and Closed-Packed Positions of Joints

JOINT	OPEN	CLOSED
Facet of spine	Midway between flexion (flex.)/extension (ext.)	Extension
Temporomandibular	Mouth slightly open	Mouth closed
Glenohumeral	55–70 degrees abduction (abd.); 30 degrees horizontal adduction (add.)	Maximum abd. and external rotation (ER)
Sternoclavicular	Anatomical	Full elevation
Acromioclavicular	Anatomical	Shoulder abd. 90 degrees
Humeroulnar	70 degrees flex.; 10 degrees supination (sup.)	Full ext. and sup.
Radiohumeral	Full ext. and sup.	90 degrees flex. and 5 degrees sup.
Superior radioulnar	70 degrees flex. and 35 degrees sup.	5 degrees sup.
Inferior radioulnar	10 degrees sup.	5 degrees sup.
Radiocarpal	10 degrees flex. and slight ulnar dev.	Max. ext.
Thumb carpometacarpal	Mid flex./ext./and abd./add.	Opposition
2nd–5th metacarpophalangeal (MCP)	Slight flex.	90 degrees flex.
1st MCP	Slight flex.	Max. ext.
1st–5th interphalangeal	Slight flex.	Max. ext.
Hip	30 degrees flex. and abd.; slight ER	IR > ext. > abd. >
Tibiofemoral	25 degrees flex.	Max. ext. and ER
Talocrural	10 degrees PF; mid inversion (inv.)/eversion (ev.)	Max. DF
Subtalar	Mid inv./ev.	Inv.
2nd–5th metatarsophalangeal	Slight flex.	Max. ext.
1st metatarsophalangeal	5–10 ext.	Max. ext.
1st–5th interphalangeal	Slight flex.	Max. ext.

(Adapted from Kaltenborn FM: Mobilization of the Extremity Joints. Oslo, Olaf Norlis Bokhandel, 1980)

at restoring joint play in extension are to be successful at the radiohumeral joint. Conversely, the direction of gliding that takes place in a joint where the convex partner is moving is opposite the direction of bone movement. At the glenohumeral joint, the motion of abduction is accompanied by an inferior glide of the convex humeral head on the concave glenoid. Therefore, as the bone movement of abduction is characterized by the limb moving superiorly, the direction of glide of the humeral head will occur opposite to that and move downward. Table 2–6 lists the common open- and closed-packed positions of joints.

References

1. Alexander JL, Fuhrer MJ: Functional Assessment of Individuals with Physical Impairments. Baltimore, Paul H Brooks, 1984
2. Beasley WC: Quantitative muscle testing: Principles and application to research and clinical services. Arch Phys Med Rehabil 42:398–425, 1961
3. Bell BD, Hoshizak TB: Relationships of age and sex with range of motion of seventeen joint actions in humans. Can J Appl Sports Sci 6:202, 1981
4. Cyriax J: Textbook of Orthopedic Medicine, 8th ed, Vol 1, Diagnosis of Soft Tissue Lesions. London, Bailliere Tindall, 1982
5. Daniels K, Worthingham C: Muscle Testing Techniques of Manual Examination, 5th ed. Philadelphia, WB Saunders, 1986
6. Frese E, Brown M, Norton B: Clinical reliability of manual muscle testing: Middle trapezius and gluteus medius muscles. J Phys Ther 67(7):1072–1076, 1987
7. Hicks JH: Mechanics of the foot: 1. The joints. J Anat 87:345, 1953
8. Jette AM: State of the art in functional status assessment. In Rothstein JM (ed): Measurement in Physical Therapy, p. 137. New York, Churchill Livingstone, 1985
9. Kaltenborn FM: Mobilization of the Extremity Joints. Oslo, Olaf Norlis Bokhandel, 1980
10. Karpovich PV, Karpovich GP: Electrogoniometer: A new device for study of joints in action. Fed Proc 18:12, 1982
11. Kendall FP, McCreary EK: Muscle Testing and Function, 3rd ed. Baltimore, Williams & Wilkins, 1983
12. Lamb R: Manual muscle testing. In Rothstein JM (ed): Measurement in Physical Therapy, pp. 47–102. New York, Churchill Livingstone, 1985
13. Lehmkuhl LD, Smith LK: Brunnstrom's Clinical Kinesiology, 4th ed. Philadelphia, FA Davis, 1983
14. Manter JT: Movements of the subtalar and transverse tarsal joints. Anat Rec 80:397, 1941
15. Miller PJ: Assessment of joint motion. In Rothstein JM (ed): Measurement in Physical Therapy, pp. 103–136. New York, Churchill Livingstone, 1985
16. Moore ML: The measurement of joint motion—Part 1: Introductory review of literature. Phys Ther Rev 29:195, 1949
17. Norkin CC, White DJ: Measurement of joint motion: A guide for goniometry. Philadelphia, FA Davis, 1985
18. Pact V, Sirotkin-Roses M, Beatus B: The Muscle Testing Handbook. Boston, Little, Brown & Co, 1984

19. Silver D: Measurement of the range of motion in joints. J Bone Joint Surg 21:569, 1923
20. Wainerdi HR: An improved goniometer for arthometry. JAMA 149:661, 1952
21. Williams M: Manual muscle testing: Development and current use. Phys Ther Rev 36:797–805, 1956
22. Zimny N, Kirk C: A comparison of methods of manual muscle testing. Clin Management Phys Ther 7(2):6–11, 1987

Bibliography

Corrigan B, Maitland GD: Practical Orthopedic Medicine. Boston, Butterworth, 1983

Gould A, Davies GJ: Orthopedic and Sports Physical Therapy. St Louis, CV Mosby, 1985
Hoppenfeld S: Physical Examination of the Spine and Extremities. New York, Appleton-Century-Crofts, 1976
Kisner C, Colby LA: Therapeutic Exercise: Foundations and Techniques. Philadelphia, FA Davis, 1985
Magee DJ: Orthopedic Physical Assessment. Philadelphia, WB Saunders, 1987
Saunders HD: Evaluation and Treatment of Musculoskeletal Disorders. Minneapolis, HD Saunders, 1982
Williams P, Warwick R (eds): Gray's Anatomy, 36th British ed. Philadelphia, WB Saunders, 1980

Posture

Chapter 3

The ability to perform a postural evaluation accurately and thoroughly requires tremendous skill on the part of the examiner, because many postural abnormalities are extremely subtle in appearance. The examiner must be able to separate the parts of the body from the whole and in turn assess the sum of the parts in reference to their interaction in the entire anatomical structure.

Correct posture consists of alignment of the body with maximal physiological and biomechanical efficiency, which minimizes stresses and strains imparted to the supporting system by the effects of gravity. In correct posture, the gravity line passes through the axes of all joints with the body segments aligned vertically. The gravity line is represented by a vertical line drawn through the body's center of gravity, located at the second sacral vertebra (S2). It is the reference point from which gravitational effects on individual body segments are assessed.

The gravity line is an ever-changing reference line that responds to the constantly altering body position during upright posture. Although the gravity line generally does not pass through all joint axes of the human body, persons with excellent posture may come close to fulfilling that criterion. Therefore, the closer a person's postural alignment lies to the center of all joint axes, the less gravitational stress is placed on the soft tissue components of the supporting system.

Assessment

Not only is it ideal to have gravitational forces passing through the center of the joint axes, it is also advantageous for the muscles, ligaments, and other soft tissue structures about the joints to be balanced. The strength and length of muscles involved in joint motion must be balanced. The balance is based on force couple (two or more translatory forces that in combination produce rotation) principles among muscles involved in the three cardinal planes of motion. When a force couple is out of balance, the segment moves off its axis of rotation, and there is faulty joint motion. The head, trunk, shoulders, and pelvic girdle are the most important segments to have in muscular and mechanical balance. They serve as the foundation from which forces are directed to the limbs.

Postural faults can be used as guidelines for identifying alterations in muscle and ligament length. For instance, round shoulders result from short or tight pectoralis major and minor muscles. Often one of the muscle groups may be tight and the antagonist elongated. For example, in lumbar lordosis the iliopsoas muscle is tight and the abdominals are stretched. Synergistic muscles around a joint may be unbalanced as well as the agonists.

The primary hip flexors may be elongated and the secondary flexors may be short. Minor alignment faults in posture limit motion and lead to tightness of muscles and other soft tissues. Muscles that are elongated often develop their maximal force in the stretched position and are weak in the normal physiological position. Kendall calls this condition stretch weakness. The body relies on the support provided by muscles and joints to minimize energy costs that further contribute to muscle imbalance and faulty posture.[3]

Alignment of body segments should be observed while the subject is standing still and during such movement as walking, to detect faulty patterns of muscle activity and joint mobility. Ideally, each segment should move in the correct sequence relative to the adjoining segment, whether movement is taking place from distal to proximal segment or vice versa. For example, timing and sequence of muscle contractions during ambulation between the hip and knee joints or between the scapula and the glenohumeral joints are required for ideal movements. The better the quality of movement and the better the alignment of gravitational forces through the joint's axes, the better is the sequence of motion. When postural alignment improves, imbalances are minimized.

This chapter presents methods of evaluating standing posture using a plumb line or a posture grid. As a guide to segmental alignment, other static postures such as sitting or getting on hands and knees and dynamic walking postures are measured by observation and palpation. Skills necessary for accurate assessment of body alignment are acquired through an understanding of kinesiology and anatomy.

Analysis

An organized, systematic approach to postural analysis involves viewing, from various perspectives, the body's anatomical alignment relative to a certain established reference line. This reference line, or gravity line, serves to divide the body into equal front and back halves and to bisect it laterally. Figures 3–1 and 3–2 demonstrate the anatomical structures that coincide with the postural reference line and the surface landmarks that coincide with established plumb lines.

In preparing to carry out postural assessment, it is important for the examiner to be aware of factors that will enhance the success and validity of the examination process:

1. The postural assessment must be performed with the subject minimally clothed, in order to ensure a clear view of the contours and anatomical landmarks used for reference. Males should be dressed only in shorts; females should wear a bra

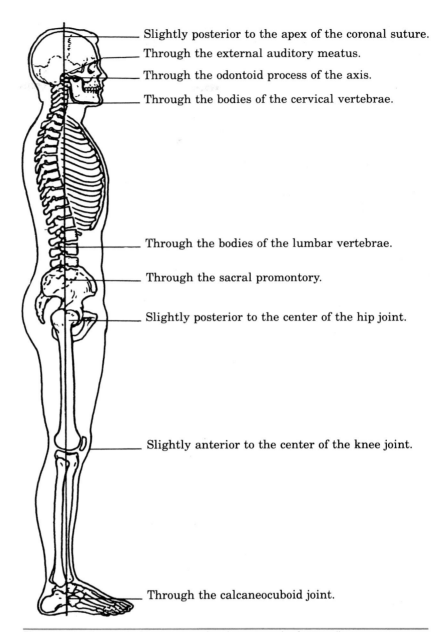

Slightly posterior to the apex of the coronal suture.

Through the external auditory meatus.

Through the odontoid process of the axis.

Through the bodies of the cervical vertebrae.

Through the bodies of the lumbar vertebrae.

Through the sacral promontory.

Slightly posterior to the center of the hip joint.

Slightly anterior to the center of the knee joint.

Through the calcaneocuboid joint.

Figure 3–1. Anatomical structures related to postural reference line.

and shorts or a two-piece bathing suit. Subjects should not wear shoes or socks during the examination.

2. The examiner should instruct the subject to assume a comfortable and relaxed posture.

3. Subjects who use orthotic support or assistive devices for activities of daily living and gait should be assessed with and without them, so that the examiner can determine the effectiveness of the devices in correcting posture.

4. The examiner should use whatever instruments are necessary to enhance the validity of the examination, including plumb lines, grids, rulers, tape measures, and goniometers.

5. The examiner should note relevant medical history and other information that may account for certain postural abnormalities. Also, any information regarding previous treatment relevant to planning a current program of management must be taken into consideration. Important information includes:

· Any history that accounts for present postural abnormalities (e.g., scoliosis, displaced fractures, congenital abnormalities).

· A complete description of present symptoms.

· All previous treatment for the presenting postural complaints, including orthopedic and neurological therapy.

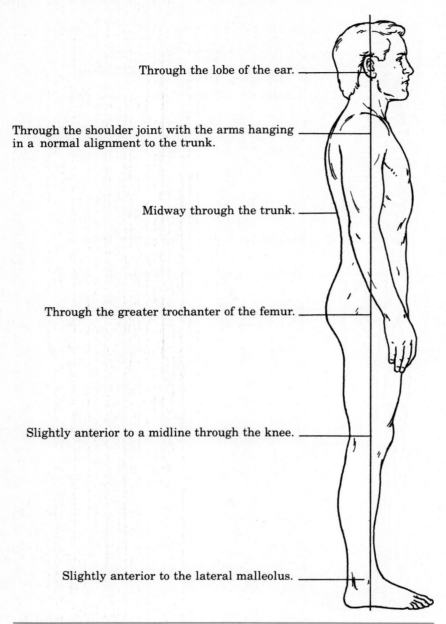

Through the lobe of the ear.

Through the shoulder joint with the arms hanging in a normal alignment to the trunk.

Midway through the trunk.

Through the greater trochanter of the femur.

Slightly anterior to a midline through the knee.

Slightly anterior to the lateral malleolus.

Figure 3–2. Surface landmarks related to dropping of plumb line.

- The upper limb dominance of the subject, which is often responsible for asymptomatic postural deviations. For example, it is common for the shoulder and scapula on the dominant side to be lower.

Postural examination is most commonly performed by assessing the body's alignment in lateral, posterior, and anterior views. It is imperative that the examiner study the alignment of the body thoroughly from head to toe in each position. The components of the postural examination are described below.

Standing Posture

Lateral View

Lateral postural assessments should be performed from both sides to detect any rotational abnormalities that might go undetected if observed from only one lateral perspective. The examiner should begin by looking at the head position relative to the previously established landmarks. Ideally, the plumb line should pass through the ear lobe and shoulder joint. A common postural abnormality is "forward head," in which the head lies anterior to the plumb line. Forward head posture is many times associated with excessive cervical lordosis and, consequently, tight cervical extensor muscles.

The cervical spine should display normal lordosis. The examiner should note an exaggerated or a flattened lordotic curve. The examiner should next look at the shoulder area of the subject for its position relative to the plumb line reference. Shoulders that fall anterior to the plumb line are referred to as rounded shoulders—a faulty posture commonly associated with excessive thoracic kyphosis and forward head. As a result, weakness of the thoracic spine extensor musculature, the middle trapezius muscle, and the rhomboid muscles is usually present. Conversely, tightness of the intercostal, the pectoralis major and minor, and the subscapularis muscles becomes apparent.

The thoracic region should demonstrate a kyphotic thoracic curve, and the gravity, or plumb, line should approximately bisect the chest. Any abnormalities of the thoracic curve should be noted. The chest should be observed for such deformities as excessive prominence or depression. One such deformity includes pectus excavatum, or funnel chest, in which the anterior thorax and sternum are depressed. Barrel chest is represented by a large rounded rib cage and an increase of the overall anteroposterior diameter. Pigeon chest, or pectus cavinatum, gives the appearance of an anterior and downward projection of the sternum.

The abdominal region is bisected by the plumb line, and the abdomen itself should be relatively flat in the adult. A protruding abdomen is often implicated in lumbar pathologies and deserves attention.

The lumbar region should be examined for a normal lordotic appearance. Excessive lumbar lordosis is associated with an anterior pelvic tilt and consequent tightness of the hip flexor musculature. Decreased lumbar lordosis is accompanied by a posterior pelvic tilt and possible hamstring muscle tightness.

In examination of the hip, the plumb line passes posterior to the hip joint creating an extension moment through the greater trochanter of the femur.

At the knee joint, the reference line should pass slightly anterior to the midline of the knee, thereby creating an extension moment. The subject should be observed for genu recurvatum, in which the plumb line will be found to lie far forward of the normal position. Conversely, a flexed knee posture secondary to bone or soft tissue limitation in the kinematic chain should also be noted, in which case the plumb line falls more posteriorly than normal.

At the ankle, the plumb line lies slightly anterior to the lateral malleolus. Deviations observed may be the result of bone or soft tissue pathology in the kinematic chain.

The feet should be examined for flat arches or supinated posture and for deformities such as hammer toes or claw toes.

Summary of Lateral View Examination of Standing Subject and Possible Findings

Head and Neck

Plumb Line. The line falls through the ear lobe to the acromion process.

Common Faults

Forward Head. The head lies anterior to the plumb line (Fig. 3–3*A*).

CAUSES
- Excessive cervical lordosis.
- Tight cervical extensor, upper trapezius, and levator scapulae muscles.
- Elongated cervical flexor muscles.

Flattened Lordotic Cervical Curve. The plumb line lies anterior to the vertebral bodies.

CAUSES
- Stretched posterior cervical ligaments and extensor muscles.
- Tight cervical flexor muscles.

Excessive Lordotic Curve. The gravity line lies posterior to the vertebral bodies (Fig. 3–3*B*).

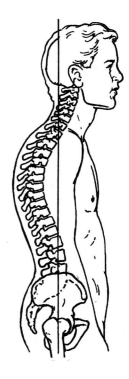

Figure 3–3. Forward head is usually accompanied by round shoulders. The external auditory meatus lies anterior to the plumb line. Cervical lordosis with accompanying forward head: The bodies of the vertebrae lie anterior to the plumb line.

CAUSES
- Vertebral bodies and joints compressed posteriorly.
- Anterior longitudinal ligament stretched.
- Tightness of posterior ligaments and neck extensor muscles.
- Elongated levator scapulae muscles.

Shoulder

Plumb Line. The line falls through the acromion process.

Common Faults

Forward Shoulders. The acromion process lies anterior to the plumb line; the scapulae are abducted (Fig. 3–4).

CAUSES
- Tight pectoralis major and minor, serratus anterior, and intercostal muscles.
- Excessive thoracic kyphosis and forward head.
- Weakness of thoracic extensor, middle trapezius, and rhomboid muscles.
- Lengthened middle and lower trapezius muscles.

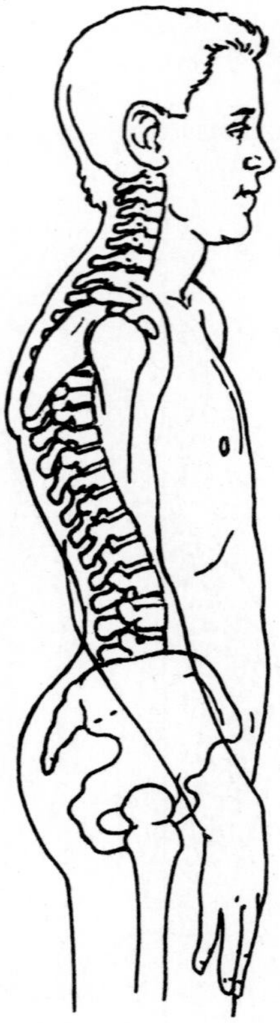

Figure 3–4. With forward, or rounded, shoulders, the acromion process of the scapula lies anterior to the plumb line.

Lumbar Lordosis. The lumbar region is flat as the subject raises arms overhead (Fig. 3–5).

CAUSES
- Tightness of the latissimus dorsi muscle and thoracolumbar fasciae.

Thoracic Vertebrae

Plumb Line. The line bisects the chest symmetrically.

Common Faults

Kyphosis. Increased posterior convexity of the vertebrae (Fig. 3–6).

CAUSES
- Compression of intervertebral disks anteriorly.
- Stretched thoracic extensors and middle and lower trapezius muscles and posterior ligaments.
- Tightness of anterior longitudinal ligament, upper abdominal, and anterior chest muscles.

Pectus Excavatum, or Funnel Chest. Depression of the anterior thorax and sternum.

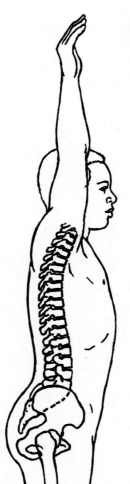

Figure 3–5. Increase in lumbar lordosis is demonstrated with the upper limbs raised above the head. Tightness of the latissimus dorsi muscle and thoracolumbar fascia prevents full shoulder joint flexion.

Causes

- Tightness of upper abdominal, shoulder adductor, pectoralis minor, and intercostal muscles.
- Bony deformities of sternum and ribs.
- Stretched thoracic extensors, middle and lower trapezius muscles.

Barrel Chest. Increased overall anteroposterior diameter of rib cage.

Causes

- Respiratory difficulties.
- Stretched intercostal and anterior chest muscles.
- Tightness of scapular adductor muscles.

Pectus Cavinatum, or Pigeon Chest. The sternum projects anteriorly and downward.

Causes

- Bony deformity of the ribs and sternum.
- Stretched upper abdominal muscles.
- Tightness of upper intercostal muscles.

Lumbar Vertebrae

Plumb Line. The line falls midway between the abdomen and back and slightly anterior to the sacroiliac joint.

Common Faults

Lordosis. Hyperextension of lumbar vertebrae (Fig. 3–7).

Causes

- Anterior pelvic tilt.
- Compressed vertebrae posteriorly.
- Stretched anterior longitudinal ligament and lower abdominal muscles.
- Tightness of posterior longitudinal ligaments and lower back extensor and hip flexor muscles.

Sway Back. Flattening of the lumbar vertebrae (the pelvis is displaced forward) (Fig. 3–8).

Causes

- Thoracic kyphosis.
- Posterior pelvic tilt.
- Stretched anterior hip ligaments—hips hyperextended.
- Compression of vertebrae posteriorly.
- Stretched posterior longitudinal ligaments, back extensors, and hip flexor muscles.

Flat Back. Flattening of the lumbar vertebrae (Fig. 3–9).

Causes

- Posterior pelvic tilt.

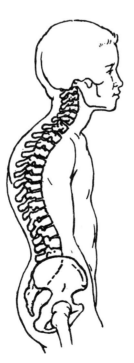

Figure 3–6. In the case of thoracic kyphosis, the thoracic vertebrae are overly flexed and the plumb line is anterior to the vertebral bodies.

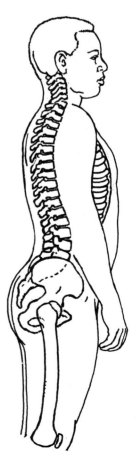

Figure 3–7. In lumbar lordosis hyperextension of the lumbar vertebrae is associated with anterior pelvic tilt and hip flexion.

- Tightness of the hamstring muscles.
- Weakness of the hip flexor muscles.
- Stretched posterior longitudinal ligaments.

Pelvis and Hip

Plumb Line.   The line falls slightly anterior to the sacroiliac joint and posterior to the hip joint through the greater trochanter, creating an extension moment.

Common Faults

Anterior Pelvic Tilt.   The anterior superior iliac spines lie anterior to the pubic symphysis (Fig. 3–10).

CAUSES
- Increased lumbar lordosis and thoracic kyphosis.
- Compression of vertebrae posteriorly.
- Stretched abdominal muscles, sacrotuberous, sacroiliac, and sacrospinous ligaments.
- Tightness of hip flexors.

Posterior Pelvic Tilt.   The symphysis pubis lies anterior to the anterior superior iliac spines (Fig. 3–11).

CAUSES
- Sway back with thoracic kyphosis.

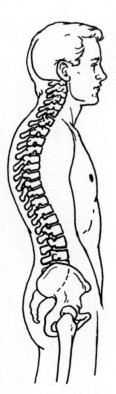

Figure 3–8.   Swayback is the manifestation of lumbar flexion with associated posterior pelvic tilt, hip extension, thoracic kyphosis, and forward displacement of the pelvis.

- Compression of vertebrae anteriorly.
- Stretched hip flexor and lower abdominal muscles and joint capsule.
- Tightness of hamstring muscles.

Knee

Plumb Line.   The line passes slightly anterior to the midline of the knee, creating an extension moment.

Common Faults

Genu Recurvatum.   The knee is hyperextended and the gravitational stresses lie far forward of the joint axis (Fig. 3–12).

CAUSES
- Tightness of quadriceps, gastrocnemius, and soleus muscles.
- Stretched popliteus and hamstring muscles at the knee.
- Compression forces anteriorly.
- Shape of tibial plateau.

Flexed Knee.   The plumb line falls posterior to the joint axis (Fig. 3–13).

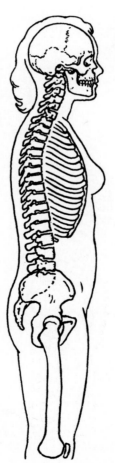

Figure 3–9.   A flat back is evidence of increased lumbar flexion with associated posterior pelvic tilt and hip extension.

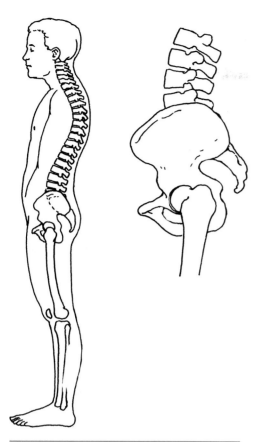

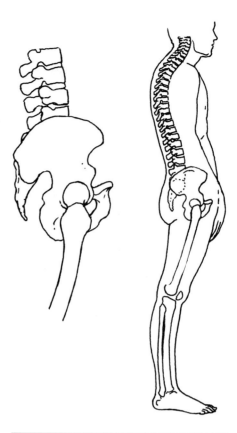

Figure 3–10. In anterior pelvic tilt the anterior superior iliac spines project anterior to a vertical line parallel with the pubic bone. Lumbar lordosis is associated with the anterior tilt.

Figure 3–11. In posterior pelvic tilt the anterior superior iliac spines are posterior to a vertical line parallel with the pubic bone.

Figure 3–12. In genu recurvatum the knees are hyperextended and the center of the joint lies posterior to the plumb line. The ankle joints are often positioned in plantar flexion.

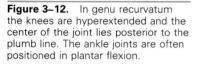

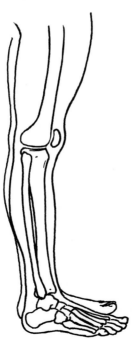

Figure 3–13. In knee flexion the axis of the knee joint lies anterior to the plumb line. This condition is not as common as genu recurvatum.

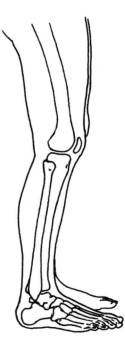

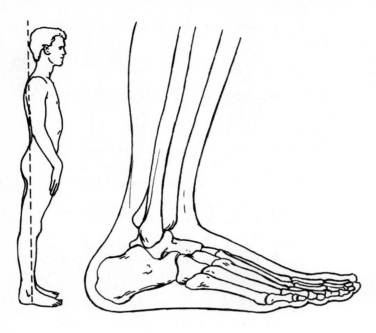

Figure 3–14. The subject with forward posture bears weight on the forefeet, and the entire body is deviated anterior to the plumb line.

CAUSES
- Tightness of popliteus and hamstring muscles at the knee.
- Stretched quadriceps and tight gastrocnemius muscles.
- Posterior compression forces.
- Bony and soft tissue limitations.

Ankle

Plumb Line. The line lies slightly anterior to the lateral malleolus aligned with the tuberosity of the fifth metatarsal (Fig. 3–14).

Common Faults

Forward Posture. The plumb line is posterior to the body; body weight is carried on the metatarsal heads of the feet.

CAUSES
- Ankles in dorsiflexion with forward inclination of the legs; posterior musculature stretched.
- Tightness of dorsal musculature.
- Posterior muscles of the trunk remain contracted.

Posterior View

In a posterior view examination, the examiner's plumb line divides the body into equal left and right halves. The following relationships are assessed.

The head should be upright, with no noticeable deviation to left or right. Lateral deviations of the head and neck may be related to torticollis or to other cervical dysfunction.

The examiner should observe the subject's shoulder height. It is considered normal to have an asymmetry in shoulder height related to hand dominance.

The scapulae are assessed for positional symmetry by observing the spines of the scapulae and the level of the inferior angles. Excessive abduction or adduction of one or both scapulae is assessed by measuring the distance from the thoracic spine to the medial scapular borders. "Winging" of the scapulae resulting from serratus anterior muscle weakness may also be evaluated from this view.

The subject's trunk is evaluated for lateral deviation to either side. Normally, the spine should lie in vertical alignment in the midline of the body.

A common cause of lateral postural deviations is scoliosis. Assessment of the subject for scoliosis is accomplished by marking the spinous processes from the second cervical vertebra to the lumbosacral junction. If a lateral curvature exists, the subject is instructed to bend forward from the trunk. Curvature that straightens with forward bending is termed *functional scoliosis,* whereas curvature that does not straighten is called *structural scoliosis.* Functional scoliosis is caused by muscle imbalances secondary to faulty posture or disease (such as cerebral palsy) and is not progressive. Structural scoliosis is progressive because of bony deformities. The thoracic region should also be examined for rib protrusions, which are commonly associated with scoliosis.

The pelvis and hip area are examined next for symmetry in levels of iliac crests, posterior superior iliac spines, gluteal folds, and greater trochanters. Asymmetries noted in this region may be associated with leg-length discrepancies, pelvic obliquities, scoliotic curves, hip pathology, or lumbar spine pathology. The examiner needs to be astute in understanding the pathomechanics and postural consequences of such pathologies so that he or she can make differential assessments accurately.

The region of the knee should be examined for varus or valgus postures. Valgus posture is one in which the distal segment deviates from the midline relative to the proximal segment. Varus posture is one in which the distal segment deviates toward the midline in relation to the proximal segment.

The tibias may be assessed for tibia varum as described in the section on biomechanical examination of the foot. The position of the Achilles tendons relative to the lower third of the leg is also observed. A medially deviated Achilles tendon is commonly found in persons with pronated postures of the foot. The foot may also be assessed for pronated or supinated postures from this view.

Summary of Posterior View Examination of Standing Subject and Possible Findings

Head and Neck

Plumb Line. The midline bisects the head through the external occipital protuberance; head is usually po-

sitioned squarely over the shoulders so that the eyes remain level.

Common Faults

Head Tilt. Subject's head lies more to one side of the plumb line (Fig. 3–15).

CAUSES
· Tightness of lateral neck flexors on one side.
· Stretched lateral neck flexors contralaterally.
· Compression of vertebrae ipsilaterally.

Head Rotated. The plumb line is to the right or left of the midline (Fig. 3–16).

CAUSES
· Tightness of the sternocleidomastoid, upper trapezius, scalene, and intrinsic rotator muscles on one side.
· Elongated contralateral rotator muscles.
· Compression and rotation of the vertebrae.

Shoulder and Scapula

Plumb Line. The line falls midway between shoulders.

Figure 3–15. In head tilt the head is deviated in the coronal plane to one side of the plumb line.

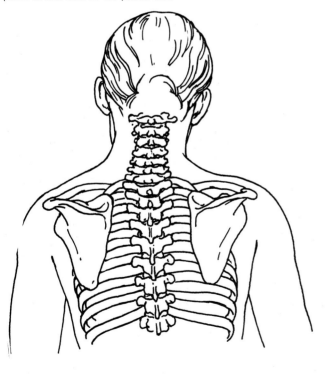

Figure 3–16. In head rotation, the head is rotated in the transverse plane to the right or left of the plumb line.

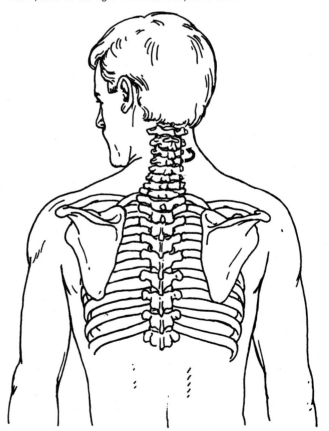

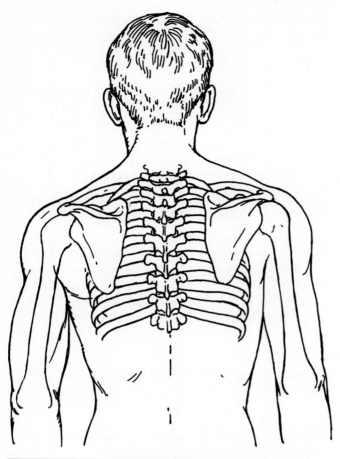

Figure 3–17. In dropped shoulder the shoulders are not level with each other in the coronal plane.

Common Faults

Dropped Shoulder.   One shoulder is lower than the other (Fig. 3–17).

CAUSES
· Hand dominance (dominant shoulder is lower).
· Lateral trunk muscles are short and hip joint is high and adducted.
· Tightness of the rhomboid and latissimus dorsi muscles.

Shoulder Elevated.   One shoulder is higher than the other.

CAUSES
· Tightness in the upper trapezius and levator scapulae muscles on one side; hypertrophy may be noticed on the dominant side.
· Elongated and weak lower trapezius and pectoralis minor muscles.
· Scoliosis of the thoracic vertebrae.

Shoulder Medial Rotation.   The medial epicondyle of the humerus is directed posteriorly.

CAUSES
· Joint limitation in lateral rotation.
· Tightness of the medial rotator muscles.

Shoulder Lateral Rotation.   The olecranon process faces posteriorly.

CAUSES
· Joint limitation in medial rotation.
· Tightness of the lateral rotators.

Figure 3–18. (*A*) In scapular adduction the medial borders of the scapulae are adducted and elevated. (*B*) In scapular abduction the medial borders of the scapulae lie laterally on the thorax. Scapular abduction is usually accompanied by rounded, or forward, shoulders.

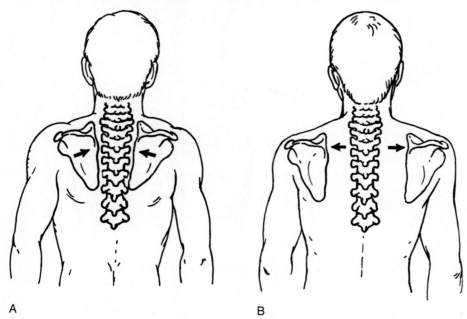

A   B

Scapulae Adducted. The scapulae are too close to the midline of the thoracic vertebrae (Fig. 3–18*A*).

CAUSES
- Shortened rhomboid muscles.
- Stretched pectoralis major and minor muscles.

Abducted Scapulae. The scapulae have moved away from the midline of the thoracic vertebrae (Fig. 3–18*B*).

CAUSES
- Tightness of the serratus anterior muscle.
- Lengthened rhomboid and middle trapezius muscles.

Winging of the Scapulae. The medial borders of the scapulae lift off the ribs (Fig. 3–19).

CAUSES
- Weakness of the serratus anterior muscle.

Trunk

Plumb Line. The line bisects the spinous process of the thoracic and lumbar vertebrae.

Common Faults

Lateral Deviation (Scoliosis). The spinous processes of the vertebrae are lateral to the midline of the trunk (Fig. 3–20).

CAUSES
- Intrinsic trunk muscles are shortened on one side.
- Contralateral intrinsic trunk muscles are lengthened.
- Compression of vertebrae on the concave side.
- Structural changes in ribs or vertebrae.
- Leg-length discrepancy and pelvic obliquity.
- Internal organ disorders.

Pelvis and Hip

Plumb Line. The line bisects the gluteal cleft, and the posterior superior iliac spines are on the same horizontal plane; the iliac crests, gluteal folds, and greater trochanters are level.

Figure 3–19. In winging of the scapula the medial border and inferior angle of the scapula are prominent and are deviated into the transverse plane.

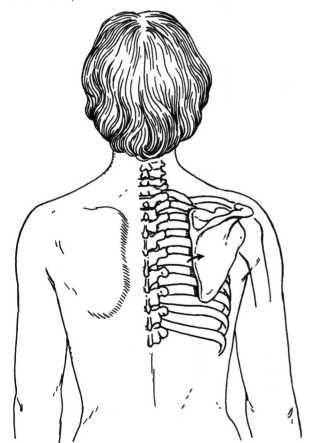

Figure 3–20. In scoliosis, the spinous processes of the vertebrae are deviated laterally from the plumb line. Uneven shoulders and pelvis are common in scoliosis.

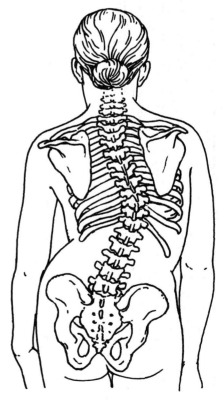

Common Faults

Lateral Pelvic Tilt.   One side of the pelvis is higher than the other (Fig. 3–21).

CAUSES
- Scoliosis with ipsilateral lumbar convexity.
- Leg-length discrepancies.
- Shortening of the contralateral quadratus lumborum.
- Tight ipsilateral hip abductor muscles on the same side and tight contralateral hip adductor muscles.
- Weakness of the contralateral abductor muscles.

Pelvic Rotation.   The plumb line falls to the right or left of the gluteal cleft.

CAUSES
- Tightness of medial rotator and hip flexor muscles on the rotated side.
- Ipsilateral lumbar rotation.

Hip Abducted.   The greater trochanter is higher on the involved side (Fig. 3–22).

CAUSES
- Tightness of hip abductor muscles.
- Tightness of contralateral hip adductor muscles.
- Weakness of contralateral hip abductors and ipsilateral adductors.

Hip Adducted.   The greater trochanter is lower on the involved side (Fig. 3–23).

CAUSES
- Tightness of the hip adductor muscles.
- Tightness of contralateral hip abductor muscles.
- Weakness of contralateral adductor and ipsilateral abductor muscles.

Knee

Plumb Line.   The plumb line lies equidistant between the knees.

Common Faults

Genu Varum.   The distal segment (leg) deviates toward the midline in relation to the proximal segment

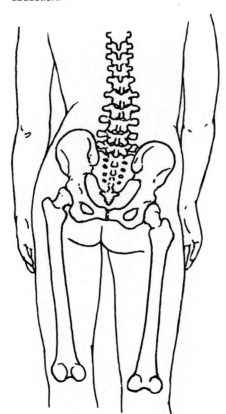

Figure 3–21.   In lateral pelvic tilt, the pelvis deviates in the coronal plane to the right (left Trendelenburg's sign). Lateral tilt of the pelvis to the right is accompanied by relative left hip adduction and right hip abduction.

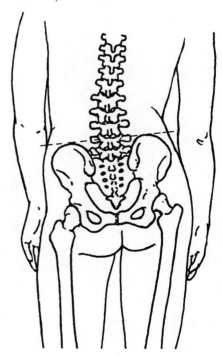

Figure 3–22.   In hip abduction (coxa vaiga) the pelvis tilts downward on the femoral head to the same side as the abducted hip.

(thigh); the knee joint lies lateral to the mechanical axis of the lower limb (Fig. 3–24).

CAUSES
- Tightness of medial rotator muscles at the hip with hyperextended knees, quadriceps, and foot everter muscles.
- Compression of medial joint structures.
- Femoral retroversion.
- Elongated lateral hip rotator muscles, popliteus, tibialis posterior.

Genu Valgum. The mechanical axis for the lower limbs is displaced laterally (Fig. 3–25).

CAUSES
- Tightness of the iliotibial band and the lateral knee joint structures.
- Femoral anteversion.
- Lengthened medial knee joint structures.
- Compression of lateral knee joint.
- Foot pronation.

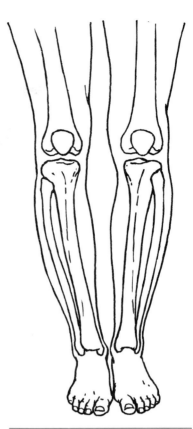

Figure 3–24. In genu varum (bowlegs) the center of the knee joint is lateral to the midline of the thigh and leg.

Figure 3–23. In hip adduction the pelvis tilts on the femoral head to the side opposite the adducted hip.

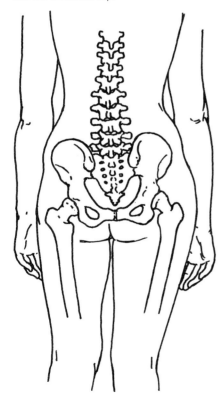

Figure 3–25. In genu valgum (knock knees) the center of the knee joint is medial to the midline of the thigh and leg.

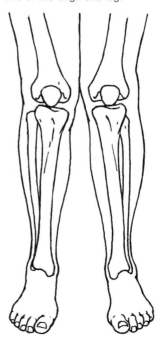

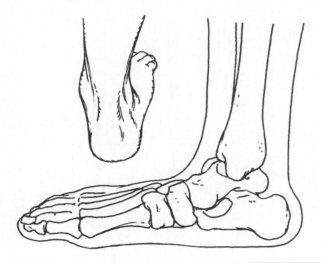

Figure 3–26. Pes planus, or flatfoot.

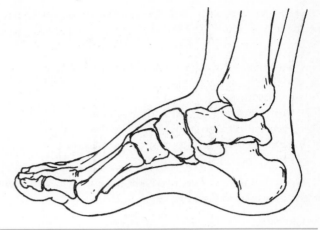

Figure 3–27. Pes cavus, or high-arched foot.

Ankle and Foot

Plumb Line. The line is equidistant from the malleoli; medially, a line (Feiss') is drawn from the medial malleous to the head of the first metatarsal bone, and the tuberosity of the navicular bone lies on the line.

Common Faults

Pes Planus (Pronated). There is a decreased medial longitudinal arch, the Achilles tendon is convex medially, and the tuberosity of the navicular bone lies below the Feiss line (Fig. 3–26).

CAUSES
- Shortened peroneal muscles.
- Elongated posterior tibial muscle.
- Stretched plantar calcaneonavicular ligament (spring).
- Structural displacement of the talus, calcaneus, and navicular bones.

Pes Cavus (Supinated). The medial longitudinal arch is high and the navicular bone lies above Feiss' line (Fig. 3–27).

CAUSES
- Shortened posterior and anterior tibial muscles.
- Elongated peroneals and lateral ligaments.

Anterior View

Relationships can be posturally assessed from an anterior view with the plumb line bisecting the body into equal left and right halves. The head and neck should lie in the midline without rotation and with no lateral deviation to either side. The mandibular region should be examined for symmetry. (See Chapter 8, "Face and Temporomandibular Joint," for specific details.) The nose, the manubrium of the sternum, the xiphoid process of the sternum, and the umbilicus should all be vertically aligned in the midline. The margins of the upper trapezius muscles should be examined for symmetry. Noticeable unilateral hypertrophy may be indicative of upper extremity dominance, while atrophy of one upper trapezius muscle may be a result of pathology or disuse. The levels of the shoulder joint should be relatively equal, but upper limb dominance may slightly affect the symmetry. The bony components of the shoulder girdle, namely the sternoclavicular joint, the clavicle, and the acromioclavicular joint, should be examined for equality and symmetry. Prominences at either joint may be attributed to effusions secondary to joint trauma or to actual bony deformation resulting from subluxation or dislocation. Protrusions along the course of the clavicle may have occurred as a result of fractures.

The examiner assessing a subject with the upper extremities in the anatomical position should note the carrying angle of the elbow. Normally, this angle is 5 to 10 degrees in males and 10 to 15 degrees in females.

The examiner should examine the pelvic and hip region for symmetry of the iliac crest heights and notice the levels of the anterior superior iliac spines. As in the posterior assessment, asymmetries may be a result of leg-length discrepancies, pelvic obliquities, scoliosis, lumbosacral pathology, or hip pathology.

The patellae should be examined for deviations such as patella alta, "winking" patellae, or excessive lateral displacement. Most of these patellar abnormalities are related to pathomechanics within the kinematic chain of the lower extremity. The fibular heads may be palpated for symmetry, the tibia examined for torsion, and the malleoli observed for equal height.

The feet may again be examined for pronation and supination. Normally when a person stands still, there is a tendency for the feet to point outward. The angle of toeing out averages 5 to 7 degrees. The feet also may be examined in this view for such deformities as hammer toes and claw toes. The great toe should also be assessed for hallux valgus.

Summary of Anterior View Examination of Standing Subject and Possible Findings

Head and Neck

Plumb Line. The line bisects the head at the midline into equal halves.

Common Faults

Lateral Tilt. See section on posterior view.

Rotation. See section on posterior view.

Mandibular Asymmetry. The upper and lower teeth are not aligned, and the mandible is deviated to one side.

CAUSES
· Tightness of the mastication muscles on one side.
· Stretched mastication muscles on the contralateral side.
· Malalignment of temporomandibular joints.
· Malalignment of teeth.

Shoulders

Plumb Line. A vertical line bisects the sternum and xiphoid process.

Common Faults

Shoulder Dropped or Elevated. See section on posterior view.

Clavicle and Joint Asymmetry

CAUSES
· Prominences secondary to joint trauma.
· Subluxation or dislocation of sternoclavicular or acromioclavicular joints.
· Clavicular fractures.

Elbows

A line bisects the upper limbs and forms an angle of 5 to 15 degrees laterally at the elbow with the elbow extended. This angle is normal and is referred to as the carrying angle.

Common Faults

Cubitus Valgus. The forearm deviates laterally from the arm at an angle greater than 15 degrees for the female and 10 degrees for the male.

CAUSES
· Elbow hyperextension.
· Distal displacement of the trochlea in relation to the capitulum of the humerus.
· Stretched ulnar collateral ligament.

Cubitus Varus. The forearm deviates medially (adducts) from the arm at an angle of less than 15 degrees for the female and 10 degrees for the male.

CAUSES
· Fracture about the elbow joint.
· Inferior displacement of the humeral capitulum.
· Stretched radial collateral ligament.

Hip

Common Faults

Lateral Rotation. The patellae angle out (Fig. 3–28).

CAUSES
· Tightness of the lateral rotators and the gluteus maximus muscles.
· Weakness of the medial rotator muscles.
· Femoral retroversion.
· Internal tibial torsion (compensated).

Medial Rotation. The patellae face inward.

CAUSES
· Tightness of the iliotibial band and the medial rotator muscles.
· Weakness of the lateral rotator muscles.
· Femoral anteversion.
· External tibial torsion (compensated).

Knee

Plumb Line. The legs are equidistant from a vertical line through the body.

Common Faults

External Tibial Torsion. Normally the distal end of the tibia is rotated laterally 25 degrees from the proximal end; excess of 25 degrees rotation is an increase in torsion and is referred to as lateral tibial torsion (toeing out) (Fig. 3–29).

CAUSES
· Tightness of the tensor fasciae latae muscle or iliotibial band.
· Bony malalignment (e.g., fracture).
· Cruciate ligament tear.
· Femoral retroversion.

Internal Tibial Torsion. The feet face directly forward or inward.

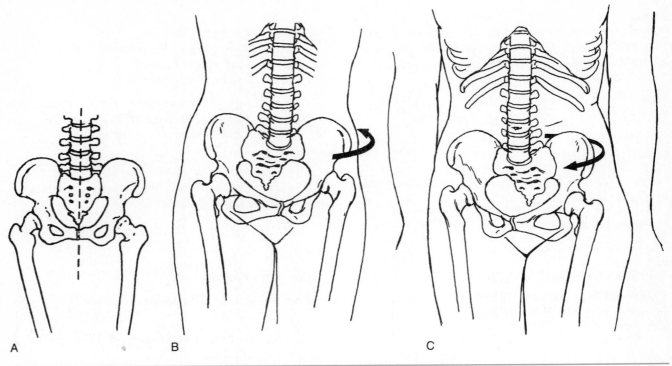

A   B   C

Figure 3–28. (A) Normal position for hips in the transverse plane; (B) Rotation of the pelvis to the right results in lateral rotation of the left hip joint. (C) Rotation of the pelvis to the left results in medial rotation of the left hip joint.

Figure 3–29. External torsion of both tibia.

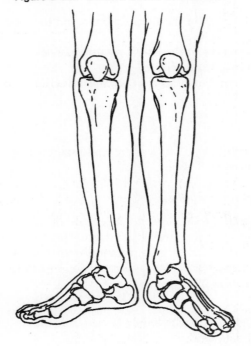

Figure 3–30. Hallux valgus.

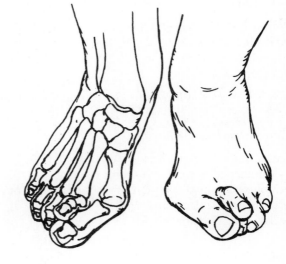

CAUSES
- Tightness of the medial hamstrings and gracilis muscles.
- Structural deformities of the tibia (traumatic or developmental).
- Anterior cruciate ligament tear.
- Femoral anteversion.
- Foot pronation.
- Genu valgus.

Ankle and Foot

Common Faults

Hallux Valgus. Lateral deviation of the first digit at the metatarsophalangeal joint (Fig. 3–30).

CAUSES
- Excessive medial bone growth of the first metatarsal head.
- Joint dislocation.
- Tight adductor hallucis muscle.
- Stretched abductor hallucis muscle.

Claw Toes. Hyperextension of the metatarsophalangeal joint and flexion of the proximal interphalangeal joints associated with pes cavus (Fig. 3–31).

CAUSES
- Tightness of the long toe flexors.
- Shortness of the toe extensor muscles.

Hammer Toes. Hyperextension of the metatarsophalangeal joints and distal interphalangeal joints and flexion of the proximal interphalangeal joints (Fig. 3–32).

CAUSES
- Shortness of the toe extensors.
- Lengthened lumbricals.

Standing on One Foot

Anteroposterior View

Trunk

Common Faults

Hip Drop. Lateral tilt to the non–weight-bearing side over 5 degrees.

CAUSE
- Weakness of the weight-bearing gluteus medius muscle.

Lateral Trunk Shift. Toward the weight-bearing side greater than 5 degrees.

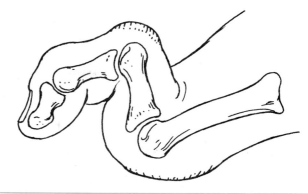

Figure 3–31. Claw toe.

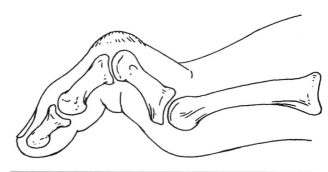

Figure 3–32. Hammer toe.

CAUSES
- Weakness of weight-bearing gluteus medius muscle.
- Pain on weight-bearing side.

Foot Pronation. See section on posterior view.

Sitting Posture

Hip and Pelvis

Observation. The pelvis assumes a posterior tilt with the posterior inferior iliac spines in the same horizontal plane as the superior pubic ramus.

Common Faults

Posterior Pelvic Tilt. The superior pubic ramus is superior to the posterior inferior iliac spines.

CAUSES
- Lumbar vertebrae flexed excessively.
- Tightness of the hamstring muscles.
- Elongated low back extensors.

Anterior Pelvic Tilt. The superior pubic ramus lies inferior to the posterior inferior iliac spine.

CAUSES
- Tightness of low back extensor muscles.
- Lengthened hip extensor muscles.
- Excessive lumbar lordosis

On Hands and Knees

Observation. The thoracic and lumbar vertebrae are level, the scapulae lie flat on the thorax, the hips are flexed 90 degrees and aligned over the knee joints, and ankles are in plantar flexion.

Common Faults

Winging of Scapulae. The vertebral border and inferior angle are lifted off the thorax.

CAUSE
- Weakness of the serratus anterior muscle.

Lumbar Lordosis. Increase in the normal curves.

CAUSES
- Weak or elongated abdominal muscles.
- Tightness of low back extensor muscles and posterior longitudinal ligaments.

Thoracic Kyphosis. Arched thoracic vertebrae.

CAUSES
- Tightness of anterior chest muscles and anterior longitudinal ligaments.
- Weakness of upper back extensor muscles.
- Vertebral deformities.

Trunk Rotation or Lateral Flexion. Deviation from the midline.

CAUSES
- Structural or functional scoliosis.
- Pelvic rotation.
- Intrinsic trunk muscle weakness.

Decreased Hip Flexion. Less than 90 degrees.

CAUSES
- Tightness of hip extensor muscles.
- Increase in lumbar flexion.
- Increase in posterior pelvic tilt.

Increased Hip Flexion. Greater than 90 degrees.

CAUSES
- Weakness of hip extensor muscles.
- Increase in lumbar lordosis.
- Increase in anterior pelvic tilt.

Hip Rotation. Not in neutral position.

CAUSES
- Tightness of rotator muscles.
- Lumbar vertebral rotation.
- Pelvic rotation left or right.

External Tibial Rotation. The foot angles outward more than 25 degrees.

CAUSES
- Tightness of iliotibial band.
- Bony deformity.

Ankle Dorsiflexion. The dorsum of the foot is not resting on the floor.

CAUSES
- Lengthened heel cord.
- Weakness of gastrocnemius and soleus muscles.
- Tightness of the dorsiflexor muscles.

Ankle Inversion. Subtalar and transtarsal joints are not in a neutral position, and the forefoot angles inward.

CAUSES
- Lengthened peroneals.
- Tightness of posterior and anterior tibial muscles.

Ankle Eversion. Subtalar and transtarsal joints are not in a neutral position and the forefoot angles outward.

CAUSES
- Lengthened anterior and posterior tibial muscles.
- Tightness of peroneals.

Gait

Observation. Dynamic posture may be evaluated by watching the subject walk; observations are organized in a methodical manner (from head to toes or vice versa).

Common Faults

Stride Length and Time Inequality. Stance phase is longer on one side.

CAUSES
- Pain.
- Lack of trunk and pelvic rotation.
- Weakness of lower limb muscles.
- Limitation of lower limb joints.
- Uncoordinated muscle control.
- Increased muscle tone.

Slow Cadence. Less than average for person's age, occupation.

CAUSES
- Generalized weakness.
- Pain or joint limitations.
- Lack of voluntary motor control.

Stance Phase. Less than 60 percent of gait cycle.

CAUSES
- Restricted plantar or dorsiflexion motion.
- Painful or restricted knee and hip joints.

Head. Erect and in the midline; for deviations, refer to discussion of standing posture.

Shoulders. Horizontal and coordinated with the arm swing; each shoulder swings reciprocally with equal motion.

Inequality

CAUSES
- Shoulder pathology.
- Generalized muscle weakness or lack of coordination.
- Emotional disturbance.

Deviations. Refer to section on standing posture.

Trunk. Erect, rotates slightly with the pelvis and shoulders; for deviations, refer to discussion of standing posture.

Pelvis. Rotates slightly in the transverse plane during the swing phase of gait; drops (laterally tilts) 4 or 5 degrees on the opposite side during the stance phase; tilts anteriorly slightly during the gait cycle, except during stance, when it is level.

Excessive Pelvic Rotation. Increased rotation in the transverse plane beyond 5 degrees.

CAUSES
- Tight hip flexor muscles on the same side.
- Limited hip joint flexion.

Excessive Pelvic Drop. Lateral tilt of the pelvis beyond 5 degrees.

CAUSES
- Weakness of the hip abductors on the stance side.
- Tightness in the quadratus lumborum on the swing side.

Posterior Pelvic Tilt. Any posterior pelvic tilt in the sagittal plane.

CAUSES
- Sway back and flat back postures.
- Tightness of the hamstring muscles.
- Weakness of the hip flexor muscles.

Anterior Pelvic Tilt. Occurring in the stance phase, a tilt in the sagittal plane beyond 5 degrees.

CAUSES
- Tightness of the hip flexor and low back extensor muscles.
- Lumbar lordosis.

Hip. Rotates medially during swing to midstance then rotates laterally through terminal stance.

Femur Medially Rotated. The hip remains medially rotated through terminal stance.

CAUSES
- Tightness of the iliotibial band.
- Weakness of the lateral rotator muscles.
- Femoral anteversion.
- Tightness of the medial rotators.

Femur Laterally Rotated. The hip remains rotated laterally during the swing phase.

CAUSES
- Tightness of the lateral rotators.
- Femoral retroversion.
- Weakness of the medial rotators.

Abduction. The base of support is wide in stance, or the subject circumducts during the swing phase.

CAUSES
- Decrease in hip flexion or dorsiflexion motion.
- Weakness in the adductor muscles.
- General body weakness.
- General lack of coordination or balance.
- Coxa vara.

Adduction. The base of support is narrowed.

CAUSES
- Increased tone in the adductor muscles.
- Genu valgum or coxa valga deformity.
- Weakness of the abductor muscles.

Flexion. Exaggerated flexion during the swing phase.

CAUSES
- Weakness in the ankle dorsiflexor muscles.
- Weakness of the hamstring muscles.
- Increased hip flexor muscle tone.

Knees. Extension of the knee at initial contact, followed by flexion at midstance, followed again by extension at terminal stance and flexion at preswing.

Hyperextension. Complete extension/hyperextension at midstance.

CAUSES
- Weakness in the quadriceps muscles.
- Spasticity in the quadriceps muscles.
- Weakness of the hamstring muscles.
- Joint deformity.

Restricted Extension. Loss of initial contact and plantar flexion.

CAUSES
- Joint disorders.

- Meniscal derangement.
- Weakness of hip extensor muscles.

Exaggerated Flexion. Increase in knee flexion during the swing and midstance phases.

CAUSES
- Increased tone in the hamstring muscles.
- Weakness of the ankle dorsiflexor muscles.
- Increased tone in the hip flexor muscles.

Genu Valgum. Patellae face inward.

CAUSES
- Femoral anteversion.
- Foot pronation.
- Tight iliotibial band.

Genu Varum. Patellae face outward.

CAUSES
- Femoral retroversion.
- Foot supination.

Ankle. Dorsiflexion at initial contact; foot flat in midstance; dorsiflexion at terminal stance and plantar flexion at preswing.

Preswing Exaggerated. Subject walks on the toes (pes equinus) or demonstrates increase in plantar flexion.

CAUSES
- Pes equinus deformity.
- Tightness in gastrocsoleus muscles.
- Increased tone in the gastrocsoleus muscles.
- Weakness in the dorsiflexor muscles.
- Knee flexion increased during stance.

Preswing Decreased. Subject lacks plantar flexion at terminal stance and preswing.

CAUSES
- Weakness of the plantar flexor muscles.
- Ankle or foot pain.

Foot Slap. Inability to maintain dorsiflexion at initial contact.

CAUSES
- Weakness of the dorsiflexor muscles.
- Lack of lower limb proprioception.

Foot Drop. Lack of adequate dorsiflexion during the swing phase.

CAUSES
- Weakness of ankle dorsiflexor muscles.
- Loss of hip extension.

Excessive Dorsiflexion. The subject walks on heels (pes calcaneus) or has increase in dorsiflexion during the swing phase of gait.

CAUSES
- Weakness of the gastrocsoleus muscle group.
- Tightness of the dorsiflexor muscles.
- Increased muscle tone in the dorsiflexors.
- Pes calcaneus deformity.

Pes Valgus. The foot turns outward and the ankle angles medially.

CAUSES
- Weakness of the posterior tibial and medial ankle ligaments.
- Pes planus deformity.
- Femoral anteversion.

Pes Varus. The ankle is angled laterally; subject walks on the lateral border of the foot.

CAUSES
- Weakness of the lateral compartment muscles.
- Increased muscle tone in the invertors of the ankle.

Foot. Weight on the lateral heel on initial contact, along the lateral border of the foot during midstance, and across the metatarsal heads during terminal stance and preswing phases.

Pronation. Decrease in the medial longitudinal arch.

CAUSES
- Hypermobility of foot.
- Femoral anteversion.
- Genu valgum.
- Weakness of dorsiflexor muscles.
- Tight heel cords.

Bibliography

Gould JA, Davies GJ: Orthopedic and Sports Physical Therapy. St Louis, CV Mosby, 1985

Kapandji IA: The Physiology of Joints, vol 3. Edinburgh, Churchill Livingstone, 1974

Kendall HO, Kendall FP: Posture and Pain. Malabar, Robert E. Krieger, 1981

Kisner C, Colby LA: Therapeutic Exercise: Foundations and Techniques. Philadelphia, FA Davis, 1985

Magee DJ: Orthopedic Physical Assessment. Philadelphia, WB Saunders, 1987

Norkin C, Levangie P: Joint Structure and Function: A Comprehensive Analysis. Philadelphia, FA Davis, 1983

Sahrmann SA: Program for Correction of Muscle Imbalance: Concepts and Principles. Boston, Continuing Education Workshop, 1986

Shoulder Complex

Chapter 4

The humerus, clavicle, scapula, and sternum comprise the shoulder girdle. The bones articulate to form three joints—sternoclavicular, acromioclavicular, and glenohumeral. The scapula also forms a physiological joint by moving on the thorax. These joints function in a closed-chain fashion: as the humerus moves in the glenoid fossa, the scapula rotates on the thorax and clavicle, and the clavicle moves on the sternum. The glenohumeral joint is a ball-and-socket synovial joint and has three degrees of freedom of movement. The sternoclavicular joint has been identified as a saddle-type synovial joint with three degrees of freedom of movement. The acromioclavicular joint is a plane synovial joint having the ability to produce motion in three planes.

The shoulder complex has developed mobility at the expense of stability. The head of the humerus hangs loosely in the glenoid fossa, and the only attachment of the upper limb to the trunk is at the sternoclavicular joint. Stabilization at the shoulder is provided by the ligaments—and primarily the tendons—of the muscle that blend into the joint capsule.

Goniometry

Shoulder

Shoulder Flexion

Motion occurs at the shoulder (glenohumeral) joint in the sagittal plane and is accompanied by motions at the sternoclavicular, acromioclavicular, and scapulothoracic joints. During glenohumeral flexion, the clavicle rises, then rotates posteriorly. To complete the range of shoulder joint flexion, the scapula rotates on the clavicle and rotates upward on the thorax approximately 60 degrees. Such accessory motions as humeral head depression, medial rotation, and posterior glide in the glenoid fossa occur simultaneously to provide smooth motion throughout the normal range. The functional range at the glenohumeral joint must include all associated motions.

Motion. Zero to 180 degrees (glenohumeral, acromioclavicular, sternoclavicular, and scapulothoracic joints).

Position. Subject lies supine, with the hips and knees flexed. The feet are flat on the table to prevent hyperextension of the lumbar vertebrae. The palm of the hand and the forearm are pronated (Fig. 4–1).

Goniometric Alignment

Axis. At the acromion process of the scapula, through the head of the humerus. *↓slightly ↗below↘in between*

Stationary Arm. Placed along the midaxillary line of the trunk in line with the greater trochanter of the femur.

Moving Arm. Placed along the lateral longitudinal midline of the humerus in line with the lateral epicondyle of the humerus.

Stabilization. The scapula should be prevented from rising and tipping posteriorly.

Precautions

- Avoid hyperextension of the lumbar vertebrae.
- Avoid abduction at the shoulder joint and elevation of the scapula. The motion occurs strictly in the sagittal plane.
- Allow medial rotation of the shoulder joint to occur at approximately 90 degrees of shoulder flexion.
- Allow for scapular and clavicular joint motion to occur at approximately 30 degrees of shoulder flexion.
- Maintain the elbow joint in extension to prevent the long head of the triceps muscle from being stretched.

Shoulder Extension and Hyperextension

Shoulder joint extension and hyperextension are the return from the flexion motion. In the sagittal plane, extension at the glenohumeral joint is accompanied by motions at the sternoclavicular, acromioclavicular, and scapulothoracic joints. When the shoulder joint is extending to the anatomical position, the scapula rotates downward and the clavicle depresses and rotates anteriorly. In hyperextension, the humerus rotates medially and glides anteriorly to complete the full functional range, while the humeral head remains depressed in the glenoid fossa.

Motion. 180 to 0 degrees of extension. *ant.* Zero to 50 degrees of hyperextension (glenohumeral, scapulothoracic, acromioclavicular, and sternoclavicular joints).

Figure 4–1. Ending position for shoulder flexion measurement.

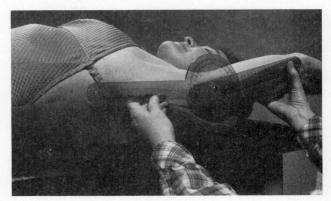

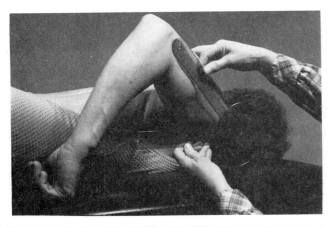

Figure 4–2. Preferred ending position for shoulder hyperextension measurement.

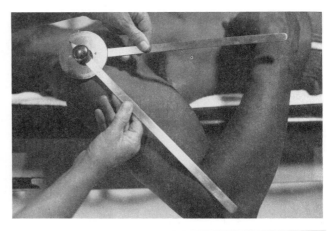

Figure 4–3. Ending position for shoulder hyperextension measurement with the subject in the supine position.

Position

- Preferred: Subject lies prone with the head comfortably positioned without a pillow. The shoulder joint is in the anatomical position with the elbow slightly flexed, and the forearm is pronated (Fig. 4–2).

  facing opp. arm

- Alternate:

  1. Subject is supine with the elbow flexed and the arm over the side of the treatment table (Fig. 4–3).

  2. Subject lies on one side with the elbow slightly flexed.

Goniometric Alignment

Axis. Slightly inferior to the acromion process of the scapula in line with the humeral head.

Stationary Arm. Placed along the midaxillary line of the trunk in line with the greater trochanter of the femur.

Moving Arm. Placed along the lateral longitudinal midline of the humerus in line with the lateral epicondyle of the humerus.

Stabilization. Stabilize the scapula.

Precautions

- Avoid flexion of the thoracic vertebrae.
- Avoid abduction of the shoulder joint.
- Keep elbow slightly flexed to prevent the biceps brachii muscle from being stretched.
- Avoid scapular adduction.
- Prevent anterior tipping and elevation of the scapula.

Shoulder Abduction

Motion of shoulder joint abduction occurs in the coronal plane. Accompanying abduction of the glenohumeral joint is clavicular elevation, followed by posterior rotation. Also, the scapula rotates upward on the thorax. The combined motions of the scapula and clavicle account for approximately 60 degrees of the movement. For the complete functional range of shoulder joint abduction to occur, there is an accompanying lateral rotation of the humerus to clear the greater tubercle under the acromion process of the scapula. The head of the humerus remains depressed in the glenoid fossa and glides inferiorly during the movement.

Motion. Zero to 180 degrees (glenohumeral, sternoclavicular, acromioclavicular, and scapulothoracic joints).

Position

- Preferred: Subject is supine with the hips and knees flexed and the feet flat on the table. The upper limb being tested is placed in the anatomical position (Fig. 4–4). The elbow joint remains extended.

Figure 4–4. Ending position for shoulder abduction measurement.

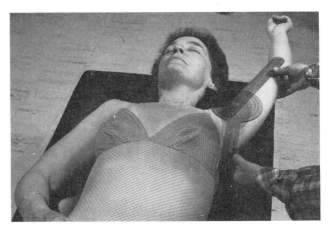

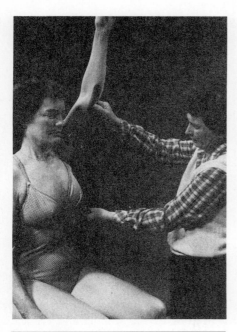

Figure 4–5. Ending position for measuring shoulder abduction from an anterior approach with the subject in a sitting position.

· Alternate: Subject sits or lies prone (Fig. 4–5).

Goniometric Alignment

Axis. Placed on the anterior portion of the acromion process of the scapula, through the center of the head of the humerus.

Stationary Arm
· Preferred: Placed on the lateral aspect of the anterior surface of the chest, parallel to the midline of the sternum.
· Alternate: Placed on the lateral aspect of the chest, parallel to the spinous process of the vertebrae.

Moving Arm
· Preferred: Placed on the anterior aspect of the arm, parallel to the midline of the humerus, in line with the medial humeral epicondyle.
· Alternate: Placed on the posterior aspect of the arm, parallel to the midline of the humerus, in line with the lateral humeral epicondyle.

Stabilization. Stabilize the thorax.

Precautions
· Avoid spine flexion toward the contralateral side.
· Avoid elevation of the scapula.
· Permit the shoulder to rotate laterally approximately 90 degrees.
· Maintain the upper limb in the coronal plane, except for the lateral rotation.

Shoulder Adduction

Adduction at the shoulder joint is measured as the return from shoulder joint abduction. The movement occurs in the coronal plane. Accompanying motions of the clavicle and the scapula occur as they return to the anatomical position during glenohumeral adduction. The humerus rotates medially and glides superiorly in the glenoid fossa until the completion of the range of motion.

Motion. From 180 degrees to 0 degrees (glenohumeral, scapulothoracic, acromioclavicular, and sternoclavicular joints).

Position
· Preferred: Subject lies supine with the knees flexed and the feet flat on the table (Fig. 4–6).
· Alternate: Subject sits.

Goniometric Alignment

Axis
· Preferred: Anterior surface of the acromion process through the head of the humerus.
· Alternate: Posterior surface of the acromion process through the head of the humerus.

Stationary Arm
· Preferred: Placed on the lateral aspect of the anterior surface of the chest, parallel to the midline of the sternum.
· Alternate: Parallel to the spinous processes of the vertebrae.

Moving Arm
· Preferred: Placed on the anterior aspect of the arm along the midline of the humerus.
· Alternate: Placed on the posterior aspect of the arm along the midline of the humerus, directed toward the olecranon process of the ulna.

Figure 4–6. Ending position for measuring shoulder adduction.

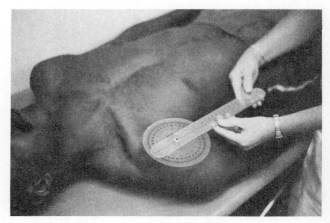

Stabilization.   Stabilize the thorax to prevent lateral spine flexion.

Precautions
- Prevent the spine from flexing ipsilaterally.
- Avoid scapular depression.
- Permit the shoulder joint to rotate medially.

Shoulder Horizontal Adduction

Horizontal adduction at the glenohumeral joint occurs in the transverse plane. The scapula abducts on the thorax, and the clavicle protracts to allow complete motion. The humeral head is depressed and glides posteriorly and laterally in the glenoid fossa.

Motion.   Zero to 120 degrees of horizontal adduction from a fully horizontally abducted position (shoulder, sternoclavicular, acromioclavicular, and scapulothor-

Figure 4–7.   Starting position for measuring horizontal shoulder adduction (from horizontally abducted position) with the subject in a sitting position.

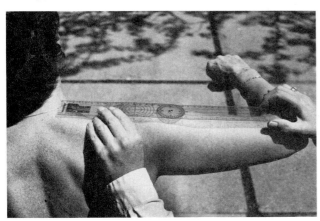

Figure 4–8.   Ending position for measuring horizontal shoulder adduction with the subject in a sitting position.

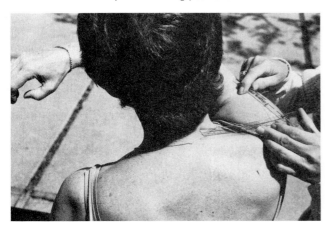

acic joints). Zero to 30 degrees of horizontal adduction from the neutral position.

Position
- Preferred: Subject sits. The shoulder joint is abducted 90 degrees and the elbow flexed 90 degrees. The shoulder joint is also positioned in neutral rotation (Figs. 4–7 and 4–8).
- Alternate:
  1. Subject sits with shoulder flexed 90 degrees and internally rotated. The elbow is flexed 90 degrees.
  2. The subject lies supine, with the shoulder and elbow positioned as described above in the preferred position (Fig. 4–9).

Goniometric Alignment

Axis.   Superiorly on the acromion process of the scapula through the head of the humerus.

Stationary Arm.   Along the midline of the shoulder toward the neck (the goniometer arm must be short). Alternate: Along the midline of the humerus in line with the lateral epicondyle of the humerus.

Moving Arm.   Along the midshaft of the humerus, in line with the lateral epicondyle of the humerus.

Stabilization.   Stabilize the thorax to prevent rotation.

Precaution
- Prevent rotation of the trunk.

Shoulder Horizontal Abduction

Horizontal abduction at the shoulder joint occurs in the transverse plane. The scapula adducts on the thorax and the clavicle retracts to allow complete motion. The hu-

Figure 4–9.   Alternate starting position for measuring horizontal shoulder adduction.

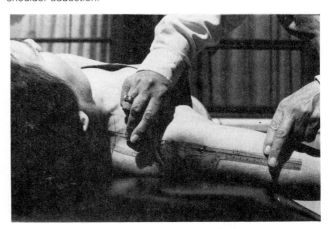

meral head remains depressed and glides anteriorly in the glenoid fossa.

Motion. Zero to 120 degrees from a fully horizontally adducted position (sternoclavicular, acromioclavicular, and scapulothoracic). Zero to 90 degrees of horizontal abduction from the neutral position.

Position. Subject sits with the shoulder joint in neutral rotation, flexed to 90 degrees, and the elbow flexed 90 degrees.

Goniometric Alignment

Axis. Superiorly on the acromion process of the scapula through the head of the humerus.

Stationary Arm. Aligned on the midline of the shoulder toward the neck. The goniometer arm must be short. Alternate: Along the midline of the humerus, in line with the lateral epicondyle of the humerus.

Moving Arm. Along the midshaft of the humerus, in line with the lateral epicondyle of the humerus (see Fig. 4–7).

Stabilization. Stabilize the thorax to prevent rotation.

Precaution
· Prevent trunk rotation.

Medial Shoulder Rotation

In the anatomical position, the motion occurs in the transverse plane. For goniometric evaluation, the shoulder joint is abducted and the elbow joint flexed 90 degrees while the subject is supine; the motion tested occurs in the sagittal plane. The evaluation position for medial rotation of the shoulder joint puts the scapula in

abduction and upward rotation. During the motion of medial rotation, the scapula adducts slightly and the humeral head glides posteriorly in the glenoid fossa.

Motion. Zero to 65 to 90 degrees.

Position
· Preferred: Subject lies supine, with the knees flexed and the feet flat on the table. The shoulder joint is abducted and the elbow flexed 90 degrees. The forearm is in midposition between supination and pronation, and is perpendicular to the table top. The full length of the humerus is supported on the table. It may be necessary to place a rolled towel under the arm to keep it level (Fig. 4–10).
· Alternate: Subject is prone with the shoulder abducted 90 degrees and the elbow flexed over the edge of the table (Fig. 4–11).

Goniometric Alignment

Axis. The olecranon process of the ulna projects through the humeral shaft toward the humeral head.

Stationary Arm. Placed parallel to the tabletop or perpendicular to the floor.

Moving Arm. Along the ulnar shaft, directed toward the styloid process of the ulna.

Stabilization. Stabilize the distal end of the humerus throughout the range of motion and the scapula and thorax toward the end of the range.

Precautions
· Keep the shoulder joint abducted 90 degrees so that the olecranon is in line with the glenoid fossa.
· Avoid flexion and extension at the shoulder joint.
· Avoid flexion of the vertebrae.
· Avoid elbow extension.

Figure 4–10. Ending position for measuring medial shoulder rotation.

Figure 4–11. Alternate ending position for measuring medial shoulder rotation with the subject prone.

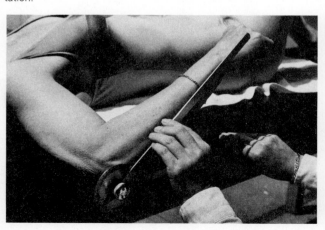

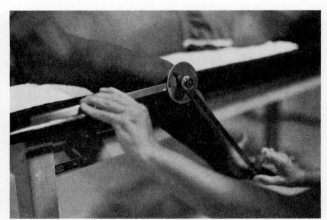

- Prevent elevation and anterior tipping of the scapula. *may have to stab. shoulder*

Ext.
Lateral Shoulder Rotation

In the anatomical position, the motion of lateral shoulder rotation occurs in the transverse plane. During goniometric evaluation, the shoulder joint is positioned in abduction and the elbow is flexed 90 degrees; therefore, the test motion occurs in the sagittal plane. When the test is conducted with the patient in the supine position, the scapula is put in abduction and upward rotation and increases slightly in both motions during lateral rotation of the glenohumeral joint. The head of the humerus is depressed in the glenoid fossa and glides anteriorly during the motion. It may be necessary to use a rolled towel or pad to keep the humerus level.

Motion. Zero to 90 degrees.

Position
- Preferred: Subject is supine, with the hips and knees flexed and the feet flat on the table. The shoulder is abducted and the elbow flexed to 90 degrees. The forearm is in midposition between supination and pronation and perpendicular to the table top, with the full length of the humerus supported. Note degree of shoulder abduction if less than 90 degrees (Fig. 4–12).
- Alternate: Subject is prone, with the shoulder abducted to 90 degrees and the elbow flexed over the edge of the table (Fig. 4–13).

Goniometric Alignment

Axis. Placed on the olecranon process of the ulna in line with the head of the humerus.

Stationary Arm. Placed parallel to the table top or perpendicular to the floor.

Moving Arm. The ulnar shaft directed toward the styloid process of the ulna.

Stabilization. Stabilize the distal end of the humerus and the scapula.

Precautions
- Keep the shoulder abducted to 90 degrees so that the olecranon is in line with the glenoid fossa.
- Avoid extension of the spine.
- Avoid extension of the elbow.
- Prevent posterior tipping of the scapula.
- Avoid flexion, extension, abduction, and adduction of the shoulder joint.

Scapula
Upward Scapular Rotation

Upward rotation of the scapula occurs in the coronal plane around an axis in the sagittal plane. The scapulothoracic joint is not a true anatomical joint but a functional one that exists between thorax, muscle, and bony scapula. In order for the scapula to rotate upward, the shoulder joint must complete a motion of abduction or flexion. Motion in this joint is seldom measured, but when it is, it is usually performed with a tape measure rather than a goniometer.

Motion. The measurement is the difference in inches between the anatomical starting position and the end position. The motion of one scapula is compared to that of the other.

Position. Subject sits with the shoulder in the anatomical position. Standing and lying prone are alternate positions (Fig. 4–14).

Figure 4–12. Ending position for measuring lateral shoulder rotation.

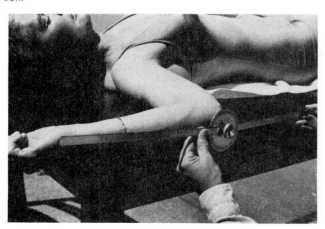

Figure 4–13. Alternate ending position for measuring lateral shoulder rotation with the subject in a prone position.

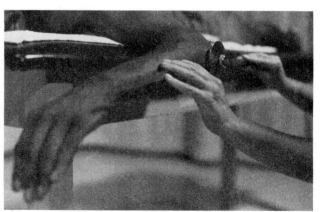

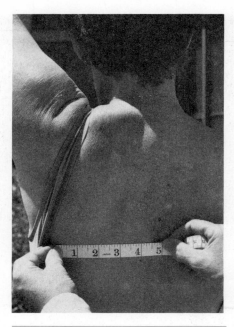

Figure 4–14. End position for measuring scapular upward rotation.

Measuring Tape
- Starting: Place the tape parallel to and in line with a line from the inferior angle of the scapula and the spinous process of the seventh thoracic vertebra (T7).
- Ending: Following motion, measure to the inferior angle of the scapula and calculate the difference in inches or centimeters. The difference between the two measurements is the amount of upward scapular rotation.

Stabilization. Stabilize the thorax.

Precaution
- Make sure the scapula does not tip.

Downward Scapular Rotation

Downward rotation occurs in the coronal plane around an axis in the sagittal plane. The scapulothoracic joint is not a true anatomical joint but a functional one necessary for complete range of motion at the shoulder joint. Downward rotation of the scapula is seldom measured.

Motion. The scapula's inferior angle moves medially when the shoulder joint is extended and adducted across the posterior trunk. The amount of motion is the difference between the starting and ending positions. It is compared with the motion in the opposite scapulothoracic joint.

Position. Subject sits with the upper limb in the anatomical position (Fig. 4–15). Alternate positions are lying prone and standing.

Measuring Tape
- Starting: Place the tape parallel to and in line with a line from the inferior angle of the scapula to the spinous process of T7.
- Ending: Following downward rotation of the scapula, using the same bony landmarks, take an end reading from the tape and calculate the difference in inches or centimeters. The total range is the difference between the two measurements.

Stabilization. Stabilize the thorax.

Precaution
- Make sure the scapula is not adducted.

Scapular Abduction

Abduction of the scapula is a translatory motion occurring in the coronal plane at the scapulothoracic joint between the thorax, muscle, and scapula when the vertebral border of the scapula moves laterally. The lateral motion of the scapula is accompanied by lateral tilt as the scapula follows the curved contour of the thorax. The starting test position is 90 degrees of shoulder abduction. The scapula is rotated slightly upward. In order for scapular abduction to occur, the shoulder joint adducts horizontally in the transverse plane.

Motion. The scapula moves laterally on the thorax as the shoulder joint moves through a complete range of horizontal adduction. The amount of motion is determined by measuring with a tape the difference between the beginning and ending points.

Figure 4–15. End position for measuring scapular downward rotation.

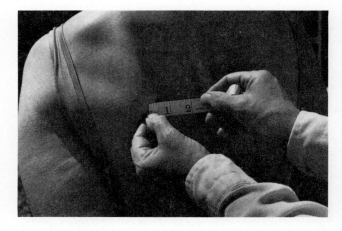

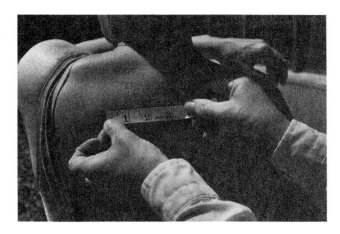

Figure 4–16.   End position for measuring scapular abduction.

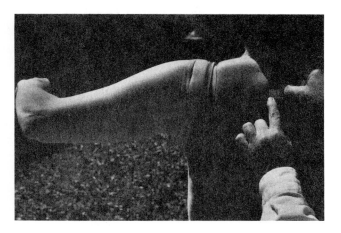

Figure 4–17.   End position for measuring scapular adduction.

Position.   Subject sits with the shoulder joint abducted and the elbow flexed 90 degrees.

Measuring Tape
- Starting: Hold the tape horizontal at the level of the root of the spine of the scapula and the thoracic vertebrae.
- Ending: Measure the difference between the beginning and end points of motion following horizontal adduction of the shoulder joint. The difference between the two measurements is the total range of scapular abduction (Fig. 4–16).

Stabilization.   Stabilize the trunk.

Precautions
- Avoid rotation of the shoulder joint.
- Avoid trunk rotation.

Scapular Adduction

The motion for scapular adduction is translatory and occurs in the coronal plane between thorax, muscle, and scapula. The motion is tested with the shoulder joint abducted 90 degrees and the scapula rotated slightly upward. The range of motion is determined when the vertebral border of the scapula moves medially toward the spinous processes of the thoracic vertebrae. Scapular adduction occurs as the shoulder joint abducts horizontally.

Motion.   The scapula moves medially during horizontal abduction of the shoulder. The range of motion is the difference between the beginning and end points of the scapula's motion.

Position.   Subject sits with the shoulder abducted 90 degrees.

Measuring Tape
- Starting: Hold the tape horizontally between the root of the spine of the scapula and the thoracic vertebrae.
- Ending: Following horizontal abduction of the shoulder joint, measure the distance between the root of the spine of the scapula and the thoracic vertebral spinous processes. The difference between the two measurements is the range of scapular adduction (Fig. 4–17).

Stabilization.   Stabilize the thorax.

Precautions
- Avoid rotation at the shoulder joint.
- Avoid trunk rotation.

Functional Muscle Testing

Upper Limb

The shoulder joint is designed to provide mobility for the upper limb, unlike the hip joints, which have developed to afford stability. Functionally upper limb motions occur in an open kinematic chain, whereas the motions of the weight-bearing lower limbs form a closed kinematic chain. Motions of the shoulder, scapula, elbow, forearm, and wrist provide mobility for the hand.

Shoulder Flexion

The motion at the glenohumeral joint is accompanied by scapular motion. The muscles that produce shoulder flexion have to overcome the weight of the upper limb and any load it carries.

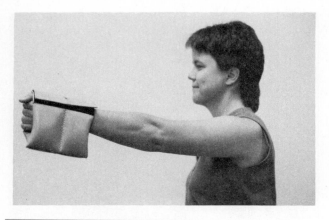

Figure 4–18. Resisted shoulder joint flexion.

Position. Subject sits, with a weight cuff attached to the wrist and the elbow extended (Fig. 4–18).

Activity. Subject lifts the weight to 90 degrees of shoulder flexion and then lowers it.

Muscles. Anterior deltoid, coracobrachialis, pectoralis major (clavicular head), and biceps brachii.

Type of Contraction
- Concentric: Raising the weight.
- Eccentric: Lowering the weight.

Resistance
- The weight of the upper limb and any load.
- Functional: 4- to 5-pound weight.

Figure 4–19. Resisted shoulder joint extension and hyperextension.

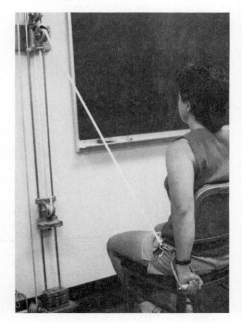

- Functionally Fair: 2-pound weight.
- Functionally Poor: Can raise upper limb only.
- Nonfunctional: Cannot raise upper limb.

Shoulder Extension and Hyperextension

The extension motion of the shoulder joint is accompanied by contraction of the scapular musculature. Usually extension movements at the shoulder joint are performed by eccentric contractions of the shoulder joint flexors. Hyperextension movements at the shoulder joint are usually formed concentrically. Pulling an object or the activity of sawing or chopping wood or pulling open a door calls for contraction of the extensor musculature.

Position. Subject sits or stands, facing an overhead wall pulley with the shoulder flexed approximately 145 degrees and the elbow extended (Fig. 4–19).

Activity. Subject pulls into hyperextension against resistance.

Muscles. Latissimus dorsi, teres major, teres minor, posterior deltoid, pectoralis major (sternal head), and long head of the triceps muscle.

Resistance
- The weight on the wall pulley.
- Functional: 4- to 5-pound weight.
- Functionally Fair: 2- to 3-pound weight.
- Functionally Poor: 1-pound weight.
- Nonfunctional: 0 weight.

Medial Shoulder Rotation

The medial rotator muscles are numerous and powerful compared with their counterparts, the lateral rotators. Also, as the shoulder rotates medially, the scapula abducts on the thoracic wall. The medial rotators at the shoulder are essential for right-handed writing, as they move the shoulder medially.

Position. Subject sits with the shoulder in the anatomical position and a weight cuff on the wrist (Fig. 4–20).

Activity. Subject places the hand in the small of the back.

Muscles. Latissimus dorsi, teres major, pectoralis major (sternal head).

Types of Contraction
- Concentric: Placing the hand on the lower back.
- Eccentric: Returning to the anatomical position.

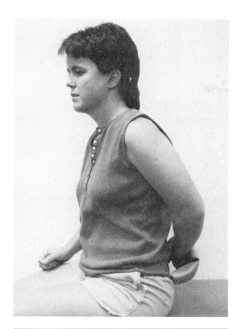

Figure 4–20. Resisted shoulder joint medial rotation.

Resistance
- The weight and the upper limb.
- Functional: 5-pound weight.
- Functionally Fair: 3- to 4-pound weight.
- Functionally Poor: 1- to 2-pound weight.
- Nonfunctional: 0 weight.

Lateral Shoulder Rotation

The lateral rotators are weak compared to the medial rotator muscles; however, they are indispensable in that they allow the hand to move laterally when it is placed anterior to the trunk, as in writing. To allow full range of lateral shoulder joint rotation, the scapula adducts on the thoracic wall.

Position. Subject sits at right angles to the wall pulley with the elbow flexed 90 degrees and the shoulder in medial rotation (Fig. 4–21).

Activity. Subject pulls into lateral rotation against resistance.

Muscles. Infraspinatus, teres minor.

Types of Contraction
- Concentric: Pulling into lateral rotation.
- Eccentric: Returning to the starting position.

Resistance
- The weight of the upper limb and the weight on the wall pulley.
- Functional: 5-pound weight.
- Functionally Fair: 3- to 4-pound weight.
- Functionally Poor: 1- to 2-pound weight.
- Nonfunctional: 0 weight.

Shoulder Abduction

The shoulder abductor muscles lie superior to the joint axis in the frontal plane. For normal abduction of the shoulder joint there must be participation in upward rotation of the scapula and lateral rotation of the glenohumeral joint. The muscles must be strong enough to overcome the weight of the upper limb and its load.

Position. Subject sits with a weight cuff on the wrist (Fig. 4–22).

Activity. Subject moves the shoulder to approximately 90 degrees in the frontal plane.

Muscles. Supraspinatus, deltoid.

Figure 4–21. Resisted shoulder joint lateral rotation.

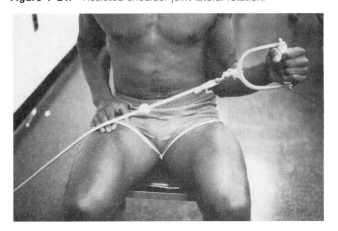

Figure 4–22. Resisted shoulder joint abduction.

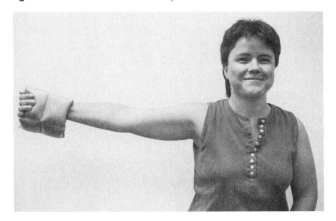

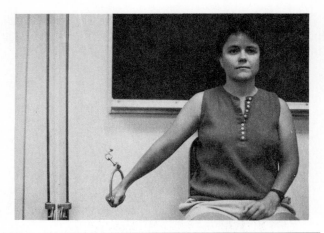

Figure 4–23. Resisted shoulder joint adduction.

Types of Contraction
- Concentric: Lifting the weight to 90 degrees.
- Eccentric: Lowering the weight to the starting position.

Resistance
- The weight of the upper limb and of the weight cuff.
- Functional: 5-pound weight.
- Functionally Fair: 3- to 4-pound weight.
- Functionally Poor: 1- to 2-pound weight.
- Nonfunctional: 0 weight.

Shoulder Adduction

Often, adduction of the shoulder joint is a return from abduction and is performed by an eccentric contraction of the shoulder abductor muscles; however, there are activities that require contraction of the adductors, such as swimming and chopping wood. In order for a coordinated movement to occur, the major and minor rhomboid muscles must contract synergistically to stabilize the scapula against the pull from the teres major muscle, which tends to rotate the scapula upward. Also, the long head of the triceps muscle must contract synergistically to offset the tendency of the latissimus dorsi muscle to displace the head of the humerus inferiorly.

Position. Subject sits at a right angle to the wall pulley with the shoulder joint abducted approximately 145 degrees (Fig. 4–23).

Activity. Subject pulls downward on the pulley.

Muscles. Teres major, latissimus dorsi, pectoralis major.

Types of Contraction
- Concentric: Pulling downward.
- Eccentric: Returning to the starting position.

Resistance
- The weight on the wall pulley.
- Functional: 5-pound weight.
- Functionally Fair: 3- to 4-pound weight.
- Functionally Poor: 1- to 2-pound weight.
- Nonfunctional: 0 weight.

Scapula

The scapula moves on the thorax between two intervening muscles, the serratus anterior and the subscapularis. The scapula is directly associated with the clavicle, and they form a closed kinematic chain. The scapula may move independently but is frequently synergistically associated with the movements at the shoulder joint.

Scapular Elevation

The scapular elevator muscles lie superior to the scapula and contract to bring the shoulder toward the ears. Usually both eccentric and concentric muscle contractions occur.

Position. Subject sits with the hands relaxed in the lap (Fig. 4–24).

Activity. Subject slowly shrugs both shoulders simultaneously.

Figure 4–24. Scapular elevation.

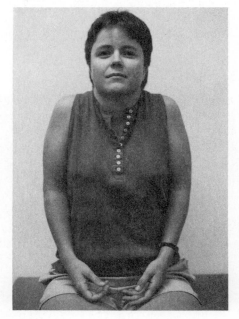

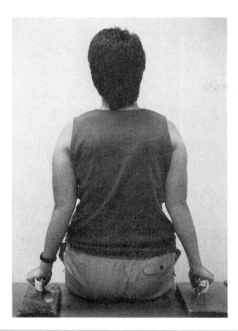

Figure 4–25. Scapular depression using sitting push-up handles.

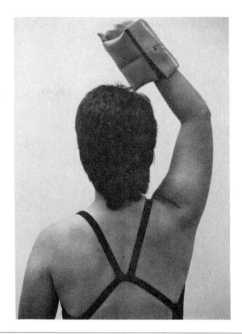

Figure 4–26. Resisted scapular upward rotation.

Muscles. Upper fibers of the trapezius, levator scapulae, major and minor rhomboids.

Types of Contraction
- Concentric: Raising the shoulders toward the ears.
- Eccentric: Controlled lowering the shoulders to the starting position.

Resistance
- Weight of the upper limbs.
- Functional: 5 repetitions.
- Functionally Fair: 3 to 4 repetitions.
- Functionally Poor: 1 to 2 repetitions.
- Nonfunctional: 0 repetitions.

Scapular Depression

Depression of the scapula is important for walking with crutches, changing positions while sitting when the lower limbs are weak, and performing wheelchair transfers. Often, with lower limb weakness, the scapulae are depressed and the musculature reverses its action. The upper limbs are stabilized and the trunk moves on the scapula.

Position. Subject sits, with the hands on the table slightly anterior and lateral to the hips. If the trunk is short, a rolled towel or push-up handles may be used (Fig. 4–25).

Activity. Subject performs sitting push-ups.

Muscles. Lower fibers of the trapezius, pectoralis major (sternal head), lower fibers of the serratus anterior, subclavius, pectoralis minor, and latissimus dorsi (indirectly through its attachment on the humerus).

Types of Contraction
- Concentric: Lifting the buttocks off the table.
- Eccentric: Lowering the buttocks onto the table.

Resistance
- Body weight.
- Functional: 5 repetitions.
- Functionally Fair: 3 to 4 repetitions.
- Functionally Poor: 1 to 2 repetitions.
- Nonfunctional: 0 repetitions.

Upward Scapular Rotation

Upward rotation of the scapula occurs during elevation of the upper limbs and accounts for approximately one third of the upper limb movement. It is a motion that aids in maintaining the glenoid fossa in an optimal position for the humeral head. Upward rotation of the scapula does not function independently of shoulder joint motions.

Position. Subject sits with the upper limb in the anatomical position and a weight cuff on the wrist (Fig. 4–26).

Activity. Subject reaches overhead to approximately 180 degrees and then lowers the arm. The scapula must be observed to rotate upward.

Muscles. Upper and lower fibers of the trapezius, lower fibers of the serratus anterior.

Types of Contraction
- Concentric: Lifting the weight.
- Eccentric: Lowering the weight.

Resistance
- The weight of the upper limb and of the weight cuff.
- Functional: 5-pound weight.
- Functionally Fair: 3- to 4-pound weight.
- Functionally Poor: 1- to 2-pound weight.
- Nonfunctional: 0 weight.

Downward Scapular Rotation

Frequently, scapular downward rotation is performed by an eccentric contraction of the upward rotators of the scapula; however, extending or adducting the shoulder joint against resistance will produce concentric contraction of the downward rotators.

Position. Subject sits with the shoulder joint abducted or flexed approximately 145 degrees facing a weighted wall pulley (Fig. 4–27).

Activity. Subject pulls down on the pulley. The scapula must be observed to rotate downward.

Muscles. Rhomboid major and minor, levator scapulae, pectoralis minor.

Figure 4–27. Resisted scapular downward rotation.

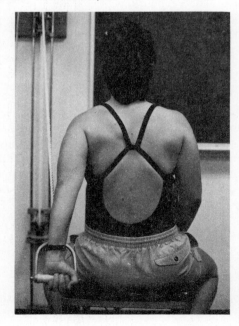

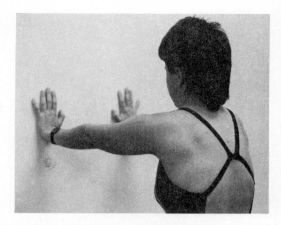

Figure 4–28. Standing push-up testing scapular abduction.

Types of Contraction
- Concentric: Pulling downward into shoulder joint adduction or extension.
- Eccentric: Allowing the pulley to return to the starting position.

Resistance
- The weight on the wall pulley.
- Functional: 5-pound weight.
- Functionally Fair: 3- to 4-pound weight.
- Functionally Poor: 1 to 2-pound weight.
- Nonfunctional: 0 weight.

Scapular Abduction

Scapular abduction may act independently of the shoulder joint, as in cupping the shoulders, but is most often used during movements of horizontal adduction and in pushing a load forward.

Position. Subject stands, facing a wall with the shoulders flexed 90 degrees and the hands on the wall (Fig. 4–28).

Activity. Subject pushes against the wall as if to perform a standing push-up.

Muscles. Serratus anterior and pectoralis minor.

Types of Contraction
- Concentric: Pushing away from the wall.
- Eccentric: Returning to the starting position.

Resistance
- Body weight.
- Functional: 5 repetitions.
- Functionally Fair: 3 to 4 repetitions.
- Functionally Poor: 1 to 2 repetitions.
- Nonfunctional: 0 repetitions.

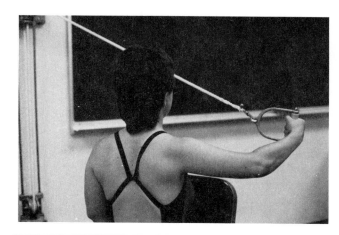

Figure 4–29. Resisted scapular adduction.

Scapular Adduction

Often the functional motion of scapular adduction is an eccentric contraction of the scapular abductors, as in a prone push-up, for example, but it may be used concentrically, particularly in combination with shoulder joint motions.

Position. Subject sits at a right angle to the wall pulley with the shoulder and elbow joints flexed 90 degrees. The subject uses a weighted wall pulley (Fig. 4–29).

Activity. Subject horizontally abducts through the full range of motion.

Muscles. Rhomboid major and minor, trapezius, levator scapulae.

Types of Contraction
· Concentric: Pulling scapulae together.
· Eccentric: Returning to the starting position.

Resistance
· The weight of the upper limbs plus the weight on the pulley.
· Functional: 5-pound weight.
· Functionally Fair: 3- to 4-pound weight.
· Functionally Poor: 1- to 2-pound weight.
· Nonfunctional: 0 weight.

Manual Muscle Testing

Upper Trapezius and Levator Scapulae

The upper trapezius and levator scapulae muscles elevate the scapula approximately 2 inches. Usually both sides are tested simultaneously, providing stabilization as well as resistance bilaterally. Simultaneous testing also provides an indication of symmetry. The neck and head must be observed for motion if a lesion is unilateral. To test isolated scapular elevation, the head is stabilized on the test side.

Palpation. Palpate the upper trapezius on the superior and posterior surface of the shoulders (Fig. 4–30). The levator scapulae is deep to the upper trapezius in the angle formed by the upper trapezius and the sternocleidomastoid muscles. To isolate the action of the levator scapulae, minimize the action of the trapezius muscle by the subject placing the hand in the small of the subject's back and shrugging the shoulders quickly within a limited range of motion (Fig. 4–31).

Figure 4–30. Palpating the upper trapezius muscle.

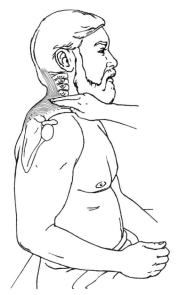

Figure 4–31. Palpating the levator scapulae muscle.

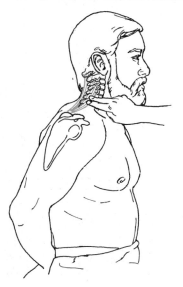

Attachments of Upper Trapezius and Levator Scapulae Muscles

Muscle	Proximal	Distal	Innervation
Upper trapezius	Superior nuchal line Ligamentum nuchae	Lateral third of clavicle and the acromion process	Spinal accessory CN XI
Levator scapulae	Transverse processes of upper four cervical vertebrae	Medial border of scapula at level of the scapular superior angle	Dorsal scapular C5 (C3 and C4)

Position

Against gravity (AG): Subject sits with the arms relaxed (Fig. 4–32).

Gravity minimized (GM): Subject is supine or prone; examiner supports upper limbs and shoulders (Fig. 4–33).

Movement.   Elevate the shoulders toward the ears.

Resistance.   Applied superiorly on the acromion process.

Stabilization.   Apply resistance to both shoulders simultaneously to offer stability or unilaterally to the posterior lateral aspect of head.

Substitutions
- Serratus anterior abducts and rotates the scapula upward, appearing to elevate it.

- Pectoralis minor anteriorly tilts the scapula, as in "round shoulders."
- Anterior, middle, and posterior scalenus muscles elevate the first and second ribs.
- Major and minor rhomboid muscles elevate the scapula, with accompanying downward rotation.

Middle Trapezius Muscle

The middle trapezius muscle adducts the scapula. The vertebral border of the scapula moves 2 inches toward the spinous processes of the thoracic vertebrae. Gravitational effects on the scapula are minimal; therefore all testing may be performed with the subject in the prone position. Results may be determined by the palpated firmness of the contraction.

Palpation.   Palpate along the medial border of the scapula near the root of the spine (Fig. 4–34).

Figure 4–32.   Muscle testing the upper trapezius and levator scapulae muscles in the AG sitting position.

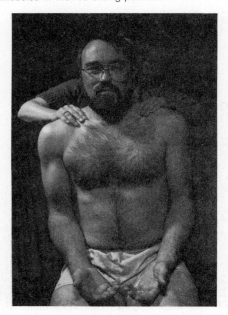

Figure 4–33.   Muscle testing the upper trapezius and levator scapulae muscles in the GM supine position.

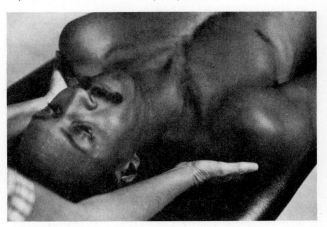

Attachments of Middle Trapezius Muscle

Muscle	Proximal	Distal	Innervation
Middle trapezius	Spinous processes of T1–T5	Superior border of scapular spine	Spinal accessory CN XI

Position

AG: Subject is prone with elbow flexed over the edge of the treatment table (Fig. 4–35).

GM: Subject sits with upper limb resting on the table shoulder joint abducted 90 degrees and elbow flexed 90 degrees. The surface must be friction free (Fig. 4–36).

Movement.   Bring scapulae together into adduction.

Resistance.   Applied to the lateral border of the scapula, pushing down and out into abduction.

Figure 4–34.   Palpating the middle trapezius muscle.

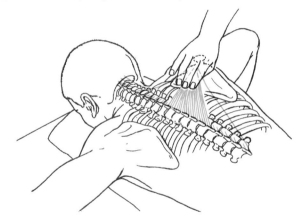

Figure 4–35.   Testing the middle trapezius muscle in the AG prone position.

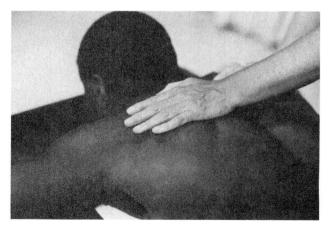

Stabilization.   Stabilize the contralateral thorax.

Substitutions

- While sitting, the subject may rotate the trunk, giving the appearance of scapular adduction.
- The posterior deltoid muscle causes horizontal abduction of the shoulder without adducting the scapula.
- Major and minor rhomboid muscles will cause the scapula to elevate and rotate downward while adducting. Do not allow the shoulder to rotate medially.
- Lower trapezius causes the scapula to depress and rotate upward.
- The rhomboids and the lower trapezius may contract synergistically to provide scapular adduction. This is monitored by palpation.
- The upper and lower fibers of the trapezius muscle contract synergistically to adduct the scapula.

Lower Trapezius Muscle

The lower fibers of the trapezius muscle produce adduction and depression of the scapula. The test range of motion is 1 to 2 inches. All grades are tested with the subject in the prone position. The upper limb is supported in an elevated position and aligned with the direction of the lower trapezius muscle fibers. Complete motion may be limited by a shortened pectoralis major

Figure 4–36.   Testing the middle trapezius muscle in the GM sitting position.

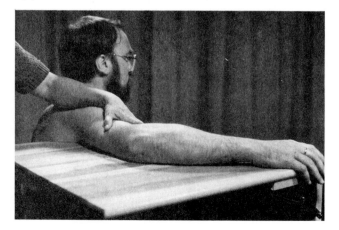

Attachments of Lower Trapezius Muscle

Muscle	Proximal	Distal	Innervation
Lower trapezius	Spinous processes of T6–T12	Apex or root, and inferiorly on the scapular spine	Spinal accessory CN XI

muscle. For 0 to P or 0 to 2 the grade is determined by the firmness of muscle contraction. The patient is unable to lift the upper limb, but the scapula may depress. If the deltoid muscle is weak, the upper limb must be manually supported. Grades of 2+ to 3− are based on how far the upper limb is lifted from the table; for grade F to N or 3 to 5 resistance is applied.

Palpation. Palpate medial to the root of the spine and the medial border of the scapula; this portion of the muscle forms a triangle (Fig. 4–37).

Figure 4–37. Palpating the lower trapezius muscle.

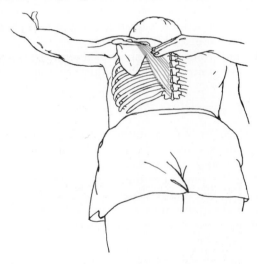

Figure 4–38. Testing the lower trapezius muscle in the AG prone position.

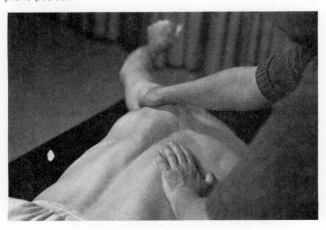

Position

AG and GM: Subject lies prone, with the shoulder abducted 130 degrees. If shoulder range of motion is limited, the upper limb may be placed over the side of the table and manually supported (Figs. 4–38 and 4–39).

Movement. Subject lifts the upper limb off the table.

Resistance. Applied to the lateral angle of the scapula in a forward and outward direction.

Stabilization. Stabilize the thorax on the opposite side.

Substitutions
- Posterior deltoid will raise the upper limb without depressing or adducting the scapula.
- Latissimus dorsi is indirectly an accessory muscle in depression of the scapula through its attachment on the humerus.
- Pectoralis major (sternal head) is indirectly

Figure 4–39. Testing the lower trapezius muscle in the GM prone position.

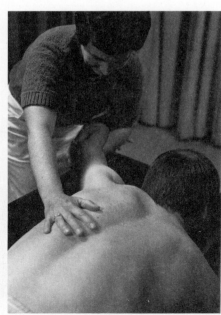

Attachments of Major and Minor Rhomboid Muscles

Muscle	Proximal	Distal	Innervation
Major rhomboid	Spinous processes of T2–5	Medial border between the root and inferior angle of the scapula	Dorsal scapular C4 and C5
Minor rhomboid	Ligamentum nuchae Spinous process of C7–T1	Medial border at root of scapula	Dorsal scapular C4 and C5

(through its attachment on the humerus) an accessory muscle for depresssion of the scapula.

Major and Minor Rhomboid Muscles

The major and minor rhomboid muscles produce the motions of scapular adduction and downward rotation. The test range consists of the inferior angle of the scapula moving approximately 1 inch toward the spinous pro-

cesses of the vertebrae. The effect of gravity on scapular motion is minimal; therefore palpation and strength measurement may be performed with the subject in the prone position.

Palpation. Place the subject's hand in the lumbar area of the back to relax the overlying trapezius muscle, and palpate beneath and along the medial border of the scapula (Fig. 4–40).

Position
AG: Subject lies prone with the hand resting on the lumbar spine (Fig. 4–41).
GM: Subject sits, with the hand resting on the lumbar spine (Fig. 4–42).

Movement. Lift the hand off the back.

Resistance. Applied to the vertebral border of the scapula, pushing into abduction and upward rotation.

Figure 4–40. Palpating the major and minor rhomboid muscles.

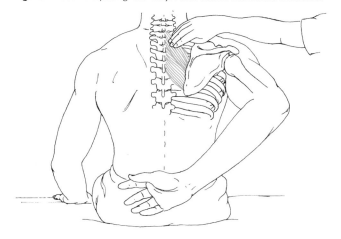

Figure 4–41. Testing the major and minor rhomboid muscles in the AG prone position.

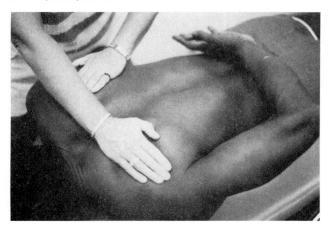

Figure 4–42. Testing the major and minor rhomboid muscles in the GM sitting position.

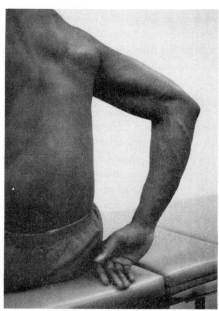

Attachments of Serratus Anterior Muscle

Muscle	Proximal	Distal	Innervation
Serratus anterior	Anterior surface of the upper eight or nine pairs of ribs	Costal surface and vertebral border of the scapula	Long thoracic C6 and 7 (C5)

Stabilization. Stabilize the thorax on the opposite side.

Substitutions
- Wrist extensors: By pressing the hand against the lumbar area of the back, the subject lifts the upper limb without moving the scapula.
- Middle trapezius adducts the scapula with no rotation.
- Posterior deltoid causes the shoulder to abduct

horizontally and may give the appearance of scapular adduction.
- Latissimus dorsi and teres major adduct and extend the shoulder with no effect on scapular rotation.
- Levator scapulae is an accessory muscle to downward scapular rotation and adduction, but it does not participate in the action unless the scapula is positioned in upward rotation.

Serratus Anterior Muscle

The serratus anterior muscle produces the motion of abduction of the scapula with accompanying upward rotation. The test range is 2 to 3 inches of the scapula sliding on the thorax. The serratus anterior muscle is a major fixator of the scapula to the thorax. Minimal weakness is difficult to detect. Standing, pushing against a wall, or performing a prone push-up may reveal "winging" of the scapula.

Palpation. Palpate along the midaxillary line adjacent to the inferior angle of the scapula (Fig. 4–43).

Position
AG: Subject lies supine with the shoulder flexed 90 degrees and the elbow joint completely flexed (Fig. 4–44).

Figure 4–43. Palpating the serratus anterior muscle.

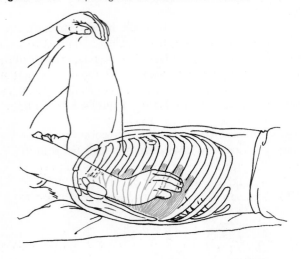

Figure 4–44. Testing the serratus anterior muscle in the AG supine position.

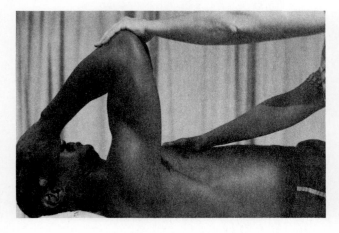

Figure 4–45. Testing the serratus anterior muscle in the GM sitting position.

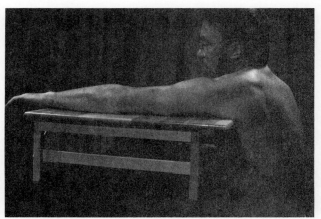

Attachments of Pectoralis Minor Muscle

Muscle	Proximal	Distal	Innervation
Pectoralis minor	Coracoid process	Second through fifth ribs	Medial and lateral pectoral C7 (C6 and C7)

GM: Subject sits with the upper limb resting on the table, the shoulder in 90 degrees of flexion, and the elbow extended (Fig. 4–45).

Movement. Reach forward or protract the shoulder joint so the scapula slides forward on the thorax.

Resistance. Applied to the elbow, pushing the scapula down into adduction.

Stabilization. Stabilize the contralateral thorax. With the subject in the sitting position, stabilize the thorax to prevent anterior displacement of the trunk.

Figure 4–46. Palpating the pectoralis minor muscle.

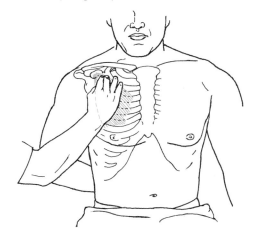

Figure 4–47. Testing the pectoralis minor muscle in the AG supine position.

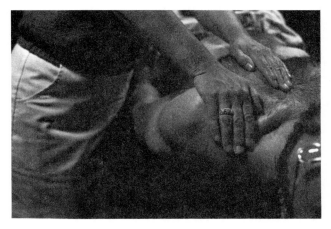

Substitutions
- In the sitting position, the subject may move the upper limb forward by flexing the vertebrae.
- Vertebral rotation of the trunk may occur while sitting.
- Pectoralis minor is an accessory muscle for scapular downward rotation and abduction.

Pectoralis Minor Muscle

The pectoralis minor muscle is tested during anterior tipping of the scapula. It is a muscle that rotates the scapula downward and assists the serratus anterior muscle during scapular abduction. The test range is approximately 10 degrees.

Palpation. Palpate inferior to the coracoid process of the scapula toward the lateral end of the clavicle. The subject is positioned with the hand resting on the lumbar region of the back to relax the pectoralis major muscle. The subject is asked to raise the hand from the lumbar region (Fig. 4–46).

Position
AG: The subject lies supine with the hand on the lumbar region of the trunk (Fig. 4–47).
GM: The subject sits with the hand resting on the small of the back (Fig. 4–48).

Movement. Tip the scapula forward, as in rounding the shoulders.

Figure 4–48. Testing the pectoralis minor muscle in the GM sidelying position.

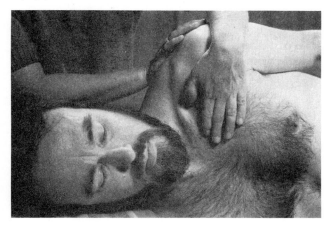

Attachments of Anterior Deltoid Muscle

Muscle	Proximal	Distal	Innervation
Anterior deltoid	Anterior and superior surfaces of lateral third of clavicle	Deltoid tuberosity of the humerus	Axillary C5 (C6)

Resistance. Applied to the acromion process, pushing into the posterior tip of the scapula.

Stabilization. Stabilize the ipsilateral thorax.

Substitutions
- In the sitting position, the subject may flex the trunk forward.
- In the supine position, the subject may flex the wrist or fingers, giving the appearance of anterior tipping of the scapula.

Figure 4–49. Palpating the anterior deltoid muscle.

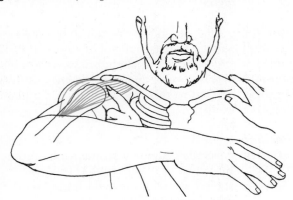

Figure 4–50. Testing the anterior deltoid muscle in the AG sitting position.

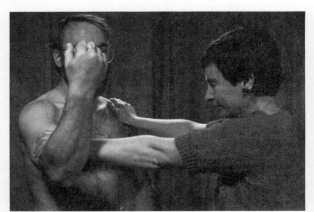

- In the sitting position the subject may hyperextend the shoulder joint.

Anterior Deltoid Muscle

The anterior deltoid muscle flexes the humerus in the sagittal plane to 180 degrees; however, the test range of motion is to 90 degrees of shoulder flexion. Another test movement for the anterior deltoid muscle is horizontal adduction at the shoulder joint. Shoulder flexion motion is accompanied by medial rotation of the humerus and upward rotation of the scapula.

Palpation. Palpate the anterior deltoid inferior to the lateral third of the clavicle. It contracts strongly during the motion of resisted horizontal adduction (Fig. 4–49).

Position
1. AG: Subject sits with the shoulder in neutral or internal rotation and the elbow flexed (Fig. 4–50).
   GM: Subject is in sidelying position with the upper limb supported and the shoulder in the neutral position, elbow flexed (Fig. 4–51).
2. AG: Subject is supine with the shoulder joint ab-

Figure 4–51. Testing the anterior deltoid muscle in the GM sidelying position.

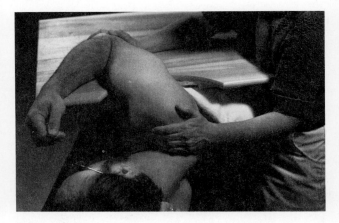

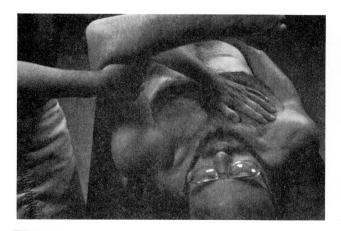

Figure 4–52. Alternate muscle test for the anterior deltoid muscle. The subject is supine performing horizontal adduction against gravity.

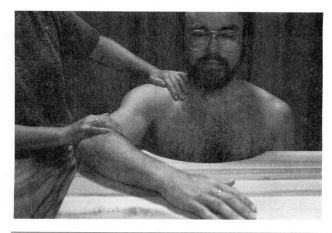

Figure 4–53. Alternate muscle test for the anterior deltoid muscle. The subject is in a GM sitting position.

ducted 90 degrees and the elbow flexed 90 degrees (Fig. 4–52).

GM: Subject sits, with the shoulder abducted and the elbow flexed 90 degrees (Fig. 4–53).

Movement
- Flex the shoulder to 90 degrees.
- Adduct shoulder horizontally to 90 degrees.

Resistance. Applied immediately proximal to the elbow, pushing down into shoulder extension or horizontal abduction.

Stabilization. Stabilize the opposite shoulder.

Substitutions
- Biceps brachii may substitute. Prevent this by not letting the subject rotate the shoulder laterally.
- Subject may elevate the shoulder and lean backward to give the appearance of shoulder flexion.
- Subject may quickly extend the shoulder, then relax, giving the appearance of shoulder flexion.
- Subject may attempt to compensate for the lack of shoulder motion by moving the scapula.
- Coracobrachialis is an accessory muscle for both shoulder flexion and horizontal adduction.
- Pectoralis major (clavicular head) is an accessory muscle for shoulder joint flexion and horizontal adduction.

Coracobrachialis Muscle

The coracobrachialis muscle is tested as a shoulder flexor if the joint is in less than 90 degrees of flexion or as a

shoulder joint extensor if the upper limb is greater than 90 degrees of flexion from the horizontal plane. The test range is usually 90 degrees of shoulder flexion with the joint in lateral rotation. The scapula rotates upward during shoulder joint motion.

Palpation. The coracobrachialis is palpated by initially identifying the short head of the biceps brachii, following the tendon proximally into the axilla to the inferior border of the pectoralis major muscle. With the shoulder flexed overhead the subject resists extension and adduction (Fig. 4–54).

Figure 4–54. Palpating the coracobrachialis muscle.

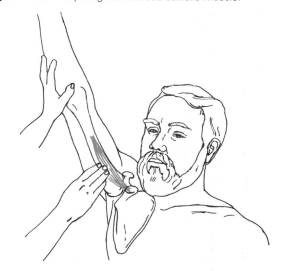

Attachments of Coracobrachialis Muscle

Muscle	Proximal	Distal	Innervation
Coracobrachialis	Coracoid process of scapula	Medial surface of midshaft of humerus	Musculocutaneous C6 (C5 and C7)

Attachments of Latissimus Dorsi Muscle

Muscle	Proximal	Distal	Innervation
Latissimus dorsi	Spinous processes of T6–12 Lumbar and sacral vertebrae Ribs 8 through 12 Thoracolumbar fascia Posterior lip of iliac crest (Occasionally) inferior angle of scapula	Medial lip of intertubercular groove of humerus	Thoracodorsal C6 and C7 (C8)

Position

AG: Subject sits, with the shoulder joint in lateral rotation, the elbow flexed (Fig. 4–55).

GM: Subject is in a sidelying position with the shoulder joint rotated laterally, the elbow flexed 90 degrees, and the forearm in pronation (Fig. 4–56).

Movement.   Flex the shoulder joint 90 degrees.

Resistance.   Applied to the anterior arm immediately proximal to the elbow joint, pushing into extension.

Stabilization.   Stabilize the opposite shoulder.

Substitutions

- Minimize the action of the biceps brachii as a shoulder joint flexor.
- Anterior deltoid also flexes at the shoulder joint.
- Subject may extend the trunk.

Figure 4–55.   Testing the coracobrachialis muscle in the AG sitting position.

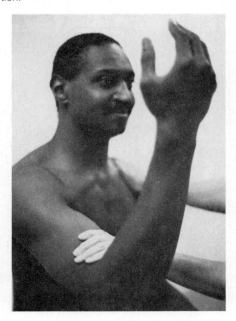

Figure 4–56.   Testing the coracobrachialis muscle in the GM sidelying position.

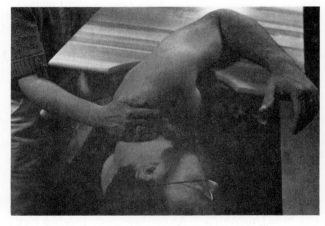

- Subject may quickly extend the shoulder joint, then relax, giving the appearance of shoulder joint flexion.
- Subject may attempt to compensate for the lack of shoulder motion by abducting and rotating the scapula upward.

Latissimus Dorsi Muscle

The latissimus dorsi, a versatile muscle of the shoulder joint, functions in medial rotation, adduction, and extension. The test motion is extension of the shoulder joint from 90 degrees of flexion to 0 degrees of extension. The shoulder is positioned in medial rotation and adduction. The scapula is allowed to rotate downward.

Palpation. Palpate along the midaxillary line on the trunk; the fiber direction is longitudinal (Fig. 4–57).

Figure 4–57. Palpating the latissimus dorsi muscle.

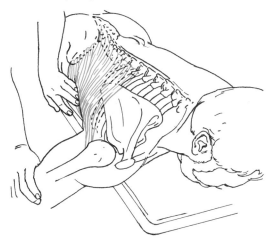

Figure 4–58. Testing the latissimus dorsi muscle in the AG prone position.

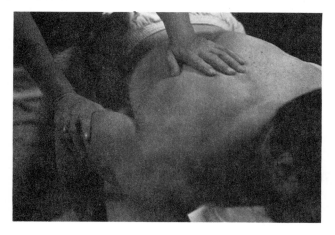

Position
AG: Subject lies prone, with the shoulder flexed and medially rotated over the edge of the table (Fig. 4–58).
GM: Subject is in a sidelying position, with upper limb supported, in 90 degrees of shoulder flexion and medial rotation, and with elbow flexed (Fig. 4–59).

Movement. Extend the shoulder, allowing the elbow to flex.

Resistance. Applied to the posterior arm just proximal to the elbow.

Stabilization. Stabilize the thorax.

Substitutions
- The scapula adducts with no shoulder motion.
- The scapula tips anteriorly and abducts.
- Teres major is an accessory muscle to shoulder joint extension and contracts against resistance.
- Posterior deltoid and pectoralis major (sternal head) are also accessory muscles for shoulder joint extension.

Teres Major Muscle

The teres major muscle is evaluated as a shoulder joint adductor or extensor. It is also a prime mover for shoulder joint medial rotation. The test motion is 90 degrees of adduction, with the shoulder joint extended and medially rotated.

Palpation. Palpate lateral to the inferior angle of the scapula; the fiber direction is horizontal (Fig. 4–60).

Figure 4–59. Testing the latissimus dorsi muscle in the GM sidelying position.

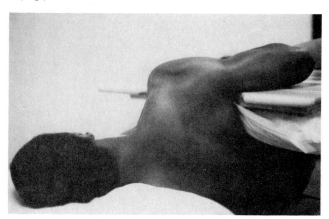

Attachments of Teres Major Muscle

Muscle	Proximal	Distal	Innervation
Teres major	Posterior surface of scapular inferior angle	Crest of lesser tubercle of humerus	Lower subscapular C6 (C7)

Position
AG: Subject lies prone with the shoulder medially rotated and the hand resting on the lower back (Fig. 4–61).
GM: The teres major muscle is not tested in a GM position, because it will contract only against resistance.

Movement.
Adduct and extend the shoulder joint.

Resistance.
Applied proximal to the elbow joint, pushing shoulder into abduction.

Figure 4–60. Palpating the teres major muscle.

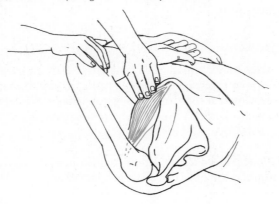

Figure 4–61. Testing the teres major muscle in the AG prone position.

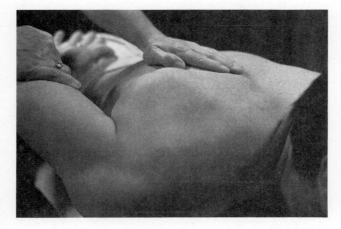

Stabilization.
Stabilize upper trunk.

Substitutions
· The scapula adducts without shoulder motion.
· The shoulder joint rotates laterally.
· Latissimus dorsi, pectoralis major, and teres minor also adduct the shoulder joint.

Supraspinatus Muscle

The supraspinatus muscle is tested during elevation of the humerus in the frontal plane to 90 degrees. The motion is normally accompanied by upward rotation of the scapula.

Palpation.
Place fingers above the spine of the scapula, with shoulder in the plane of the scapula, which is approximately 30 degrees into the sagittal plane from the frontal plane (Fig. 4–62).

Position
AG: Subject sits with the shoulder in neutral rotation and the elbow flexed (Fig. 4–63).

Figure 4–62. Palpating the supraspinatus muscle.

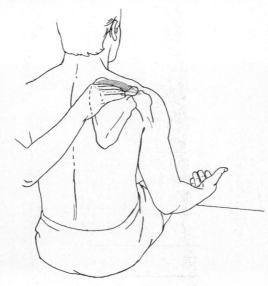

Attachments of Supraspinatus Muscle

Muscle	Proximal	Distal	Innervation
Supraspinatus	Supraspinatus fossa	Superior surface of greater tubercle of humerus	Suprascapular C5 (C4 and C6)

GM: Subject is supine with upper limb supported, shoulder in neutral rotation, and elbow flexed (Fig. 4–64).

Movement. Ask the subject to deduct the shoulder joint within a 30° range.

Resistance. Applied to the lateral arm immediately proximal to the elbow.

Stabilization. Stabilize the opposite shoulder.

Substitutions
- Prevent substitution by biceps brachii by not letting the shoulder rotate laterally.
- Serratus anterior may elevate the acromion process, giving the appearance of shoulder abduction.
- Scapular elevation and lateral flexion of the trunk to the opposite side may give the appearance of shoulder abduction.
- Trunk flexes to the opposite side.
- Deltoid abducts the shoulder joint.

Middle Deltoid Muscle

The three portions of the deltoid muscle are tested during shoulder joint abduction in the coronal plane. The anterior and posterior portions are also tested as horizontal adductors and horizontal abductors, respectively. The test range of motion for the middle deltoid muscle is 90 degrees. The motion is accompanied by upward scapular rotation.

Palpation. Palpate laterally and inferior to the acromion process (Fig. 4–65).

Figure 4–63. Testing the supraspinatus muscle in the AG sitting position.

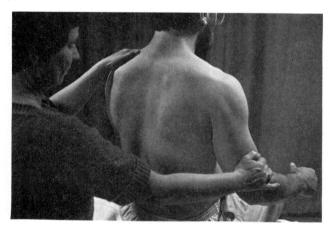

Figure 4–64. Testing the supraspinatus muscle in the GM supine position.

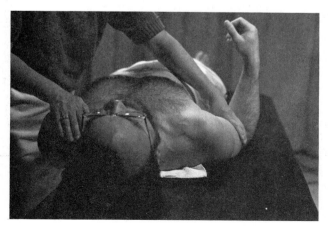

Figure 4–65. Palpating the middle portion of the deltoid muscle.

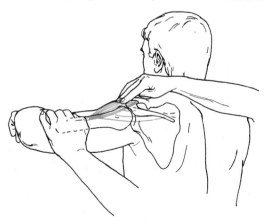

Attachments of Middle Deltoid and Posterior Deltoid Muscles

Muscle	Proximal	Distal	Innervation
Middle deltoid	Superior lateral surface of the acromion process of the scapula	Deltoid tuberosity of the humerus	Axillary C5 (C6)
Posterior deltoid	Inferior lip of spine of scapula	Deltoid tuberosity of the humerus	Axillary C5 (C6)

Position

AG: Subject sits with the shoulder joint in neutral and the elbow flexed 90 degrees (Fig. 4–66).

GM: Subject is supine with the upper limb supported and the elbow flexed 90 degrees (Fig. 4–67).

Movement. Abduct shoulder to 90 degrees in the coronal plane.

Resistance. Applied to the lateral arm immediately proximal to the elbow.

Stabilization. Stabilize the opposite shoulder.

Substitutions

· Prevent substitution by biceps brachii by keeping the shoulder joint in neutral rotation.
· Supraspinatus is also a shoulder joint abductor.
· Serratus anterior may abduct the scapula, giving the appearance of shoulder abduction.
· Trunk flexion to the same side.

Posterior Deltoid Muscle

The posterior portion of the deltoid muscle produces the test motion of shoulder horizontal abduction in the transverse plane from a flexed position. The starting position is 90 degrees of shoulder flexion. The shoulder moves into 120 degrees of abduction in the transverse plane.

Palpation. Palpate below and lateral to the spine of the scapula, crossing the shoulder joint posteriorly (Fig. 4–68).

Position

AG: Subject is prone with the shoulder flexed over the edge of the table and the elbow relaxed (Fig. 4–69).

GM: Subject sits with the upper limb supported on a table, the shoulder and elbow flexed 90 degrees (Fig. 4–70).

Movement. Horizontal abduction from 90 degrees of shoulder flexion to 120 degrees of abduction.

Figure 4–66. Testing the middle deltoid muscle in the AG sitting position.

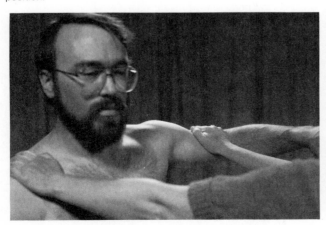

Figure 4–67. Testing the middle deltoid muscle in the GM supine position.

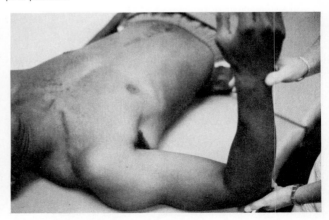

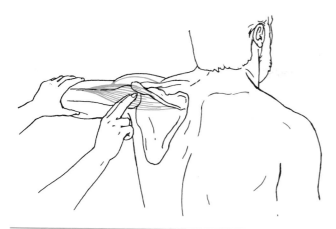

Figure 4–68. Palpating the posterior portion of the deltoid muscle.

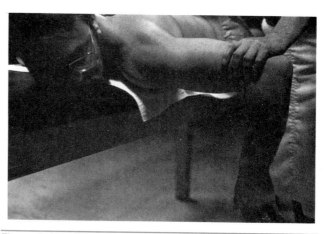

Figure 4–69. Testing the posterior deltoid muscle in the AG prone position.

Resistance. Applied to the posterior arm immediately proximal to the elbow.

Stabilization. Stabilize the scapula on the same side.

Substitutions
- Adduction of the scapula without horizontally abducting the shoulder can occur.
- In the GM position, the trunk may rotate and the subject may throw the upper limb posteriorly, giving the appearance of horizontal adduction. Prevent this motion by stabilizing the trunk.
- Long head of the triceps is an accessory muscle; movement may be attempted by extending the elbow.

Pectoralis Major Muscle

The pectoralis major muscle is tested during horizontal adduction of the shoulder joint, in which the shoulder is positioned in 90 degrees of abduction. Motion occurs in the transverse plane toward 90 degrees of shoulder joint flexion.

Palpation. Palpate the pectoralis major (clavicular) muscle immediately inferior to the medial end of the clavicle. Sternal portion of the pectoralis major is palpated in the anterior axillary fold, against a resistance into extension and adduction (Fig. 4–71).

Position
AG: Subject is supine with shoulder in neutral rotation and 90 degrees of abduction with elbow flexed (Figs. 4–72 and 4–73).
GM: Subject sits with shoulder in neutral rotation and 90 degrees of abduction, elbow flexed 90 degrees, and upper limb supported (Fig. 4–74).

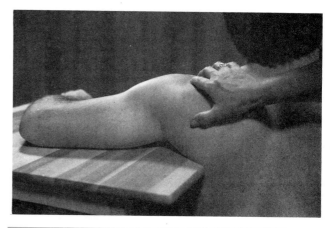

Figure 4–70. Testing the posterior deltoid muscle in the GM sitting position.

Movement. Horizontal adduction from 90 degrees of abduction to 90 degrees of flexion, moving toward the opposite shoulder.

Resistance. Applied to the antero-medial arm immediately proximal to the elbow.

Stabilization. Stabilize the contralateral shoulder or the ipsilateral trunk.

Substitutions
- Prevent the subject from twisting the trunk and throwing the upper limb using momentum by stabilizing the trunk.
- Anterior deltoid is an accessory muscle to the motion of horizontal adduction.
- Coracobrachialis and biceps brachii are accessory muscles to the motion of horizontal adduction.

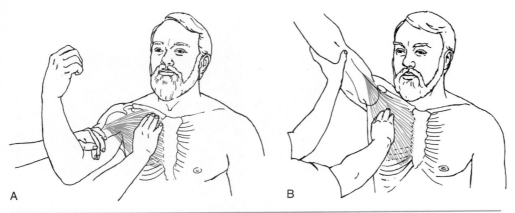

Figure 4–71.   Palpating the pectoralis major muscle: (*A*) Clavicular portion; (*B*) sternal portion.

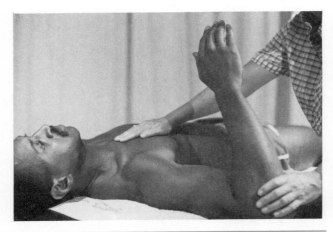

Figure 4–72.   Testing the clavicular head of the pectoralis major muscle in the AG supine position.

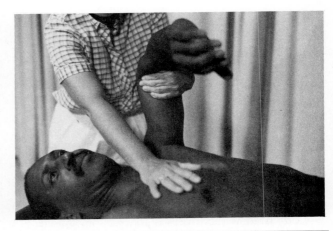

Figure 4–73.   Testing the sternal head of the pectoralis major muscle in the AG supine position.

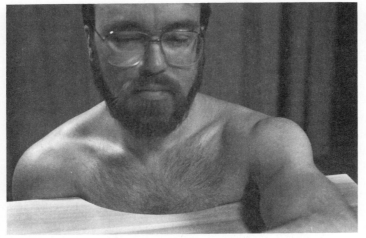

Figure 4–74.   Testing both heads of the pectoralis major muscle in the GM sitting position.

Attachments of Pectoralis Major Muscle (Clavicular and Sternal)

Muscle	Proximal	Distal	Innervation
Pectoralis major (clavicular)	Anterior surface of medial half of clavicle	Inferior crest of greater tubercle of humerus	Lateral and medial pectoral C6 (C5)
Pectoralis major (sternal)	Anterior surface of sternum, costal cartilages of upper six pairs of ribs	Superior crest of greater tubercle of humerus	Lateral and medial pectoral C7 and C8 (T1)

Attachments of Subscapularis Muscle

Muscle	Proximal	Distal	Innervation
Subscapularis	Subscapular fossa of the scapula	Lesser tubercle of humerus	Upper and lower subscapular C6 (C5 and C7)

Subscapularis Muscle

The subscapularis muscle is tested during the movement of medial rotation of 60 degrees, with the shoulder joint positioned in 90 degrees of abduction and the elbow flexed over the edge of the table. A towel roll or the examiner's hand may be placed under the test elbow for comfort. Motion may be limited by tightness of the lateral rotators of the shoulder.

Palpation. Palpate with subject inclined forward, so that the scapula abducts (slides forward) on the thorax by the weight of the arm. Place fingers on the costal surface of the scapula, beyond the latissimus dorsi muscle. Ask for medial rotation of the shoulder (Fig. 4–75).

Position
AG: Subject is prone with the shoulder abducted and the elbow flexed over the edge of the table (Fig. 4–76).
GM: Subject is prone with the shoulder flexed over the edge of the table (Fig. 4–77).

Movement. Medial rotation of the shoulder joint to 60 degrees.

Figure 4–75. Palpating the subscapularis muscle.

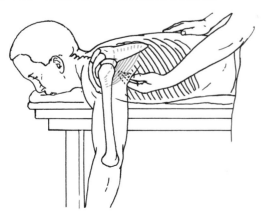

Figure 4–76. Testing the subscapularis muscle in the AG prone position.

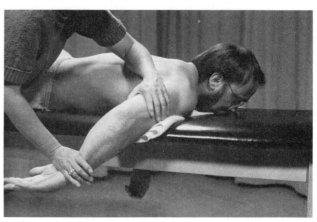

Attachments of Infraspinatus and Teres Minor Muscles

Muscle	Proximal	Distal	Innervation
Infraspinatus	Infraspinatus fossa of scapula	Posterior on greater tubercle	Suprascapular C5 (C6)
Teres minor	Upper portion of lateral border of scapula	Inferior on posterior aspect of greater tubercle of humerus	Axillary C5 (C6)

Resistance. Applied immediately proximal to the wrist on the anterior surface of the forearm.

Stabilization. Stabilize the humerus and thorax with your hand and forearm.

Substitutions
· Prevent abduction of the scapula by stabilizing it.
· The subject may use momentum by laterally rotating the shoulder joint followed by relaxation, giving the appearance of medial rotation.
· Pronation of the forearm may give the appearance of medial rotation.
· Pectoralis major, teres major, and latissimus dorsi muscles are also medial rotators of the shoulder joint.

Figure 4–77. Testing the subscapularis muscle in the GM prone position.

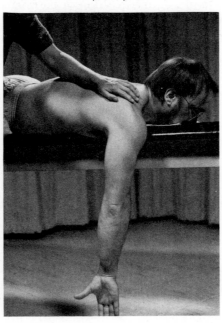

Infraspinatus and Teres Minor Muscles

The infraspinatus and the teres minor muscles produce the motion of lateral rotation of the shoulder joint through the test range of 90 degrees. For grades AG, the shoulder is abducted 90 degrees with the arm resting on the table and the elbow flexed 90 degrees. For grades GM, the shoulder is flexed over the edge of the table. A rolled towel or the examiner's hand is placed under the elbow joint for comfort.

Palpation. With subject in a prone position with the shoulder abducted and the elbow flexed over the edge of the table, palpate inferior to the spine of the scapula for the infraspinatus and along the lateral border of the scapula superior to the inferior angle of the scapula for the teres minor muscle. The two are often indistinguishable (Fig. 4–78).

Position
AG: Subject lies prone with the elbow flexed over the edge of the table (Fig. 4–79).
GM: Subject lies prone with the shoulder flexed over the edge of the table (Fig. 4–80).

Movement. Rotate the shoulder laterally 90 degrees.

Resistance. Applied immediately proximal to the wrist on the extensor surface of the forearm.

Stabilization. Stabilize the humerus and the thorax.

Substitutions
· Posterior deltoid can cause shoulder hyperextension.
· Supination of the forearm may give the appearance of lateral rotation.
· Subject may use momentum of medial rotation giving the appearance of lateral rotation.
· Posterior deltoid is an accessory muscle to the motion of lateral rotation.

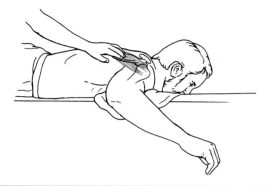

Figure 4–78. Palpating the infraspinatus and teres minor muscles.

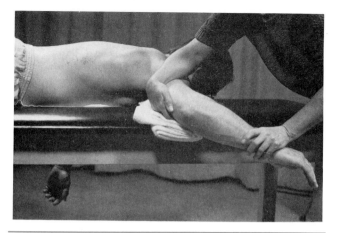

Figure 4–79. Testing the infraspinatus and teres minor muscles in the AG prone position.

Clinical Tests

Palpation

Palpation of the following structures and skeletal landmarks is essential to provide the examiner with complete, accurate information relative to assessment of pathology in the shoulder complex.

1. The scapula may be examined from behind the subject as well as from the side. Landmarks to be included in palpation are the inferior angle, spine of the scapula, vertebral border, acromion process, and coracoid process.
2. The clavicle may be examined from the front by palpating the lateral end where it articulates with the acromion and the medial end where it articulates with the manubrium of the sternum.
3. The proximal humerus should be assessed by palpating the greater tuberosity, lesser tuberosity, and the bicipital groove, which transmits the tendon of the long head of the biceps brachii muscle.

In assessing musculoskeletal pathology involving the shoulder, it is necessary for the examiner to be able to palpate the tendons of the rotator cuff musculature in addition to the tendon of the long head of the biceps brachii muscle.

1. The supraspinatus tendon is palpated at the anterolateral tip of the shoulder. The subject should be supine or half-sitting with the hand tucked behind the ipsilateral hip. This position causes the shoulder to move into an internally rotated position, thereby bringing the supraspinatus tendon nearer the surface for ease of palpation (Fig. 4–81).

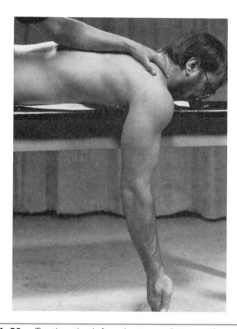

Figure 4–80. Testing the infraspinatus and teres minor muscles in the GM prone position.

2. The infraspinatus tendon is palpated with the subject prone on elbows and the weight shifted over the shoulder being examined. The shoulder is in a position of horizontal adduction, which brings the infraspinatus out for ease in palpation and treatment. The examiner palpates the spine of the scapula, follows it laterally to the posterior acromion, and then drops just inferiorly to locate the infraspinatus tendon (Fig. 4–82).
3. The tendon of the long head of the biceps brachii can be palpated between the greater and

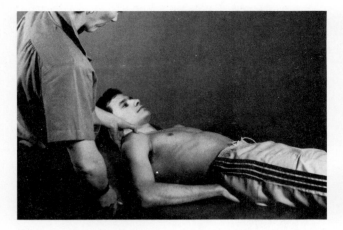

Figure 4–81. Palpating the supraspinatus tendon.

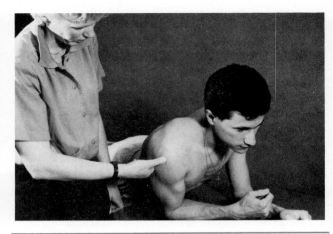

Figure 4–82. Palpating the infraspinatus tendon.

lesser tuberosities, where it lies within the bicipital (intertubercular) groove (Fig. 4–83).

Active and Passive Movements

The motions to be assessed both actively and passively at the shoulder complex include:

1. Sternoclavicular joint:
   a. Elevation.
   b. Depression.
   c. Protraction.
   d. Retraction.
2. Scapulothoracic joint:
   a. Elevation.
   b. Depression.
   c. Abduction.
   d. Adduction.
   e. Upward rotation.
   f. Downward rotation.
3. Glenohumeral joint:
   a. Flexion.
   b. Extension.
   c. Abduction
   d. Adduction.
   e. Internal rotation.
   f. External rotation.
   g. Horizontal abduction.
   h. Horizontal adduction.

Contractile Testing

The contractile testing that should be performed at the shoulder includes:

1. Flexion.
2. Extension.
3. Abduction.

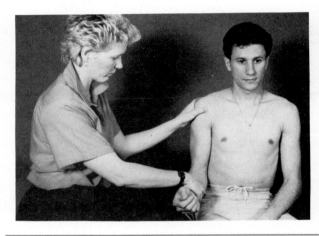

Figure 4–83. Palpating the tendon of the long head of the biceps.

4. Adduction.
5. Internal rotation.
6. External rotation.
7. Horizontal abduction.
8. Horizontal adduction.

Special Tests

Apley's Scratch Tests

Indication. Apley's tests are designed to provide the examiner with a quick, nonspecific functional assessment of shoulder girdle mobility.

Method

Abduction and External Rotation. The subject is instructed to touch with the hand the superior medial border of the scapula on the contralateral side (Fig. 4–84).

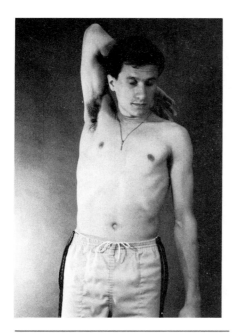

Figure 4–84. Apley's scratch test (abduction and external rotation).

Adduction and Internal Rotation. The subject is asked to bring the tested arm behind the back and touch the inferior angle of the opposite scapula with the hand (Fig. 4–85).

Results. The ability to perform these tests demonstrates good functional ability of the glenohumeral com-

plex. These tests are highly correlated to a person's ability to do basic activities of daily living, including combing hair and reaching a wallet in the back pocket. Difficulty in assuming these positions indicates limitations somewhere in the glenohumeral complex.

Speed's Test

Indication. Speed's test is designed to evaluate the integrity of the long head of the bicep's tendon.

Method. The subject flexes the shoulder against the examiner's resistance while keeping the elbow extended and forearm supinated (Fig. 4–86).

Results. Pain localized to the area of the bicipital groove indicates a positive test for bicipital tendon pathology, usually inflammation.

Drop Arm Test

Indication. The drop arm test is used as an adjunctive technique in the assessment of a rotator cuff tear, specifically of the supraspinatus contractile unit.

Method. The subject either stands or sits and is instructed to completely abduct the shoulder. The subject is asked to slowly lower the upper limb from the fully abducted position back to the original position (Fig. 4–87).

Results. The ability to control the lowering of the upper limb back to an adducted position represents a

Figure 4–85. (*A* and *B*). Adduction and internal rotation in Apley's scratch test.

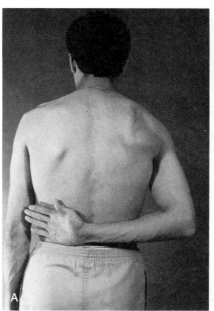
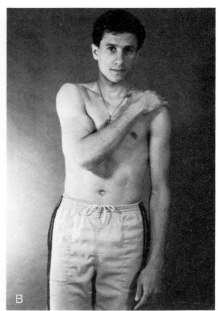

negative test for involvement of the supraspinatus tendon. A positive result is confirmed when, as the subject lowers the upper limb, it drops uncontrollably to the side from the abducted position of approximately 90 degrees.

Apprehension Test

Indication. The apprehension test is indicated in suspected cases of shoulder subluxation or dislocation.

Method. The subject lies supine on the examining table. The examiner passively abducts the shoulder to approximately 90 degrees and then superimposes shoulder external rotation (Fig. 4–88A). The examiner should be careful to support the joint anteriorly in subjects who,

by virtue of medical history or previous dislocations, are predisposed to shoulder instability.

Results. The combination of excessive shoulder abduction and external rotation is a common mechanism of injury in shoulder dislocation. As the combined motions of abduction and external rotation are initiated, the subject reacts by sensing that dislocation is about to occur and demonstrates a facial expression of apprehension (Fig. 4–88B) accompanied by resistance to further motion of the shoulder.

Painful Arc Syndrome

Indication. Painful arc should be detected during the course of a peripheral joint assessment. The arc is pri-

Figure 4–86. Speed's test.

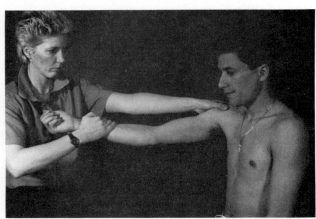

Figure 4–87. Drop arm test.

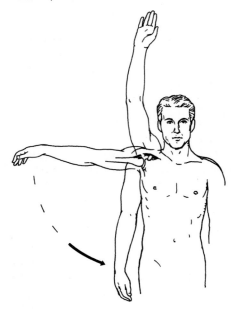

Figure 4–88. (*A*) Shoulder apprehension test. (*B*) A look of apprehension on patient's face is a positive finding.

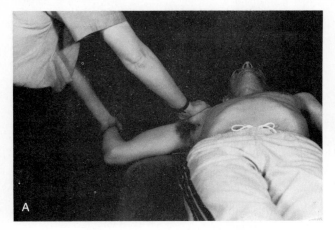

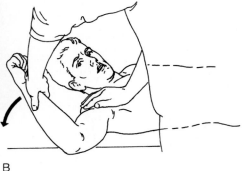

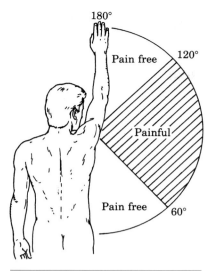

Figure 4–89. Painful arc.

marily found in the motion of shoulder joint abduction, although flexion may also demonstrate this defect. The pain associated with this syndrome is mechanical, resulting from pinching of structures between the acromial arch and the coracoacromial ligament.

Method. Usually no pain is associated with abduction of the shoulder until approximately 70 to 90 degrees, at which point the greater tuberosity must pass beneath the coracoacromial arch in order to complete full, painless abduction (Fig. 4–89). Inflamed structures in the suprahumeral space or faulty biomechanics compromise an already restricted area allowed for smooth motion. As a result, structures are pinched, creating pain that may continue through the range until approximately 120 degrees. At this point, the pinched structures have passed under the coracoacromial arch, thereby allowing painfree movement through the completion of shoulder abduction.

Results. The subject experiences no pain–pain–no pain in the range of motion of the shoulder. A painful arc may be evident during passive or active motion.

Yergason's Test

Indication. Yergason's test is done to evaluate for bicipital tendinitis in the bicipital groove.

Method. The subject may be examined while sitting or standing (Fig. 4–90). The elbow is stabilized against the trunk as it is held in 90 degrees of flexion. The examiner resists forearm supination from a fully pronated position while simultaneously resisting external rotation.

Results. Pain experienced by the subject during the resisted muscle contraction or tenderness to palpation of the bicipital groove represents a positive test. During the

test, the bicipital tendon may pop out of the groove, possibly indicating a tear of the transverse humeral ligament. A more definitive means of assessing the transverse humeral ligament is described below.

Transverse Humeral Ligament Test

Indication. The transverse humeral ligament test may be beneficial in assessing the integrity of the transverse humeral ligament, which is responsible for stabilizing the biceps tendon in the bicipital groove.

Method. The subject's shoulder is actively or passively placed in abduction and external rotation (Fig. 4–91A and B). In this position, the examiner palpates the tendon in the bicipital groove while internally and externally rotating the subject's shoulder.

Results. The biceps tendon palpated popping in and out of the groove during the motions of rotation indicates a positive result for a tear of the ligament.

Ludington's Test

Indication. Ludington's test is performed in suspected cases of rupture of the long head of the biceps brachii.

Method. The subject clasps the hands on the top of the head, allowing the interlocked grip to support the weight of the upper extremities (Fig. 4–92). The subject is then directed to contract and relax the biceps brachii muscle alternately, while the examiner palpates the biceps tendon proximally in the bicipital groove.

Figure 4–90. Yergason's test.

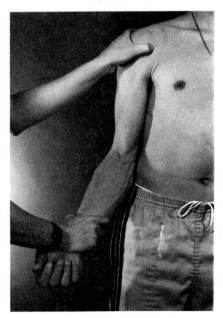

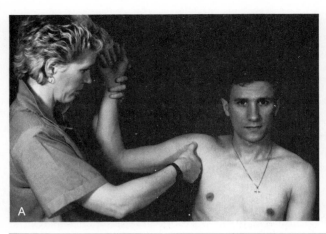 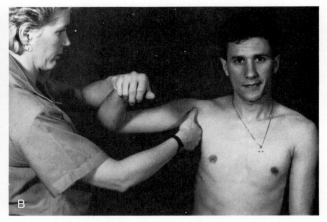

Figure 4–91. Transverse humeral ligament test. (*A*) Starting position; (*B*) end position.

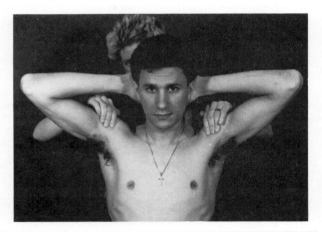

Figure 4–92. Ludington's test.

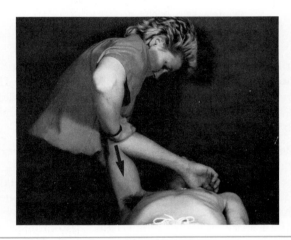

Figure 4–93. Posterior apprehension test.

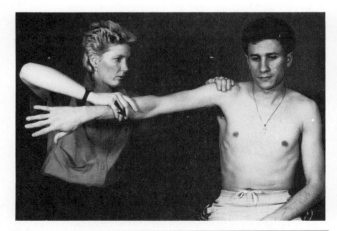

Figure 4–94. Supraspinatus test.

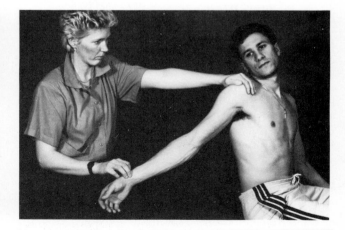

Figure 4–95. Adson's maneuver.

Results. Palpation of the unaffected biceps tendon during contraction is possible, while no palpable contraction is evident on the involved side. This finding is typical of a rupture of the long head of the biceps brachii.

Posterior Apprehension Test

Indication. The posterior apprehension test is used in the assessment of posterior dislocation of the shoulder.

Method. The subject lies supine, with the shoulder flexed and internally rotated and with the elbow flexed and resting on the trunk (Fig. 4–93). A posterior force is transmitted by the examiner through the subject's elbow.

Results. A look of apprehension and resistance to further movement constitute a positive result indicative of posterior dislocation.

Supraspinatus Test

Indication. A suspected tear within the supraspinatus contractile unit is the indication for the supraspinatus test.

Method. The subject sits with the shoulder in 90 degrees of abduction and the glenohumeral joint in neutral rotation. The examiner provides resistance to shoulder abduction in this position. Next, the subject's shoulder is rotated internally (so that the thumbs point toward the floor) and horizontally adducted 30 degrees (Fig. 4–94). The examiner again resists shoulder abduction looking for pain or weakness.

Results. A positive test is represented by pain or weakness during resisted abduction of the shoulder.

Tests For Thoracic Outlet Syndrome

Adson's Maneuver

Indication. Adson's maneuver, a thoracic outlet test, is used to rule out compression of the neurovascular bundle secondary to a cervical rib or abnormalities of scalene musculature.

Method. The subject's head is extended and rotated toward the side being tested. The examiner palpates the radial pulse while extending and externally rotating the shoulder (Fig. 4–95). The subject is instructed to take a deep breath and hold it while the examiner continues to palpate the pulse.

Results. A diminution or disappearance of the radial pulse is a positive result for thoracic outlet syndrome.

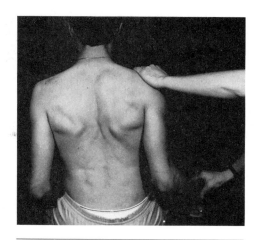

Figure 4–96. Costoclavicular syndrome test.

Costoclavicular Syndrome Test

Indication. The costoclavicular syndrome test is used when compromise of the thoracic outlet might be attributed to entrapment of the subclavian artery and brachial plexus as they pass between the clavicle and the first rib.

Method. The examiner palpates the radial pulse and continues to do so while depressing and retracting the subject's shoulder complex (Fig. 4–96).

Results. A positive result is the same as that for Adson's maneuver, above.

Hyperabduction Syndrome Test

Indication. The hyperabduction syndrome test is done in cases of suspected thoracic outlet syndrome due to entrapment of subclavian vessels and the brachial plexus beneath the tendon of the pectoralis minor and the coracoid process.

Method. The upper limb being tested is placed and maintained in a position of shoulder hyperabduction as the examiner palpates the radial pulse (Fig. 4–97).

Results. Positive results are the same as those for Adson's maneuver.

Halstead's Maneuver

Indication. Halstead's maneuver is utilized to assess for thoracic outlet syndrome.

Method. The subject hyperextends the head and rotates it away from the side being tested (Fig. 4–98). The subject's radial pulse is palpated as the examiner exerts a downward traction force on the upper limb being assessed.

Results. Diminution or absence of the radial pulse represents a positive result.

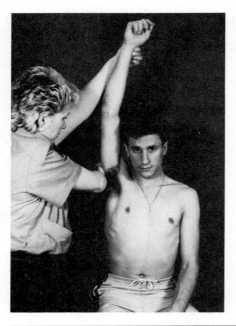

Figure 4–97. Hyperabduction syndrome test.

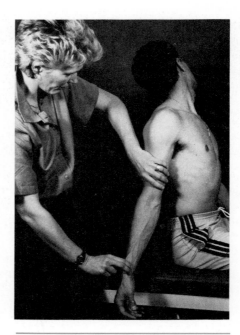

Figure 4–98. Halstead's maneuver.

Allen's Test

Indication. Allen's test is performed in order to confirm or rule out thoracic outlet syndrome.

Method. The subject's shoulder is abducted 90 degrees with the elbow flexed 90 degrees (Fig. 4–99). The examiner palpates the radial pulse as the subject is instructed to rotate the head away from the tested side.

Results. A positive result is noted if the radial pulse weakens or disappears when the subject rotates the head.

Impingement Tests

Neer's Test

Indication. Neer's test is indicated in suspected cases of shoulder impingement.

Method. The examiner passively and forcibly flexes the subject's shoulder forward, thereby jamming the greater tuberosity against the anteroinferior surface of the acromion process (Fig. 4–100).

Figure 4–99. Allen's test.

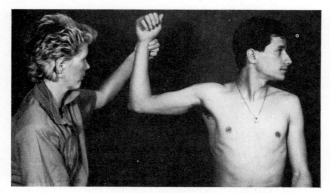

Figure 4–100. Neer's test.

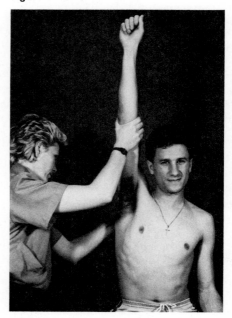

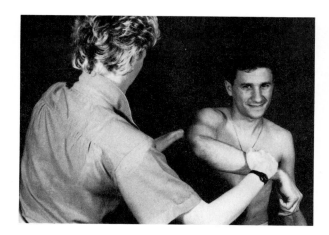

Figure 4–101. Hawkins' test.

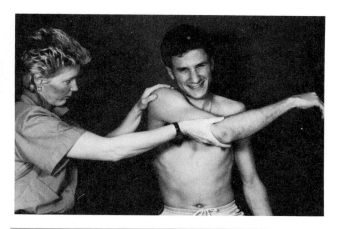

Figure 4–102. Impingement sign.

Results. A positive test result is indicated by the subject's pain, which may register on the face. It is the long head of the biceps brachii tendon that is pinched during this maneuver.

Hawkins' Test

Indication. Hawkins' test is used in assessing impingement pathology of the shoulder.

Method. The subject's shoulder and elbow joints are flexed to 90 degrees. The examiner then forcibly internally rotates the shoulder (Fig. 4–101).

Results. A positive test result is similar to positive results for Neer's test. The structure most often involved with this maneuver is the supraspinatus tendon.

Impingement Sign

Indication. The impingement sign test is useful in assessing impingement of the shoulder.

Method. The subject sits while the examiner passively and forcibly horizontally adducts the shoulder from a starting position of 90 degrees of flexion (Fig. 4–102).

Results. Previous testing criteria also apply here for confirmation of a positive test result. The involved structure associated with this particular test is the long head of the biceps brachii tendon.

Joint Play (Accessory Movements)

Scapulothoracic Joint

Superior Glide (Fig. 4–103*A*)

Restriction. Elevation.

Open-Packed Position. Anatomical position.

Positioning. The subject is in the sidelying position with the test scapula uppermost. The examiner stands at the side of the table facing the subject and stabilizes the upper limb with the distal forearm and the body. Intrinsic stabilization is also provided by the position of the subject and location of the scapula.

Movement. The therapist uses one hand to mobilize the scapula by holding the inferior angle at the web space. The other hand grasps the superior aspect of the scapula by cupping the acromion process. The scapula moves in a superior direction.

Inferior Glide (Fig. 4–103*B*)

Restriction. Depression.

Positioning. The subject is in a sidelying position with the scapula being treated uppermost. The examiner stands at the side of the table facing the subject and stabilizes the upper limb being tested with the distal forearm and the body. Intrinsic stabilization is also provided by the subject's position and the location of the scapula.

Movement. One of the therapist's hands acts to mobilize the scapula by holding the inferior angle with the web space. The other hand grasps the superior aspect of the scapula by cupping over the acromion. The scapula moves in an inferior direction.

Lateral Glide (Fig. 4–104*A*)

Restriction. Abduction.

Positioning. As for inferior glide.

Movement. As for inferior glide, except that the scapula moves in a lateral direction.

Medial Glide (Fig. 4–104*B*).

Restriction. Adduction.

Positioning. As for inferior glide.

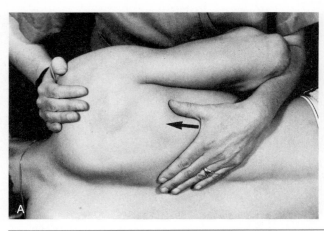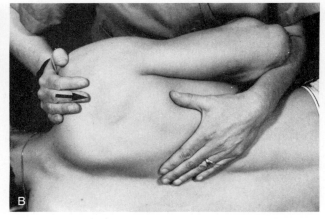

Figure 4–103.   (A) Superior and (B) inferior glide of the scapula.

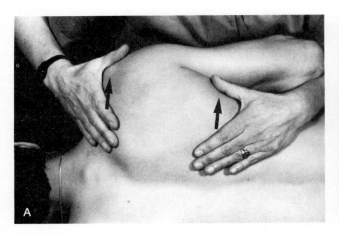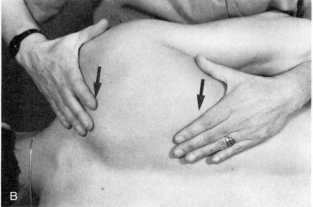

Figure 4–104.   (A) Lateral and (B) medial glide of the scapula.

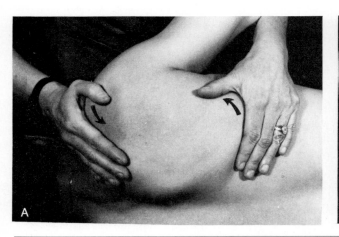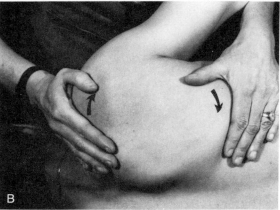

Figure 4–105.   (A) Lateral and superior glide of the scapula. (B) Medial and inferior glide.

Movement. As for inferior glide, except that the scapula is moved in a medial direction.

Lateral and Superior Glide (Fig. 4–105*A*)

Restriction. Abduction and upward rotation.

Positioning. As for inferior glide.

Movement. As for inferior glide, except that the scapula is moved laterally and superiorly, the therapist primarily controlling the motion at the inferior angle.

Medial and Inferior Glide (Fig. 4–105*B*)

Restriction. Adduction and downward rotation.

Positioning. As for inferior glide.

Movement. As for inferior glide, except that the scapula is moved medially and inferiorly with the therapist primarily controlling the motion at the inferior angle.

Glenohumeral Joint

Distraction (Lateral) (Fig. 4–106)

Restriction. General hypomobility.

Open-Packed Position. 55 to 70 degrees abduction; 30 degrees horizontal adduction.

Positioning. The subject lies supine; a strap is applied to stabilize the scapula. The web space of the mobilizing hand is placed high in the axilla with the forearm placed across the body. The other limb is used only to support the subject's upper limb and maintain the resting position.

Movement. The mobilizing hand in the axilla imposes a lateral distracting force to the humeral head, thereby moving it away from the glenoid fossa.

Inferior Glide (Fig. 4–107)

Restriction. Abduction.

Positioning. The subject lies supine; a strap is applied to stabilize the scapula. The therapist places the web space of the mobilizing hand superiorly around the humeral head. The other limb is used only to support the subject's upper limb and maintain the resting position.

Movement. The mobilizing hand applies an inferiorly directed force to the subject's humeral head.

Posterior Glide (Fig. 4–108)

Restriction. Internal rotation.

Positioning. The subject lies supine; a stabilizing wedge is placed along the spine of the scapula extending to the acromion process. The mobilizing hand is placed anteriorly over the humeral head with the ulnar border as close to the joint space as possible. The other hand is

Figure 4–106. Distraction of the glenohumeral joint.

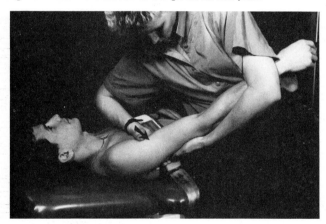

Figure 4–107. Inferior glide of the humerus.

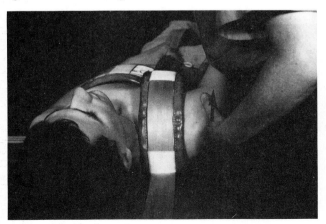

Figure 4–108. Posterior glide of the humerus.

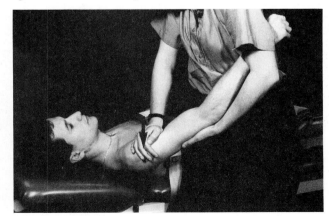

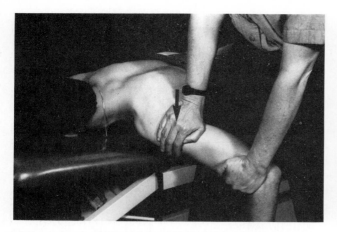

Figure 4–109. Anterior glide of the humerus.

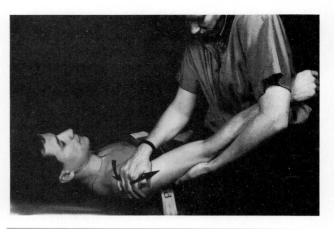

Figure 4–110. Posterior inferior glide of the humerus.

used to support the patient's upper limb and to maintain the resting position.

Movement. The mobilizing hand applies a posterior force to the subject's humeral head.

Anterior Glide (Fig. 4–109)

Restriction. External rotation.

Positioning. The subject lies prone; a stabilizing wedge is placed beneath the coracoid process. The mobilizing hand is placed posteriorly over the humeral head, with the ulnar border of the hand as close to the joint space as possible. The other hand is used to support the subject's upper limb and to maintain the resting position.

Movement. The mobilizing hand applies an anterior force to the subject's humeral head.

Posterior Inferior Glide (Fig. 4–110)

Restriction. Flexion.

Positioning. The subject lies supine; a stabilizing wedge is placed along the spine of the scapula extending

to the acromion process. A strap is also applied to stabilize the scapula and trunk. The mobilizing hand is placed over the superior anterior humeral head with the ulnar border of the hand as close to the joint space as possible.

Movement. The mobilizing hand applies a posterior inferior force to the subject's humeral head. This movement is best described as a scooping of the joint so that the motion describes a **C** shape.

Acromioclavicular Joint

Ventrolateral Glide (Fig. 4–111)

Restriction. General hypomobility.

Open-Packed Position.. Anatomical.

Positioning. The subject may be seated or prone for this test. The stabilizing hand of the therapist is placed around the acromion process, humeral head, and coracoid process. The thumb of the mobilizing hand is placed on the posterior aspect of the lateral clavicle. An alternate position is to place the heel of the mobilizing hand

Figure 4–111. Two methods of performing ventrolateral glide of the clavicle.

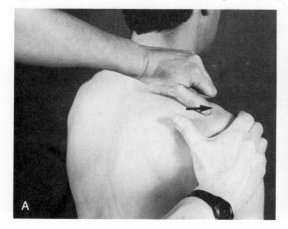

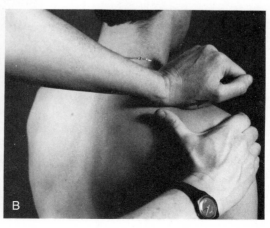

A

B

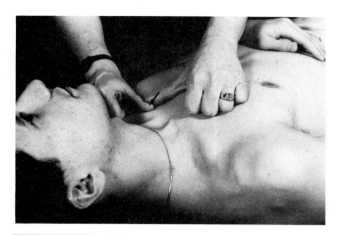

Figure 4–112. Superior glide of the clavicle.

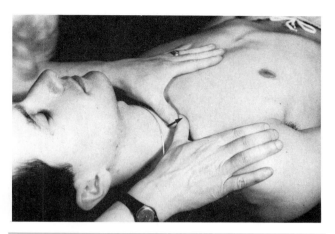

Figure 4–113. Inferior glide of the clavicle.

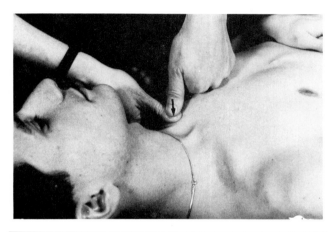

Figure 4–114. Posterior glide of the clavicle.

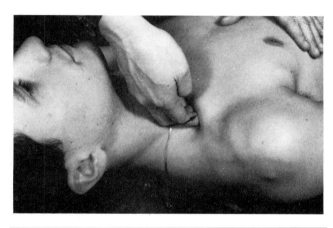

Figure 4–115. Anterior glide of the clavicle.

posteriorly on the lateral aspect of the clavicle (Fig. 4–111*B*).

Movement. A ventrolateral force is applied to the posterior aspect of the lateral clavicle.

Sternoclavicular Joint

Superior Glide (Fig. 4–112)

Restriction. Depression.

Open-Packed Position. Anatomical.

Positioning. The subject lies supine. The therapist places the palmar surface of one thumb on the inferior aspect of the medial clavicle. The other thumb is placed on top, providing reinforcement to the mobilizing thumb.

Movement. A superior force is applied to the inferior surface of the medial clavicle.

Inferior Glide (Fig. 4–113)

Restriction. Elevation.

Positioning. The subject lies supine. The therapist places the palmar surface of one thumb on the superior aspect of the medial clavicle. The other thumb is placed on top, providing reinforcement to the mobilizing thumb.

Movement. An inferior force is applied to the superior surface of the medial clavicle.

Posterior Glide (Fig. 4–114)

Restriction. Retraction.

Positioning. The subject lies supine. The therapist places the palmar surface of one thumb on the anterior aspect of the medial clavicle. The other thumb is placed on top, providing reinforcement to the mobilizing thumb.

Movement. A posterior force is applied to the anterior surface of the medial clavicle.

Anterior Glide (Fig. 4–115)

Restriction. Protraction.

Table 4–1. Summary of Joint Play of the Shoulder Complex

GLIDE	RESTRICTION	FIXED BONE	MOVING BONE
Scapulothoracic Joint			
Superior	Elevation	Thorax	Scapula
Inferior	Depression	Thorax	Scapula
Lateral	Abduction or protraction	Thorax	Scapula
Medial	Adduction or retraction	Thorax	Scapula
Upward rotation	Upward rotation	Thorax	Scapula
Downward rotation	Downward rotation	Thorax	Scapula
Distraction	General hypomobility	Thorax	Scapula
Glenohumeral Joint			
Distraction	General hypomobility	Glenoid	Humerus
Anterior	External rotation	Glenoid	Humerus
Posterior	Internal rotation	Glenoid	Humerus
Inferior	Abduction	Glenoid	Humerus
Posteroinferior	Flexion	Glenoid	Humerus
Anteroinferior	Extension	Glenoid	Humerus
Dorsolateral	Horizontal adduction	Glenoid	Humerus
Acromioclavicular Joint			
Ventrolateral	General hypomobility	Acromion process	Clavicle
Sternoclavicular Joint			
Superior	Depression	Manubrium	Clavicle
Inferior	Elevation	Manubrium	Clavicle
Ventral	Protraction	Manubrium	Clavicle/disc
Dorsal	Retraction	Manubrium	Clavicle/disc

Positioning. The subject lies supine. The therapist hooks the palmar surface of the distal phalanges of digits two and three around the superior clavicle, reaching as far onto the posterior surface as possible.

Movement. An anterior force is applied to the posterior surface of the medial clavicle.

Table 4–1 provides a summary of joint play of the shoulder complex.

Bibliography

Backhouse KM, Hutchings RT: Color Atlas of Surface Anatomy. Baltimore, Williams & Wilkins, 1986

Corrigan B, Maitland GD: Practical Orthopedic Medicine. Boston, Butterworth, 1983

Daniels L, Worthingham C: Muscle Testing Techniques of Manual Examination. Philadelphia, WB Saunders, 1986

Gould JA III, Davies G (eds): Orthopedic and Sports Physical Therapy. St Louis, CV Mosby, 1985

Hollinshead WH, Jenkins DB: Functional Anatomy of the Limbs and Back. Philadelphia, WB Saunders, 1981

Hoppenfeld S: Physical Examination of the Spine and Extremities. New York, Appleton-Century-Crofts, 1976

Kaltenborn M: Mobilization of the Extremity Joints. Oslo, Bygdoy Alle, 1980

Kendall FP, McCreary EK: Muscle Testing and Function. Baltimore, Williams & Wilkins, 1983

Kessler R, Hertling D: Management of Common Musculoskeletal Disorders. Philadelphia, Harper & Row, 1983

Kisner C, Colby LA: Therapeutic Exercise: Foundations and Techniques. Philadelphia, FA Davis, 1985

Magee J: Orthopedic Physical Assessment. Philadelphia, WB Saunders, 1987

Maitland GD: The Peripheral Joints: Examination and Recording Guide. Adelaide, Australia, Virgo Press, 1973

Mellion B: Sports Injuries and Athletic Problems. Philadelphia, Hanley & Belfus, 1988

Norkin CC, White DJ: Measurement of Joint Motion: A Guide to Goniometry. Philadelphia, FA Davis, 1985

Saunders H: Evaluation, Treatment, and Prevention of Musculoskeletal Disorders. Minneapolis, H Duane Saunders, 1985

Schneider RC, Kennedy JC, Plant ML: Sports Injuries: Mechanisms, Prevention, and Treatment. Baltimore, Williams & Wilkins, 1985

Turek SL: Orthopedics: Principles and Their Application, Vol 2. Philadelphia, JB Lippincott, 1984

Williams P, Warwick R (eds): Gray's Anatomy, 36th British ed. Philadelphia, WB Saunders, 1980

Elbow and Forearm Complex

Chapter 5

The elbow joint, an intermediate joint between the shoulder and the hand, permits lengthening and shortening of the upper limb. It is a structurally stable joint and with its musculature is designed primarily to position the hand. It allows the hand to be brought close to the face for eating or placed at a distance for reaching. Many of the muscles that act on the wrist and shoulder cross the elbow joint, aid in providing stability, and enhance the function of the hand.

The elbow joint moves in one plane of motion around a single axis. The motions produced at the elbow joint are flexion and extension. The head of the radius articulates with the capitulum of the humerus. The ulna articulates with the trochlea of the humerus. The axis of motion is transverse in a plane through the trochlea and the capitulum. The trochlea extends more distally than the capitulum; therefore when the elbow is extended and the forearm supinated, the forearm deviates laterally in relation to the humerus. This deviation accounts for what is termed the carrying angle. The axis lies immediately distal to the lateral and medial epicondyle of the humerus.

The radius and ulna are connected both proximally and distally. The two joints act together and form a uniaxial joint producing the motion of supination and pronation. Most of the motion occurs because the radius rotates on the ulna. When the two bones are parallel, the forearm is supinated. When the radius crosses over the ulna, the forearm is pronated. The hand follows the movement of the radius. The axis of motion of the radioulnar joints is vertical through the head of the radius (proximally) and through the head of the ulna (distally), permitting one degree of freedom of motion.

Goniometry

Elbow Flexion — towel under upper arm

The elbow is a double-hinge joint. The test motion occurs in the sagittal plane, between the radius moving on the humeral capitulum and the trochlear notch of the ulna on the olecranon fossa. As motion occurs the head of the radius glides anteriorly on the capitulum. A roll is placed under the humerus to keep it level with the glenoid fossa.

Motion.   0 to 145 degrees into flexion.

Position.   Subject lies supine, with the arm parallel to the lateral midline of the trunk and the forearm in the anatomical position. The arm is positioned as close to the trunk as feasible.

Goniometric Alignment (Fig. 5–1)

Axis.   Over the lateral epicondyle of the humerus.

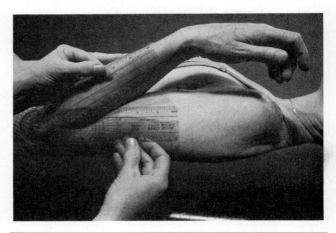

Figure 5–1.   End position for elbow joint flexion.

Stationary Arm.   Placed along the lateral midline of the humerus in line with the acromion process of the scapula.

Moving Arm.   Placed along the lateral midline of the radius in line with the styloid process of the radius.

Stabilization.   The distal end of the humerus is stabilized.

Precautions
- Prevent shoulder joint flexion.
- Note position of the forearm if not in the anatomical position.

Elbow Extension and Hyperextension

Elbow extension, the return from elbow joint flexion, occurs in the sagittal plane between radius and humerus and ulna and humerus. As the motion occurs, the head of the radius glides in a posterior direction. Hyperextension of the elbow joint is often accompanied by an increase in the carrying angle, particularly in females. The amount of motion available is determined by the articulation between the ulnar olecranon process and the fossa of the humerus.

Motion.   145 to 0 degrees (note any hyperextension).

Position.   Subject lies supine with the arm parallel to the lateral midline of the trunk and the forearm supinated.

Goniometric Alignment (Fig. 5–2)

Axis.   On the lateral epicondyle of the humerus.

Stationary Arm.   Placed along the lateral midline of the humerus in line with the acromion process of the scapula.

Supination often falls short of 90° → Hcan pronate

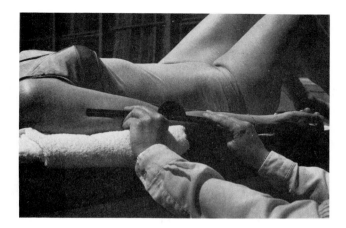

Figure 5–2. End position for elbow joint extension.

Moving Arm. Placed along the lateral midline of the radius in line with the styloid process of the radius.

Stabilization. The humerus is stabilized.

Precautions
- Prevent shoulder joint flexion.
- Note position of the forearm if not in the anatomical position.

Radioulnar Pronation

In the anatomical position, the pronation motion occurs in the transverse plane, but in the test position the motion occurs in the coronal plane. The forearm is posi-

tioned midway between supination and pronation with the elbow flexed to 90 degrees. Motion occurs between the head of the radius spinning on the capitulum of the humerus and on the radial notch of the ulna. The distal end of the radius glides over the head of the ulna at the inferior radioulnar joint. In this position, the radius is crossed over the ulna. Minimal motion of abduction of the ulna accompanies pronation at the proximal joint, and none occurs at the inferior radioulnar joint.

Motion. 0 to 90 degrees from midforearm position into full pronation.

Position
- Preferred: Subject sits or lies supine with the elbow flexed to approximately 90 degrees and the arm held close to the side of the trunk. The forearm is positioned midway between supination and pronation.
- Alternate: The subject is in the preferred position holding a pencil vertically in the hand.

Goniometric Alignment (Figs. 5–3 to 5–6)

Axis → moves → just circle that goniometer arms are flat ↓ means they have 0°
- Preferred: Lateral to the ulnar styloid process.
- Alternate: 3rd metacarpal head, citing the 3rd metacarpal and between the radioulnar joints.

Stationary Arm
- Preferred: Placed at the level of the dorsal aspect of the wrist and parallel to the long axis of the

Figure 5–3. Starting position for radioulnar joint pronation.

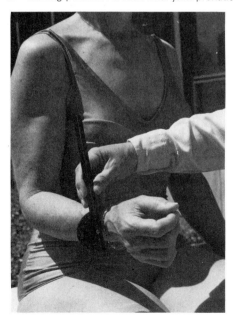

Figure 5–4. End position for radioulnar joint pronation.

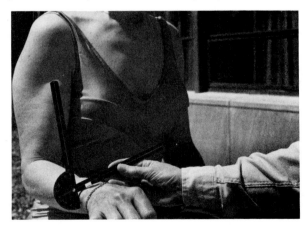

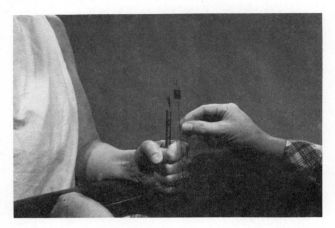

Figure 5–5. Alternate starting position for radioulnar joint pronation.

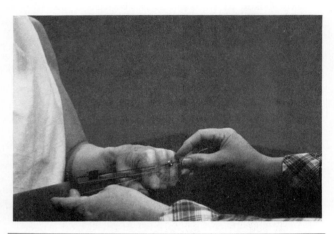

Figure 5–6. Alternate end position for radioulnar joint pronation.

humerus, with the protractor directed away from the trunk at the level of the wrist.
- Alternate: Placed perpendicular to the table top.

Moving Arm
- Preferred: Placed across the dorsum of the wrist on a line between and proximal to the styloid processes of the radius and the ulna.
- Alternate: Placed parallel to the long axis of the pencil. The subject must have good to normal grip.

Stabilization. Stabilize the distal end of the humerus.

Precautions
- Keep the elbow close to the side of the trunk.
- Avoid shoulder abduction and medial rotation.
- Avoid lateral flexion of the trunk toward the opposite side.

- Avoid wrist and finger motion when using the alternate method of measuring.

Radioulnar Supination

The test motion of supination at the radioulnar joints occurs in the coronal plane. The pivoting motions exist between the head of the radius on the capitulum of the humerus and the proximal ulna. Distally, the radius glides over the head of the ulna until the two bones lie parallel. The shoulder and elbow joints are positioned as for pronation.

Motion. 0 to 90 degrees into supination.

Position
- Preferred: Subject sits or lies supine, with the elbow flexed to 90 degrees and the arm held close to the side. The forearm is positioned midway between supination and pronation.
- Alternate: Same as preferred position, except that the subject holds a pencil in the vertical position. Good grip is essential.

Goniometric Alignment (Figs. 5–7 to 5–10)

Axis
- Preferred: Placed on the medial side of the distal forearm in line with the styloid process of the ulna.
- Alternate: Placed at the distal end of the third metacarpal, projecting up between the radioulnar joints same as in pronation.

Stationary Arm
- Preferred: Placed on the anterior surface of the wrist parallel to the anterior long axis of the humerus.
- Alternate: Placed parallel to and over the long axis of the pencil or perpendicular to the table top.

Moving Arm
- Preferred: Placed on the anterior surface of the wrist, just proximal to the styloid processes at the most flattened area proximal to the wrist.
- Alternate: Aligned parallel to and over the long axis of the pencil.

Stabilization. The humerus is stabilized.

Precautions
- Avoid lateral flexion of the trunk to the same side as the measurement.
- Avoid adduction and lateral rotation of the shoulder joint.

- Avoid wrist and finger motions when using the alternate test method.

Functional Muscle Testing

Elbow

The elbow links the shoulder and forearm. It allows the forearm to assume any position by shortening or lengthening the upper limb. This ability allows the hand to be brought close to the face for eating or placed at a distance equal to the length of the upper limb from the trunk. The elbow joint may also provide stability for skilled movements of the hand.

Elbow Flexion

The elbow flexor muscles work to their best advantage with the elbow flexed to 90 degrees. They are composed of more type II muscle fibers, which are designed for speed of movement rather than for stability at the elbow. The brachioradialis muscle, attached distally on the radius, is used more for producing a compression force, and thus, provides more stability.

Position. Subject sits with the upper limb in the anatomical position (Fig. 5–11).

Activity. Subject brings the hand with a weight placed in it to the mouth.

Figure 5–7. Starting position for radioulnar joint supination.

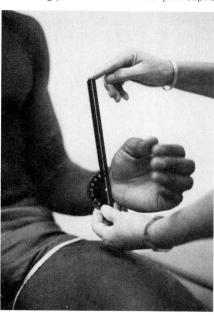

Figure 5–8. End position for radioulnar joint supination.

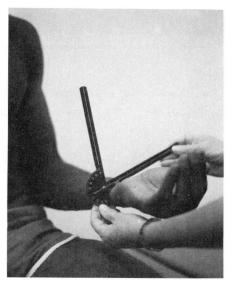

Figure 5–9. Alternate starting position for radioulnar joint supination.

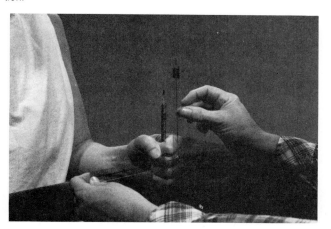

Figure 5–10. Alternate end position for radioulnar joint supination.

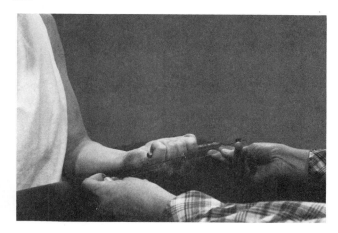

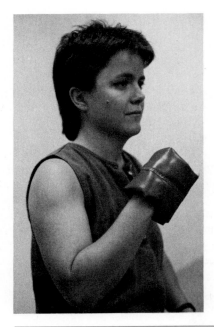

Figure 5–11. Resisted elbow joint flexion.

Muscles. Biceps brachii, brachialis, brachioradialis.

Types of Contraction
- Concentric: Bringing the hand to the mouth.
- Eccentric: Returning the hand to the starting position.

Resistance
- The weight of the forearm and hand, plus a weight, offers the resistance.
- Functional: 5-pound weight.
- Functionally Fair: 3- to 4-pound weight.
- Functionally Poor: 1- to 2-pound weight.
- Nonfunctional: 0 weight.

Elbow Extension

Often elbow extension is accomplished by an eccentric contraction of the elbow flexors. The medial head of the triceps brachii muscle contracts concentrically without resistance; the other two heads contract only during resistance. The triceps brachii muscle is much more powerful when the shoulder and elbow joints are flexed. These muscles act as extensors or flexors of the elbow joint in a closed kinematic chain such as a prone push-up. They act as a synergist to prevent elbow flexion during forearm supination.

Position
- Preferred: Subject stands facing a wall with the shoulders flexed to 90 degrees.

- Alternate: Subject lies prone with the hands on the treatment table and the body in a push-up position.

Activity
- Preferred: The subject pushes against the wall.
- Alternate: The subject performs prone push-ups.

Muscles. Triceps and anconeus.

Types of Contraction
- Eccentric: Lowering the trunk toward the wall or table between the hands.
- Concentric: Pushing up to the starting position.

Resistance
- The body weight offers the resistance.
- Functional: 5 repetitions.
- Functionally Fair: 3 to 4 repetitions.
- Functionally Poor: 1 to 2 repetitions.
- Nonfunctional: 0 repetitions.

Forearm

The musculature of the forearm is functionally assessed with the elbow in a flexed position that stabilizes the arm. In this way, movement may occur in the forearm without interference from shoulder joint rotation.

Forearm Supination

The supinator muscle is usually assisted by the biceps brachii during any supinated motion against resistance or speed, particularly with the elbow flexed.

Position. Subject stands or sits facing a closed door.

Activity. Subject, by turning the palm upward, turns the doorknob to open the door (Fig. 5–12).

Figure 5–12. Resisted radioulnar joint supination.

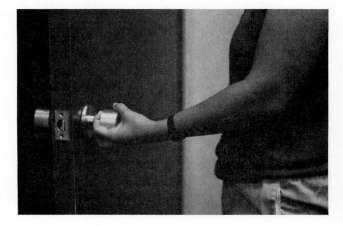

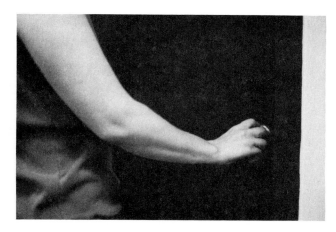

Figure 5–13.   Resisted radioulnar joint pronation.

Muscles.   Supinator, biceps brachii.

Type of Contraction
· Concentric: Turning the doorknob.

Resistance
· The doorknob offers the resistance.
· Functional: 5 repetitions.
· Functionally Fair: 3 to 4 repetitions.
· Functionally Poor: 1 to 2 repetitions.
· Nonfunctional: 0 repetitions.

Forearm Pronation

The pronator musculature is weak compared with its counterpart, the supinator muscles. During resistive activities that require pronation, the shoulder joint usually abducts and rotates medially to add power to the movement. Pronation is used for loosening a right-handed screw and pouring from a pot.

Position.   Subject stands or sits, facing a closed door.

Activity.   Subject, by turning the palm downward, turns the doorknob to open the door. (Fig. 5–13).

Muscles.   Pronator teres, pronator quadratus.

Type of Contraction
· Concentric: Turning the doorknob.

Resistance
· The doorknob offers the resistance.
· Functional: 5 repetitions.
· Functionally Fair: 3 to 4 repetitions.
· Functionally Poor: 1 to 2 repetitions.
· Nonfunctional: 0 repetitions.

Manual Muscle Testing

Biceps Brachii, Brachialis, and Brachioradialis Muscles

The biceps brachii muscle is tested during the motion of elbow flexion to 90 degrees from complete extension. Against-gravity (AG) grades are determined with the subject sitting, and gravity-minimized (GM) evaluation may be done with the subject in a sidelying, supine, or sitting position. The forearm is positioned in supination. The biceps brachii also flexes the shoulder joint, and if the shoulder joint were allowed to rotate laterally, the biceps brachii would assist in shoulder joint abduction. The brachioradialis muscle participates in the motion of elbow flexion only if resistance is applied or if the motion is performed rapidly.

Palpation

Biceps brachii.   With the forearm in a supinated position, palpate the arm anteriorly for the muscle belly or the cubital fossa for the tendon of insertion; each head may be palpated proximally on the arm. The long head is on the anterior surface of the humerus, lateral to the lesser tuberosity; the short head is medial on the arm, directed toward the coracoid process (Fig. 5–14).

Brachialis.   With the forearm pronated to minimize the action of the biceps, place fingers either lateral or medial to the common biceps tendon immediately proximal to the cubital fossa and push the relaxed biceps to one side. Flex the elbow with as little effort as possible, and feel the contraction of the brachialis deep to the biceps tendon (Fig. 5–15).

Brachioradialis.   With the forearm in midposition between supination and pronation and the elbow in 90 degrees of flexion, apply resistance. The muscle is super-

Figure 5–14.   Palpation for the biceps brachii muscle.

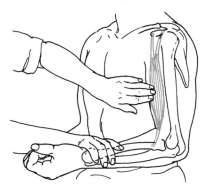

Attachments of Biceps Brachii, Brachialis, and Brachioradialis Muscles

Muscle	Proximal	Distal	Innervation
Biceps brachii			
Long head	Supraglenoid tubercle of scapula	Tuberosity of radius and bicipital aponeurosis	Musculocutaneous C6 (C5)
Short head	Coracoid process apex	Same as above	Same as above
Brachialis	Distal half of anterior surface of humerus	Tuberosity and coronoid process of ulna	Musculocutaneous small branch of radial C6 (C5)
Brachioradialis	Proximal two thirds of lateral supracondylar ridge of humerus	Base of styloid process of radius	Radial C6 (C6 and 7)

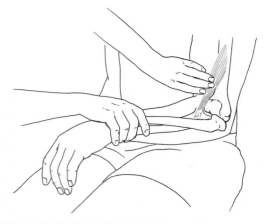

Figure 5–15. Palpation for the brachialis muscle.

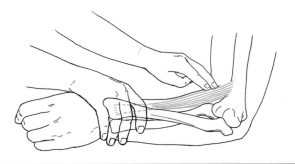

Figure 5–16. Palpation for the brachioradialis muscle.

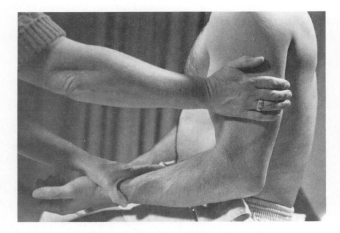

Figure 5–17. AG sitting position, testing the three anterior arm muscles simultaneously.

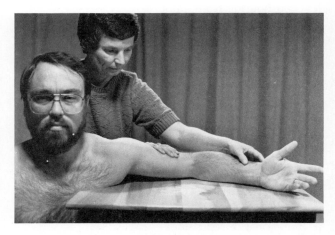

Figure 5–18. GM sitting position, testing the three anterior arm muscles simultaneously.

ficial and can be palpated along its course. It forms the lateral border of the cubital fossa. It is best felt just lateral to the biceps tendon at the level of or proximal to the elbow (Fig. 5–16).

Position
- AG: Subject is sitting, with the upper limb in the anatomical position (Fig. 5–17).
- GM: Subject is sitting, with the arm supported in 90 degrees of abduction, shoulder in neutral rotation, elbow extended, and the forearm supinated (Fig. 5–18).

Movement.   Flex elbow to 90 degrees with the forearm in supination.

Resistance.   Applied immediately proximal to the wrist on the anterior forearm.

Stabilization.   The arm is stabilized.

Substitutions
- The patient may extend the shoulder, causing passive flexion of the elbow.
- The patient may quickly extend the elbow and relax it, giving the appearance of flexion.
- Pronator teres causes the forearm to pronate as flexion occurs.
- Wrist and finger extensors and flexors originating from both the medial and lateral epicondyles can cause substitute motions.

Triceps Brachii (Long, Lateral, and Medial Heads), Anconeus Muscles

The triceps and anconeus muscles produce the movement of elbow extension from complete elbow flexion. The test range is 145 degrees of elbow extension. Resistance must be applied to palpate for contraction of the long and lateral heads of the triceps muscle. The medial head contracts any time during elbow extension.

Palpation

Triceps brachii.   The proximal portion of the long head is felt as it emerges beneath the posterior deltoid muscle. The lateral head, the strongest, is felt distal to the posterior deltoid muscle. The medial head is covered by the other two heads but is felt distal on the posterior arm on either side of the common triceps tendon (Figs. 5–19 to 5–21).

Anconeus.   Between the lateral epicondyle and the olecranon process of the ulna, it is deep to the tendinous sheath of the triceps.

Figure 5–19.   Palpation for the long head of the triceps brachii muscle.

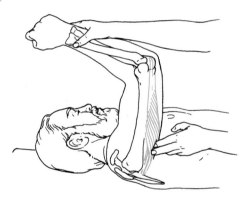

Figure 5–20.   Palpation for the lateral head of the triceps brachii muscle.

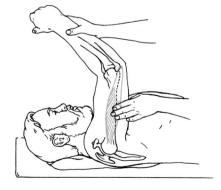

Figure 5–21.   Palpation for the medial head of the triceps brachii muscle.

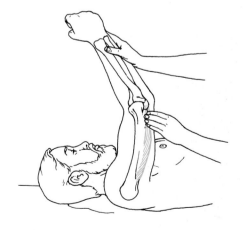

Attachments of Triceps Brachii and Anconeus Muscles

Muscle	Proximal	Distal	Innervation
Triceps brachii			
Long head	Infraglenoid tubercle of scapula	Olecranon process of ulna	Radial C7 and 8 (C6)
Lateral head	Lateral and proximal surface of upper one half of humeral shaft above radial groove	Olecranon process of ulna	Radial C7 and 8 (C6)
Medial head	Distal two thirds of medial and posterior aspects of humerus below radial groove	Olecranon process of ulna	Radial C7 and 8 (C6)
Anconeus	Lateral humeral epicondyle	Lateral surface of ulnar olecranon process and upper posterior shaft of ulna	Radial C7 and 8 (C6)

Position
- AG: Subject lies supine with the shoulder flexed 90 degrees and the elbow fully flexed (Fig. 5–22).
- GM: Subject sits with the shoulder supported in 90 degrees of abduction and medial rotation with the elbow flexed and the forearm neutral (Fig. 5–23).

Movement. Extend elbow from 145 degrees of flexion.

Resistance. Applied immediately proximal to the wrist on the posterior forearm.

Stabilization. The arm is stabilized.

Substitutions
- Subject may further flex the shoulder, causing passive extension of the elbow.
- Subject may quickly increase flexion of the elbow, giving the appearance of extension.

Figure 5–22. AG supine position; testing the three heads of the triceps brachii muscle simultaneously.

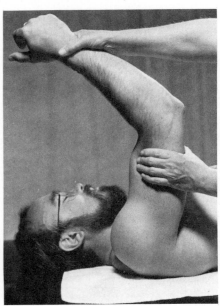

Figure 5–23. GM sitting position; testing the three heads of the triceps brachii muscle.

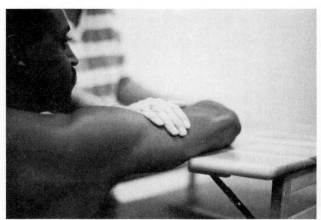

Attachments of Supinator Muscle

Muscle	Proximal	Distal	Innervation
Supinator	Lateral epicondyle of humerus, radial collateral and annular ligaments, and supinator crest of ulna	Lateral surface of upper third of radial shaft	Radial C6 (C5)

- In the GM position, subject may abduct the shoulder joint.

Supinator Muscle

The supinator muscle produces the movement of supination at the radioulnar joints. With a starting position in full pronation, the full range is 180 degrees.

Palpation.   The supinator is a deep muscle, extending under the common extensor muscles from the lateral epicondyle. Relax the wrist and finger extensors and push them laterally. Place fingers under extensor muscles as much as possible (Fig. 5–24).

Position
- AG: Subject sits with the arm at the side of the trunk and the elbow flexed 90 degrees (Fig. 5–25).
- GM: Subject sits with the shoulder supported in 90 degrees of flexion, the elbow flexed 90 degrees, and the forearm perpendicular to the table (Figs. 5–26 and 5–27).

Movement.   From full pronation to full supination in the GM position and from full pronation to neutral forearm position for AG position.

Resistance.   Applied immediately proximal to the wrist into pronation.

Stabilization.   The arm is stabilized with the elbow close to the trunk.

Substitutions
- Subject may flex trunk laterally toward the same side and adduct the shoulder.
- Brachioradialis supinates from a completely pronated position to neutral.
- Subject may laterally rotate the shoulder joint and move elbow across chest.

Pronator Teres, Pronator Quadratus Muscles

The pronator teres and pronator quadratus muscles produce the motion of pronation at the radioulnar joints from the starting position of supination. The complete range of motion for pronation is 180 degrees.

Figure 5–24.   Palpation for the supinator muscle.

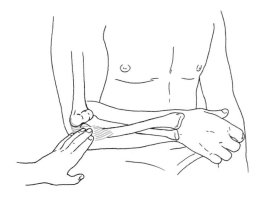

Figure 5–25.   AG sitting position; testing the supinator muscle.

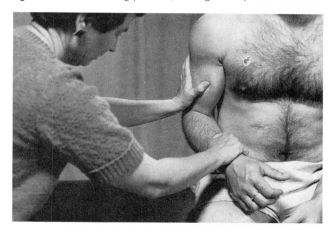

Palpation

1. Palpate the pronator teres on the medial surface of the cubital fossa; the fibers run laterally to the radius (Fig. 5–28).
2. The pronator quadratus muscle is too deep to be palpated.

Position

- AG: Subject sits, with the arm against the trunk and the elbow flexed to 90 degrees (Fig. 5–29).
- GM: Subject sits, with the shoulder and elbow flexed to 90 degrees and the forearm perpendicular to the table (Figs. 5–30 and 5–31).

Movement. In the GM position the motion is from full supination to full pronation. AG, it is from full supination to neutral, midway between supination and pronation.

Resistance. Applied immediately proximal to the wrist into supination.

Figure 5–26. GM prone position; testing the supinator muscle.

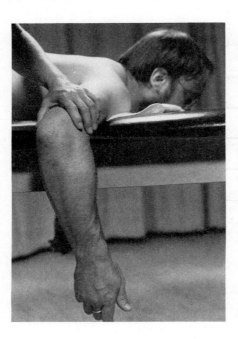

Figure 5–27. Alternate GM sitting position; testing the supinator muscle.

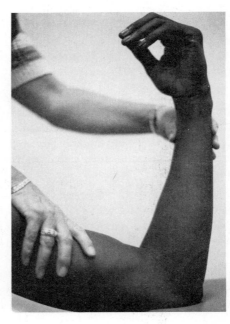

Figure 5–28. Palpation for the pronator teres muscle.

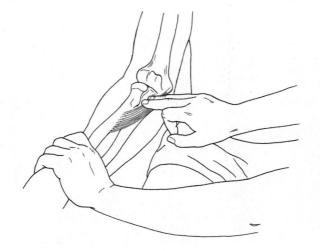

Figure 5–29. AG sitting position; testing the pronator teres muscle.

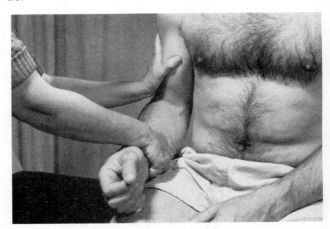

Attachments of Pronator Teres and Pronator Quadratus Muscles

Muscle	Proximal	Distal	Innervation
Pronator teres	Proximal portion of medial epicondyle of humerus and medial side of coronoid process of ulna	Midradial shaft on lateral side	Median C7 (C6)
Pronator quadratus	Anterior surface and distal quarter of ulna	Anterior surface and distal quarter of radius	Median C8 (T1)

Stabilization. Stabilize the arm, keeping the elbow next to the trunk.

Substitutions
- Subject may flex trunk to contralateral side, abduct and medially rotate the shoulder.
- The end range may be completed by wrist flexors.

Clinical Tests

Palpation

In examining the elbow and forearm complex, the examiner needs to be familiar with the location of various bony and soft tissue landmarks. The structures that should be examined in the patient evaluation are:

1. Medial epicondyle of the humerus.
2. Lateral epicondyle of the humerus.
3. Groove that transmits the ulnar nerve.
4. Lateral supracondylar ridge of the humerus.
5. Olecranon process of the ulna.
6. Radial head.
7. Cubital fossa.
8. Common flexor origin on the medial epicondyle.
9. Proximal attachments of the wrist extensor musculature.
10. Radial styloid.
11. Ulnar styloid.
12. Ulnar head.
13. Lister's tubercle on the dorsal radius, which transmits the extensor pollicis longus tendon.

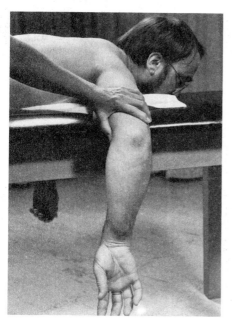

Figure 5–30. GM prone position; testing the pronator teres muscle.

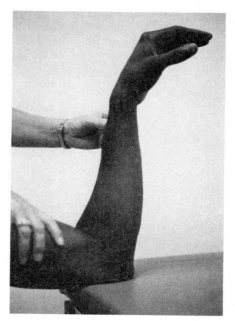

Figure 5–31. Alternate GM sitting position; testing the pronator teres muscle.

Active and Passive Movements and Contractile Testing

The motions to be assessed during active and passive movement of the elbow and forearm joints include:

1. Elbow flexion.
2. Elbow extension.
3. Forearm supination.
4. Forearm pronation.

Contractile testing includes:

1. Elbow flexion.
2. Elbow extension.
3. Forearm supination.
4. Forearm pronation.

Special Tests

Reflex Testing

Biceps Brachii Reflex

Indication. The biceps brachii reflex test is used to assess the integrity of the reflex innervated by the C5 nerve root.

Method. The subject's forearm is placed over the examiner's opposite forearm, so that the weight of the subject's arm and forearm is borne by the examiner. The elbow being assessed is positioned in some degree of flexion. The examiner supports the subject's arm along the medial elbow, places the thumb distally on the biceps brachii tendon, and depresses the tendon (Fig. 5–32). With the triangular end of the reflex hammer, the examiner strikes the thumbnail, depressing the tendon. For all reflex tests, it is imperative that the subject be relaxed.

Results. A normal response is one in which there is a flexion response of the elbow comparable to that on the uninvolved side. Unsuccessful attempts to elicit the reflex are an indication that there may be pathological involvement of the C5 nerve root. An excessive response may be an indication of an upper motor neuron lesion, whereas a diminished response may reflect lower motor neuron involvement.

Brachioradialis Reflex

Indication. The brachioradialis reflex test is used to assess the integrity of the C6 nerve root.

Method. The subject's upper limb is positioned as described for the biceps brachii reflex. Using the broad side of the hammer, the examiner strikes the radial side of the forearm just above the styloid process over the brachioradialis tendon (Fig. 5–33).

Results. A normal reflex will elicit a response of elbow flexion. Absent, depressed, or exaggerated movement indicates involvement of the C6 nerve root.

Triceps Reflex

Indication. The triceps reflex is associated with function of the C7 nerve root.

Method. The subject's position is the same as described previously. Using the triangular end of the hammer, the examiner taps the triceps tendon just proximal to the olecranon process (Fig. 5–34).

Results. The normal reflex response is elbow extension. Abnormalities of this reflex indicate the possibility of a lesion of the C7 nerve root.

Tests for Ligament Instability

Valgus Stress Test

Indication. The valgus stress test is used to assess the stability of the medial (ulnar) collateral ligament.

Figure 5–32. Testing the biceps tendon reflex.

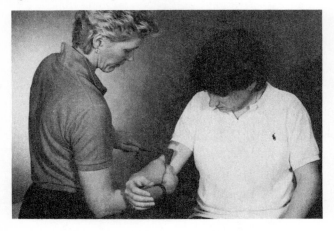

Figure 5–33. Testing the brachioradialis tendon reflex.

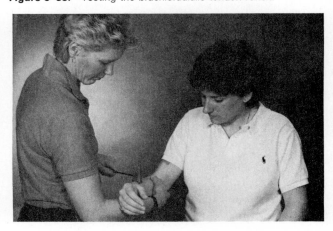

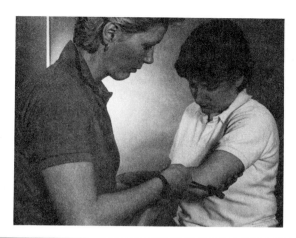

Figure 5–34. Testing the triceps tendon reflex.

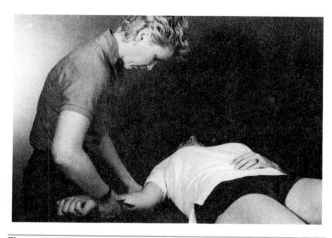

Figure 5–35. Valgus stress test.

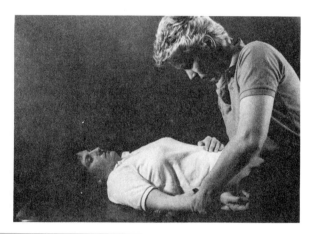

Figure 5–36. Varus stress test.

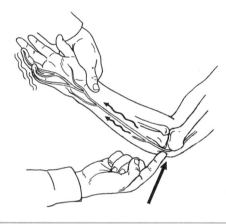

Figure 5–37. Tinels sign. This tests for ulnar nerve entrapment.

Method. The subject's elbow is positioned in slight flexion with the forearm supinated. The examiner places one hand on the lateral aspect of the elbow joint and the other medially on the midportion or distal forearm (Fig. 5–35). The examiner then imparts a valgus force to the elbow by pulling the forearm away from the body, using the elbow as a fulcrum.

Results. The test is positive if the subject experiences pain or if gapping is felt or seen along the medial aspect of the elbow. The uninvolved side is tested as a base for comparison.

Varus Stress Test

Indication. The varus stress test assesses the stability of the lateral (radial) collateral ligament.

Method. The subject's elbow is slightly flexed and the forearm is supinated. One of the examiner's hands is positioned on the medial aspect of the elbow joint, while the other is placed along the radial forearm, either at

midshaft or distally (Fig. 5–36). A varus force is applied by adducting the forearm relative to the arm, using the elbow as a fulcrum.

Results. Pain or gapping of the lateral aspect of the joint is a positive sign. The uninvolved side is compared.

Tinels Sign

Indication. Tinels sign at the elbow is designed to assess the integrity of the ulnar nerve where it lies in the ulnar groove between the olecranon process and the medial epicondyle. If there is a compromise of the ulnar nerve in this area, it may be reflected in a positive result.

Method. The examiner taps the ulnar nerve where it lies in the ulnar groove (Fig. 5–37).

Results. A tingling sensation within the distribution of the ulnar nerve in the forearm and hand constitutes a positive result.

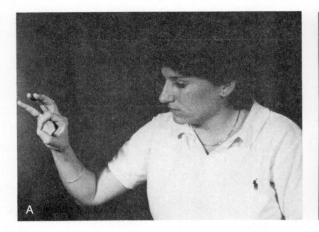
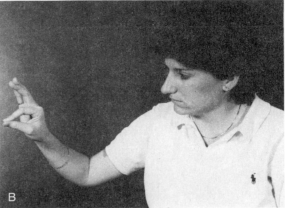

Figure 5–38. (A) Pinch grip test. Normal response is the ability to pinch the tip of the thumb to the tip of the index finger. (B) Lesion of the anterior interosseous nerve results in pinching of the pads of the distal phalanges of the thumb and index finger rather than the tips.

Pinch Grip Test

Indication. The pinch grip test assesses the possibility of a lesion in the anterior interosseous nerve (branch of the median nerve), which may be the result of entrapment of the nerve where it passes between the two heads of the pronator teres.

Method. The subject is asked to pinch the tip of the thumb to the tip of the index finger (Fig. 5–38A).

Results. If the subject is unable to pinch tip to tip, but instead pinches by approximating the pads of the distal phalanges, the test result is considered positive (Fig. 5–38B).

Tests for Lateral Epicondylitis (Tennis Elbow)

Method 1

Indication. Method 1 test is designed to detect inflammation in the musculature originating on and around the lateral epicondyle by imposing stress through contraction.

Method. The forearm is pronated and the elbow is slightly flexed. The examiner resists wrist extension and finger extension in various ways (Fig. 5–39A–C). The testing positions include:

1. Wrist extension and radial deviation to assess the extensor carpi radialis longus and brevis.
2. Wrist extension and ulnar deviation to assess the extensor carpi ulnaris.
3. Finger extension to assess the extensor digitorum.

Results. A positive result is sudden pain in the origin of the muscles being contracted. Because the extensor carpi radialis brevis is often involved in pathology, it is important to differentiate this structure from the exten-

sor carpi radialis longus by palpating and by recognizing the specific site of pain. In involvement of the extensor carpi radialis longus, pain is felt above the lateral epicondyle, where it originates on the supracondylar ridge. Conversely, the extensor carpi radialis brevis responds with localization of pain at its origin on the lateral epicondyle.

Method 2

Indication. Method 2 identifies inflammation in the extensor musculature of the wrist and hand originating on and about the lateral epicondyle. It requires stressing the musculature by elongation or stretching.

Method. The examiner extends the elbow and causes the subject's forearm to pronate while simultaneously flexing and deviating the wrist toward the ulna (Fig. 5–39D). It is important that these motions be performed to the end ranges of motion to ensure complete stretching of the extensor musculature.

Results. A positive result is pain elicited at or near the lateral epicondyle. The specific tendon can be found in the manner described in the previous test. The position of the patient for this test may also be utilized in treatment as flexibility conditioning.

Test for Medial Epicondylitis (Golfer's Elbow)

Method 1

Indication. Method 1 is used to assess inflammation of the common flexor tendons of the wrist by stressing the musculature with contraction.

Method. The subject is positioned with the elbow in slight flexion and the forearm supinated (Fig. 5–40A). The examiner then resists flexion of the wrist.

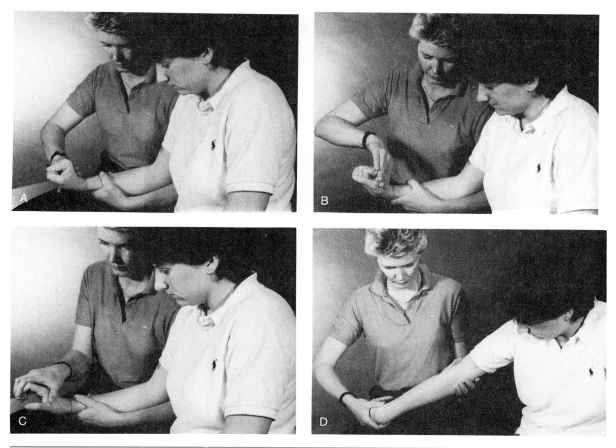

Figure 5–39. (*A–C*) Contractile testing of the wrist extensor musculature. (*D*) Flexibility testing of the wrist extensor musculature.

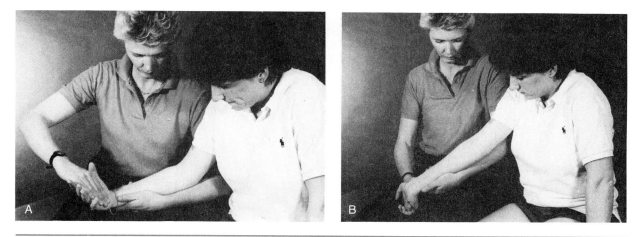

Figure 5–40. (*A*) Contractile testing of the wrist flexor musculature. (*B*) Flexibility testing of the wrist flexor musculature.

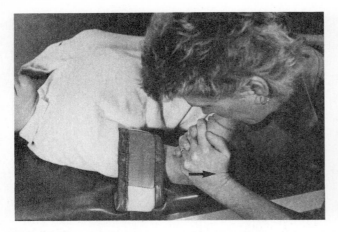

Figure 5–41. Distraction of the humeroulnar joint.

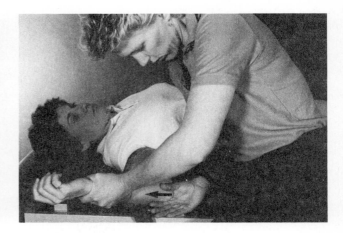

Figure 5–42. Anterior glide of the ulna.

Results. Pain in the region of the medial epicondyle is a positive result. It is impossible clinically to identify the specific flexor muscle involved because of the common origin.

Method 2

Indication. Method 2 is used to identify inflammation of the common flexor tendons about the elbow by imposing stress through stretching.

Method. The subject's forearm is fully supinated while the examiner places the elbow and wrist in maximal extension (Fig. 5–40B).

Results. Pain over the medial epicondyle indicates a positive test result. As in Method 1, localization of the specific flexor tendon involved is not possible. This position may be used in flexibility training of the affected structures.

Joint Play (Accessory Movements)

Humeroulnar Joint

Distraction (Fig. 5–41)

Restriction. General hypomobility.

Open-Packed Position. 70 degrees of flexion; 10 degrees of forearm supination.

Positioning. Subject lies supine, with a stabilizing strap across the distal humerus. The therapist bends forward, using proper body mechanics, and rests the subject's distal forearm on the shoulder. The therapist then grips the proximal forearm close to the joint space.

Movement. The therapist leans backward creating a distraction force on the joint.

Anterior Glide (Fig. 5–42)

Restriction. Flexion.

Positioning. Subject lies supine with the shoulder abducted and externally rotated. A stabilization strap or table stabilizing pad is positioned at the distal humerus. The therapist places the humeroulnar joint in the resting position and places the web space of the mobilizing hand around the olecranon process with the thumb and index fingers along the long axis of the ulna. The other hand placed around the distal forearm acts to maintain the resting position and to support the subject's limb.

Movement. The mobilizing hand delivers an anterior force to the joint by moving the ulna distally along its long axis.

Medial Glide (Fig. 5–43)

Restriction. Flexion and extension.

Positioning. Subject lies supine with a strap stabilizing the distal humerus. The therapist places the mobilizing hand proximally on the radial side of the forearm and supports the subject's forearm by holding the distal forearm.

Movement. The therapist delivers a medially directed force through the radial side of the proximal forearm.

Lateral Glide (Fig. 5–44)

Restriction. Flexion and extension.

Positioning. Subject lies supine, with a strap stabilizing the distal humerus. The therapist places the mobilizing hand proximally on the ulnar side of the forearm and supports the subject's forearm by holding the distal forearm.

Movement. The therapist delivers a laterally directed force through the ulnar side of the proximal forearm.

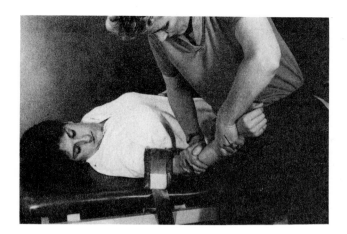

Figure 5–43.   Medial glide of the ulna.

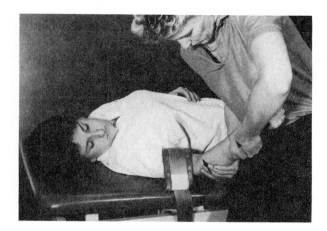

Figure 5–44.   Lateral glide of the ulna.

Radiohumeral Joint

Dorsal Glide (Fig. 5–45)

Restriction.   Extension.

Open-Packed Position.   Full elbow extension; full forearm supination.

Positioning.   Subject lies supine, with the upper limb stabilized by the table. The therapist grips the distal humerus and proximal ulna, thereby providing additional stabilization. The thenar eminence of the opposite hand is placed anteriorly on the proximal radius, close to the joint space.

Movement.   The therapist imposes a dorsal force on the anterior surface of the proximal radius.

Ventral Glide (Fig. 5–46)

Restriction.   Flexion.

Positioning.   Same as for dorsal glide, except the distal phalanges of digits two through five are placed posteriorly along the proximal radius.

Movement.   The therapist imposes a ventral (anterior) force to the posterior surface of the proximal radius.

Superior Radioulnar Joint

Ventral Medial Glide (Fig. 5–47)

Restriction.   Forearm supination.

Open-Packed Position.   70 degrees of elbow flexion; 35 degrees of forearm supination.

Positioning.   Subject may be either seated or supine with the table acting to stabilize the limb. One hand of the therapist grips the distal humerus and proximal ulna, thereby providing additional stabilization. The thenar eminence of the opposite hand is placed anteriorly on the proximal radius, close to the joint space. The distal phalanges of digits two through five are placed posteriorly along the proximal radius.

Movement.   The therapist imposes a ventral medial force to the posterior surface of the proximal radius.

Figure 5–45.   Dorsal glide of the radius.

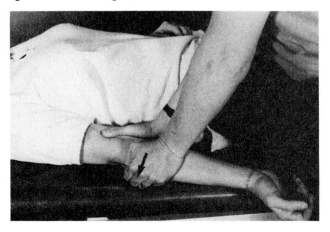

Figure 5–46.   Ventral glide of the radius.

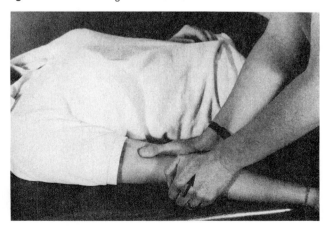

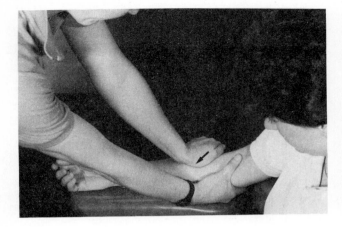

Figure 5–47. Ventral medial glide of the radius.

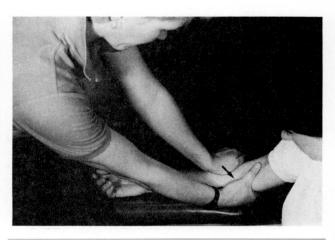

Figure 5–48. Dorsal lateral glide of the radius.

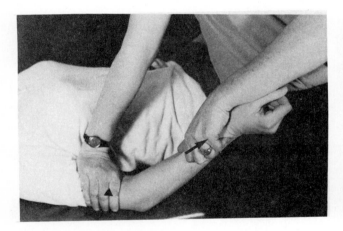

Figure 5–49. Distraction or distal glide of the radius.

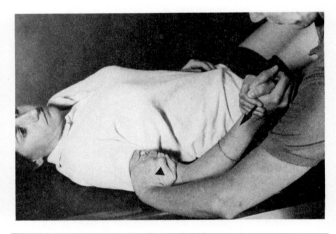

Figure 5–50. Compression or proximal glide of the radius.

Dorsal Lateral Glide (Fig. 5–48)

Restriction. Forearm pronation.

Positioning. Same as for ventral medial glide.

Movement. The therapist imposes a dorsal lateral force to the anterior surface of the proximal radius.

Distraction (Fig. 5–49)

Restriction. Proximal positional fault of the radius.

Positioning. Patient is supine or seated. One hand of the therapist acts to stabilize the distal humerus, while the other grasps the distal radius.

Movement. The therapist pulls the radius distally along its long axis, thereby creating a distraction force to the proximal radius. The positional fault is corrected not only at the superior radioulnar joint but at the radiohumeral joint as well.

Compression (Fig. 5–50)

Restriction. Distal positional fault of the radius.

Positioning. Same as for distraction glide.

Movement. The therapist moves the radius proximally along its long axis, thereby creating a compression force to the proximal radius. The positional fault is corrected not only at the superior radioulnar joint but at the radiohumeral joint as well.

Inferior Radioulnar Joint

Ventral Medial Glide (Fig. 5–51)

Restriction. Forearm pronation.

Open-Packed Position. 10 degrees of forearm supination.

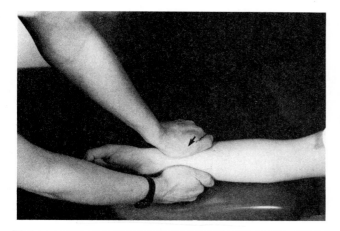

Figure 5–51. Ventral medial glide of the radius.

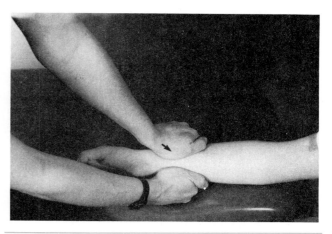

Figure 5–52. Dorsal lateral glide of the radius.

Positioning. Subject is either supine or seated. One hand of the therapist acts to stabilize the distal ulna. The mobilizing hand is placed with the thenar eminence on the anterior surface of the distal radius, and the distal phalanges of digits two through five on the posterior surface of the distal radius.

Movement. The therapist imparts ventral medial force to the posterior surface of the distal radius.

Dorsal Lateral Glide (Fig. 5–52)

Restriction. Forearm supination.

Positioning. Same as for ventral medial glide.

Movement. The therapist produces a dorsal lateral force on the anterior surface of the distal radius.

Table 5–1 provides a summary of joint play of the elbow and forearm joints.

Table 5–1. Summary of Joint Play of the Elbow and Forearm Joints

GLIDE	RESTRICTION	FIXED BONE	MOVING BONE
Humeroulnar Joint			
Distraction	General hypomobility	Humerus	Ulna
Ventral	Flexion	Humerus	Ulna
Medial	Flexion-extension	Humerus	Ulna
Lateral	Flexion-extension	Humerus	Ulna
Radiohumeral Joint			
Distraction	General hypomobility	Humerus	Radius
Ventral	Flexion	Humerus	Radius
Dorsal	Extension	Humerus	Radius
Superior Radioulnar Joint			
Ventral medial	Supination	Ulna	Radius
Dorsal lateral	Pronation	Ulna	Radius
Distraction	Proximal positional fault	Ulna	Radius
Compression	Distal positional fault	Ulna	Radius
Inferior Radioulnar Joint			
Ventral medial	Pronation	Ulna	Radius
Dorsal lateral	Supination	Ulna	Radius

Bibliography

Backhouse KM, Hutchings RT: Color Atlas of Surface Anatomy. Baltimore, Williams & Wilkins, 1986

Daniels L, Worthingham C: Muscle Testing Techniques of Manual Examination. Philadelphia, WB Saunders, 1986

Gould A III, Davies G (eds): Orthopedic and Sports Physical Therapy. St Louis, CV Mosby, 1985

Hollinshead WH, Jenkins DB: Functional Anatomy of the Limbs and Back. Philadelphia, WB Saunders, 1981

Hoppenfeld S: Physical Examination of the Spine and Extremities. New York, Appleton-Century-Crofts, 1976

Kaltenborn M: Mobilization of the Extremity Joints. Oslo, Bygdoy Alle, 1980

Kendall FP, McCreary EK: Muscle Testing and Function. Baltimore, Williams & Wilkins, 1983

Kessler R, Hertling D: Management of Common Musculoskeletal Disorders. Philadelphia, Harper & Row, 1983

Kisner C, Colby LA: Therapeutic Exercise: Foundations and Techniques. Philadelphia, FA Davis, 1985

Magee J: Orthopedic Physical Assessment. Philadelphia, WB Saunders, 1987

Maitland GD: The Peripheral Joints: Examination and Recording Guide. Adelaide, Australia, Virgo Press, 1973

Norkin CC, White DJ: Measurement of Joint Motion: A Guide to Goniometry. Philadelphia, FA Davis, 1985

Saunders H: Evaluation, Treatment, and Prevention of Musculoskeletal Disorders. Minneapolis, H Duane Saunders, 1985

Williams P, Warwick R (eds): Gray's Anatomy, 36th British ed. Philadelphia, WB Saunders, 1980

Wrist
and Hand

Chapter 6

The wrist and hand are complex structures that are dependent on the entire upper limb. The hand is necessary for such delicate activities of daily living as sewing and painting, as well as such powerful ones as hammering. Loss in the proximal upper limb may translate into diminished function of the hand.

The wrist joint is formed by the distal end of the radius, the proximal carpal bones (scaphoid and lunate), and the articular disc of the ulna and the triquetrum. The joint moves in two planes of motion and is called a condyloid synovial joint. Intercarpal motions occur during wrist joint flexion, extension, abduction, and adduction. The intercarpal joints are plane joints. The axis for flexion and extension is transverse (from medial to lateral) and is located at the level of the capitate bone. The axis for radial deviation (abduction) and ulnar deviation (adduction) is transverse anteriorly and posteriorly, also through the capitate.

In the hand the distal row of carpal bones articulates with the metacarpals. These joints, called saddle joints, have little or no movement except in the first and fifth digits. The base of the first metacarpal articulates with the trapezium and allows three degrees of freedom of motion. The joint is capable of flexion, extension, abduction, adduction, and opposition. The metacarpophalangeal joints of the medial four digits are condyloid joints and permit flexion, extension, abduction, and adduction motions. The first digit's metacarpophalangeal joint is like an interphalangeal joint of the medial four digits, which are hinge joints, permitting only flexion and extension.

Goniometry

Wrist

Wrist Flexion

The majority of wrist flexion occurs at the radiocarpal joint in the sagittal plane between the radius and the scaphoid and lunate bones. Movement of wrist flexion also occurs between the intercarpals and the head of the ulna and the articular disc. As the wrist joint flexes, the proximal row of carpal bones glides in a posterior direction on the distal end of the radius. The fingers are held loosely in extension to allow complete range of motion at the wrist joint.

Motion. 0 to 90 degrees from the anatomical wrist position into flexion.

Position
- Preferred: Subject sits with the forearm supported on the table in pronation. The elbow joint is flexed 90 degrees, the wrist is in the neutral position, and the fingers are extended.

- Alternate:
1. Subject sits with the elbow flexed. The forearm is in a position between supination and pronation. Fingers are held loosely in extension.
2. Subject lies supine with the elbow flexed. The forearm and wrist are positioned as above.

Goniometric Alignment (Figs. 6–1 to 6–3)

Axis
- Preferred: Placed distal to the styloid process of the ulna, the axis shifts slightly distally following movement.
- Alternate: Placed over the capitate bone.
- Alternate: Placed on the styloid process of the radius.

Stationary Arm
- Preferred: Placed parallel to and over the lateral midline of the ulna, in line with the olecranon process.
- Alternate: Placed along the midline of the dorsal surface of the forearm.
- Alternate: Placed along the radial shaft in line with the head.

Moving Arm
- Preferred: Along the lateral midline of the fifth metacarpal.
- Alternate: Placed on the midline of the dorsal surface of the third metacarpal.
- Alternate: Placed on the midline of the second metacarpal.

Stabilization. The forearm is stabilized.

Precautions
- Make sure fingers stay relaxed during measurement.
- Avoid radial and ulnar deviation of the wrist joint.
- Avoid depression of the fifth metacarpal.

Figure 6–1. End position for wrist flexion.

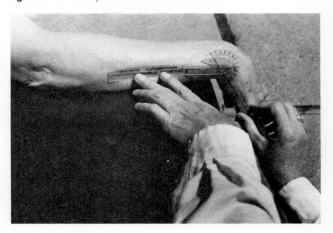

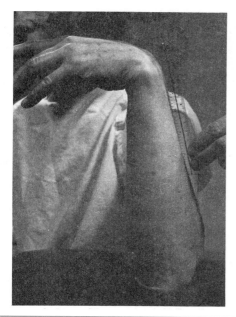

Figure 6–2. Alternate end position for wrist flexion with the goniometer placed on the posterior surface of the joint.

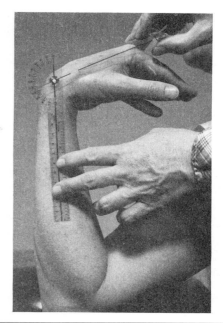

Figure 6–3. Alternate end position for wrist flexion with the placement of the goniometer on the lateral aspect of the joint.

Wrist Extension and Hyperextension

Wrist extension and hyperextension occur in the sagittal plane at the radiocarpal and intercarpal joints. As the wrist moves into extension the proximal row of carpal bones glide anteriorly. Wrist extension is the return from flexion. Wrist flexion and extension can be measured on the radial or ulnar side of the hand, but the measurements of the two sides will vary because of anatomical structure of the wrist and the cupping of the hand on the ulnar side. If measured on the radial side, the second metacarpal is used as the distal landmark.

Motion. 90 to 0 degrees of extension, and about 70 degrees of hyperextension.

Position. Same as for wrist flexion, with the fingers held loosely in flexion.

Goniometric Alignment (Figs. 6–4 to 6–6)

Axis
- Preferred: Placed distal to the styloid process of the ulna; the axis will shift slightly proximally by the end of the movement.
- Alternate: Placed distal to the styloid process of the radius.
- Alternate: Placed over the capitate bone.

Stationary Arm
- Preferred: Parallel to and over the lateral midline of the ulna, in line with the olecranon process.

- Alternate: Parallel to and over the long axis of the radius, in line with the radial head.
- Alternate: Placed along the midline of the anterior of the forearm.

Moving Arm
- Preferred: Along the long axis of the fifth metacarpal.

Figure 6–4. End position for wrist joint extension and hyperextension.

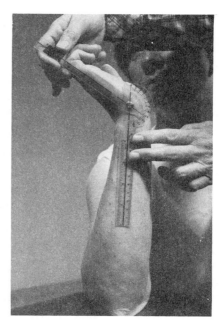

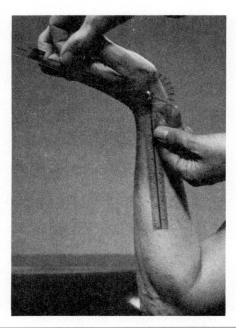

Figure 6–5. Alternate end position for wrist extension and hyperextension with the goniometer placed on the lateral aspect of the joint.

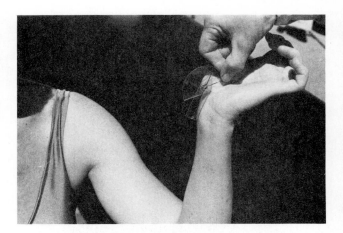

Figure 6–6. Alternate end position for wrist extension and hyperextension with the goniometer placed on the anterior surface of the joint.

- Alternate: Along the long axis of the second metacarpal.
- Alternate: Placed on the midline of the palm in line with the third metacarpal.

Stabilization. The forearm is stabilized.

Precautions
- Avoid extension of the fingers.
- Avoid radial and ulnar deviation at the wrist joint.
- Prevent cupping of the fifth metacarpal.
- Range of motion will vary according to the position of the goniometer. Always place consistently on each subject.

Wrist Radial Deviation (Abduction)

In the anatomical position, the motion of radial deviation at the wrist occurs in the coronal plane. The test position produces movement in the transverse plane. The motion occurs between the radius and the proximal row of carpal bones and between the intercarpals. The distal row of carpals moves radially, and the proximal row glides ulnarly on the distal end of the radius during wrist abduction.

Motion. 0 to 25 degrees of radial deviation.

Position
- Preferred: Subject sits with the elbow flexed and forearm pronated on the table. The forearm and

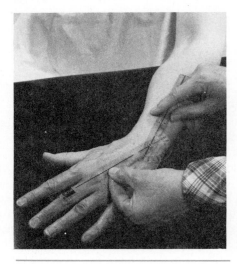

Figure 6–7. End position for radial deviation (abduction) of the wrist.

hand are supported on the table top with the wrist in a neutral position.
- Alternate: The subject lies supine.

Goniometric Alignment (Fig. 6–7)

Axis. Placed on the dorsal surface of the wrist over the capitate bone. – drop postradius & ulnar

Stationary Arm. Placed along the dorsal midline surface of the forearm.

Moving Arm. Placed on the midline of the dorsal surface of the third metacarpal bone.

Stabilization. The forearm is stabilized.

Precautions
- Avoid flexion or extension of the wrist.

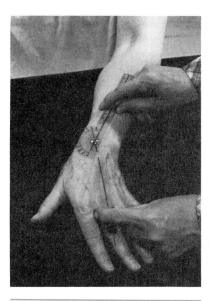

Figure 6–8. End position for ulnar deviation (adduction) of the wrist.

• Avoid pronation or supination of the forearm.
• Do not use the third digit as a point of reference.

Wrist Ulnar Deviation (Adduction)

In the test position, the motion occurs in the transverse plane. The motion occurs between the intercarpal bones and the radiocarpal joint. When ulnar deviation occurs the distal carpal bones move in an ulnar direction, and at the end of the range the proximal row of carpal bones glides radially on the distal end of the radius.

Motion. 0 to 35 degrees of ulnar deviation from the neutral position of the wrist joint.

Position. Subject sits with the elbow flexed to 90 degrees, the forearm pronated on the table and the hand supported.

Goniometric Alignment (Fig. 6–8)

Axis. Placed over the capitate.

Stationary Arm. Placed along the midline of the dorsal surface of the forearm.

Moving Arm. Placed on the midline of the dorsal surface of the third metacarpal.

Stabilization. The forearm is stabilized.

Precautions
• Avoid flexion and extension of the wrist joint.

• Avoid pronation and supination of the radioulnar joints.
• Do not use the third digit as the point of reference.

Metacarpophalangeal Joints (Digits 2 to 5)

Metacarpophalangeal Joint Flexion

The hand is in a neutral position with the forearm in midposition between supination and pronation. In the anatomical position the motion occurs in the sagittal plane, but in the test position the motion occurs in the transverse plane. The motion occurs between the metacarpals and the proximal phalanx of each of the fingers. As the motion occurs, the base of the phalanx glides in an anterior direction.

If the patient has edema or bony joint changes and the arms of the goniometer cannot be placed accurately, alternate measurements may be made. A ruler measurement may be made from the tip of each finger to the distal carpal crease. Tracings, x-rays, or photographs may also be used. A goniometer with short arms or a goniometer designed for the digits is recommended for measurements.

Motion. 0 to 90 degrees of flexion while maintaining the interphalangeal joints in extension.

Position. Subject is sitting, with the elbow flexed to 90 degrees, the forearm supported in the midposition, and the wrist and fingers in the anatomical position.

Goniometric Alignment (Fig. 6–9)

Axis. Placed on the dorsal surface of the metacarpophalangeal joint.

Figure 6–9. End position for metacarpophalangeal joint flexion.

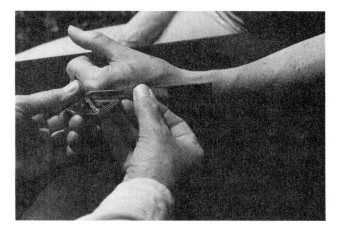

Stationary Arm. Placed on the midline of the dorsal surface of the metacarpal of the joint being measured.

Moving Arm. Placed on the midline of the dorsal surface of the proximal phalanx of the joint being measured.

Stabilization. The metacarpals are stabilized.

Precautions
· Hold the fingers loosely in extension.
· Hyperextend the wrist slightly.
· Avoid metacarpophalangeal joint abduction and adduction.

Metacarpophalangeal Joint Extension and Hyperextension

Extension of the metacarpophalangeal joint is the return of flexion, and hyperextension occurs beyond the neutral (0) position. As the proximal phalanx moves into extension and hyperextension, the base glides in a posterior direction.

Motion. 90 to 0 degrees for extension and 0 to 30 degrees for hyperextension, with the interphalangeal joints held loosely in flexion.

Position. Subject sits with elbow and shoulder flexed and forearm in midposition between supination and pronation. The wrist remains in the anatomical position.

Goniometric Alignment (Fig. 6–10)

Axis. Placed over the palmar aspect of the metacarpophalangeal joint being measured.

Stationary Arm. Placed along the palmar midline shaft of the metacarpal being measured.

Moving Arm. Placed along the palmar midline shaft of the proximal phalanx being measured.

Stabilization. The metacarpals are stabilized.

Precautions
· Keep the fingers relaxed in a flexed position.
· Keep the wrist in the anatomical position.

Metacarpophalangeal Joint Abduction

In the test position, metacarpophalangeal joint abduction motion occurs in the transverse plane. The metacarpophalangeal joints are maintained in an extended position. The second digit (index finger) moves in a radial direction from the third digit (middle finger), and the fourth and fifth digits (ring and little fingers) move in an ulnar direction from the middle finger. The proximal phalanx glides in the same direction on the head of the metacarpal.

Motion. 0 to 20 degrees of metacarpophalangeal joint abduction (movement away from the middle finger).

Position. Subject sits with the elbow joint flexed and the wrist joint in a neutral position. The forearm and hand are supported in a pronated position.

Goniometric Alignment (Fig. 6–11)

Axis. Placed over the dorsal midline of the metacarpophalangeal joint to be tested.

Stationary Arm. Placed over the dorsal midline of the metacarpal being tested.

Moving Arm. Placed over the dorsal midline of the proximal phalanx of the joint being tested.

Stabilization. The metacarpal is stabilized.

Figure 6–10. End position for metacarpophalangeal joint extension and hyperextension.

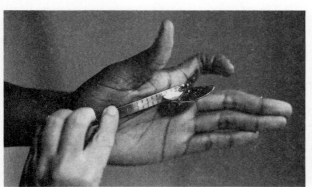

Figure 6–11. End position for metacarpophalangeal joint abduction.

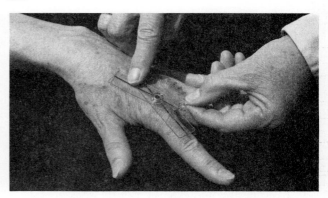

Precautions
- Prevent wrist motions.
- Avoid flexion at the metacarpophalangeal joint.

Metacarpophalangeal Joint Adduction

Adduction at the metacarpophalangeal joints is the return from abduction. The test position allows the motion to be in the transverse plane. The second digit (index finger) moves in an ulnar direction, and the fourth and fifth digits (ring and little fingers) move radially toward the third digit. The base of the proximal phalanx adducts on the head of the metacarpal and glides in the same direction as the motion.

Motion. 0 to 20 degrees at the metacarpophalangeal joints.

Position. Subject sits with the elbow joint flexed, the forearm pronated, and the wrist and fingers in a neutral position. The forearm and hand are supported. The third digit (middle finger) is positioned to allow 20 degrees of motion to occur from the anatomical position.

Goniometric Alignment (Fig. 6–12)

Axis. Placed dorsally over the metacarpophalangeal joint being measured.

Stationary Arm. Placed over the dorsal midline of the metacarpal being measured.

Moving Arm. Placed over the dorsal midline of the proximal phalanx of the finger being measured.

Stabilization. The metacarpals are stabilized.

Precautions
- Prevent wrist motion.
- Avoid metacarpophalangeal joint flexion.

Figure 6–12. End position for metacarpophalangeal joint adduction.

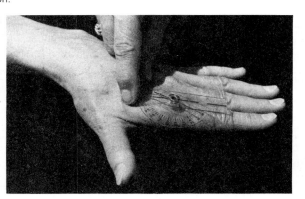

Proximal Interphalangeal Joint Flexion

Flexion at the proximal metacarpophalangeal joints occurs in the sagittal plane when in the anatomical position. In the test position the motion occurs in the transverse plane. As the middle phalanx flexes on the proximal one, it glides in an anterior direction.

Motion. 0 to 120 degrees for flexion.

Position. Subject sits, with elbow flexed and forearm supported on the table in the midposition between supination and pronation. The wrist is slightly hyperextended.

Goniometric Alignment (Fig. 6–13)

Axis. Placed over the dorsal aspect of the proximal interphalangeal joints.

Stationary Arm. Placed along the dorsal midline of the proximal phalanx.

Moving Arm. Placed along the dorsal midline of the middle phalanx.

Stabilization. The proximal phalanx is stabilized.

Precaution
- Prevent wrist flexion.

Interphalangeal Joint Extension and Hyperextension

Interphalangeal joint extension motion is the return from flexion. The base of the middle phalanx glides in a posterior direction as the joint moves into extension.

Motion. 120 to 0 degrees for extension and 0 to 10 degrees for hyperextension.

Figure 6–13. End position for proximal interphalangeal joint flexion.

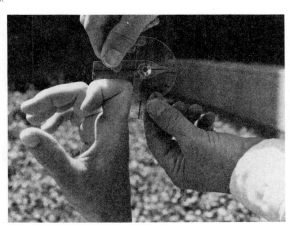

Position. Subject sits, with elbow flexed and forearm supported on the table in the midposition between supination and pronation. The wrist joint is in the anatomical position, and the digits are relaxed in flexion.

Goniometric Alignment (Fig. 6–14)

Axis. Placed over the palmar aspect of the joint being measured.

Stationary Arm. Placed over the midline of the palmar aspect of the proximal phalanx.

Moving Arm. Placed over the midline of the palmar aspect of the middle phalanx.

Stabilization. The proximal phalanx is stabilized.

Precaution
• Prevent wrist hyperextension.

Figure 6–14. End position for proximal interphalangeal joint extension.

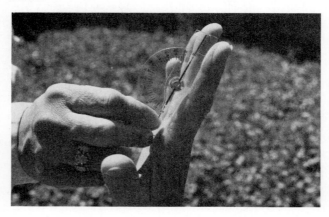

Figure 6–15. End position for distal interphalangeal joint flexion.

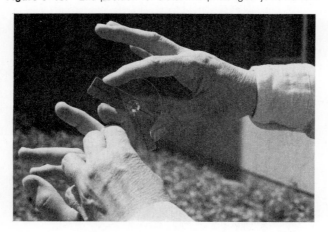

Distal Interphalangeal Joint Flexion

Distal interphalangeal flexion occurs between the middle and distal phalanges. As flexion of the distal interphalangeal joint occurs, the base of the distal phalanx glides in an anterior direction.

Motion. 0 to 80 degrees of distal interphalangeal joint flexion with the proximal interphalangeal joint positioned in slight flexion.

Position. Subject sits with elbow flexed and forearm in midposition between supination and pronation. The forearm and hand are supported on the table. The wrist is slightly hyperextended.

Goniometric Alignment (Fig. 6–15)

Axis. Placed over the dorsal surface of the joint being measured.

Stationary Arm. Placed over the dorsal midline shaft of the middle phalanx of each digit.

Moving Arm. Placed over the dorsal midline shaft of each distal phalanx.

Stabilization. The middle phalanx of each digit is stabilized.

Precaution
• Allow the wrist to remain slightly hyperextended.

Distal Interphalangeal Joint Extension

Distal interphalangeal joint extension motion is the return from flexion of the distal interphalangeal joints. During the motion the base of the distal phalanx glides in a posterior direction on the head of the middle phalanx.

Motion. 80 to 0 degrees of extension, and 0 to 10 degrees of hyperextension at the distal interphalangeal joints.

Position. Subject sits with elbow flexed and forearm supported in midposition between supination and pronation. The wrist joint is in the anatomical position.

Goniometric Alignment (Fig. 6–16)

Axis. Placed over the palmar midpoint of the joint being measured.

Stationary Arm. Placed over and parallel to the midline of the palmar surface of the middle phalanx.

Moving Arm. Placed over and parallel to the midline of the palmar surface of the distal phalanx.

Stabilization. The middle phalanx of each digit is stabilized.

Precaution
• Keep wrist and metacarpophalangeal joints properly aligned.

Thumb Carpometacarpal Joint Flexion

[handwritten: measure thumb w) tape measure & to what pt. lacks]

In the test position, the flexion at the carpometacarpal joint occurs in the transverse plane between the first metacarpal and the trapezium. The first metacarpal moves across the palm of the hand, and the base glides ulnarly.

Motion. 0 to 15 degrees at the carpometacarpal joint (allow the first metacarpal to slide over the second metacarpal).

Position. Subject sits with the elbow joint flexed and the forearm supinated and supported. The wrist, fingers, and thumb joints are in the anatomical position.

Goniometric Alignment (Fig. 6–17)

Axis. Placed over the palmar surface of the first carpometacarpal joint.

Stationary Arm. Placed along the long axis of the radial shaft.

Moving Arm. Placed along the long axis of the first metacarpal shaft.

Stabilization. The carpal bones are stabilized.

Precautions
• Prevent wrist flexion and ulnar deviation.
• Prevent thumb opposition.

Thumb Carpometacarpal Joint Extension and Hyperextension (Radial Abduction)

In the anatomical position, extension at the carpometacarpal joint occurs in the coronal plane; in the test position, however, the motion occurs in the transverse plane. During the motion the base of the first metacarpal glides radially in the same direction as the motion on the trapezium bone.

Motion. 0 to 70 degrees of extension at the metacarpal joint. The thumb is extended in the plane of the palm.

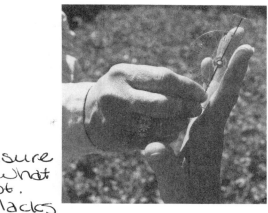

Figure 6–16. End position for distal interphalangeal joint extension.

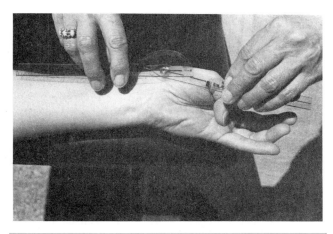

Figure 6–17. End position for first digit carpometacarpal joint flexion.

Position. Subject sits with the elbow flexed and the forearm pronated and supported. The wrist and fingers remain in the anatomical position.

Goniometric Alignment (Figs. 6–18 and 6–19)

Axis
• Preferred: Placed over the dorsal aspect of the carpometacarpal joint of the thumb.
• Alternate: Placed over the palmar aspect of the carpometacarpal joint of the thumb.

Stationary Arm
• Preferred: Placed dorsally on the midline of the radius.
• Alternate: Placed over the anterior midline of the radius.

Moving Arm
• Preferred: Placed on the midline of the dorsal surface of the first metacarpal bone.

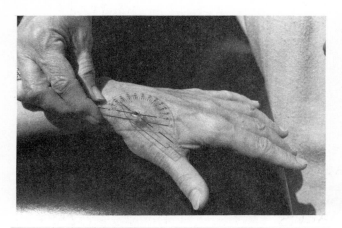

Figure 6–18. End position for carpometacarpal joint extension.

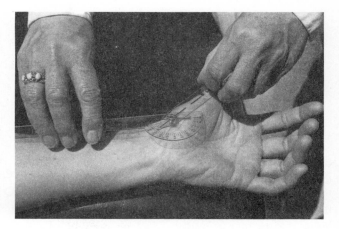

Figure 6–19. Alternate end position for carpometacarpal joint extension.

• Alternate: Placed over the lateral midline of the first metacarpal bone.

Stabilization. The carpal bones are stabilized.

Precautions
• Prevent thumb flexion or abduction.
• Prevent radial deviation of the wrist joint.

Thumb Carpometacarpal Joint Opposition

The motion of opposition is a combination of flexion, abduction, and medial rotation between the first metacarpal and the trapezium. The movement of rotation occurs as the thumb moves toward the base or tip of the fifth finger. A ruler or tape measure is used to determine the distance between the fifth finger and the thumb when complete motion is not obtained. Normally the thumb pad touches the fifth finger and the thumbnail faces away from the palm.

Motion. The distance is between the tip of the fifth finger and the thumb. The pad of the thumb approaches the base of the fifth fingers.

Position. Subject sits with elbow flexed and forearm supported in supination. The wrist and finger joints are in the anatomical position.

Measurement. When motion is limited, the ruler is placed from the tip of the thumb to the tip or base of the fifth finger. The distance recorded is the deficit in complete range of motion (Figs. 6–20 and 6–21).

Stabilization. The metacarpal and fingers not involved in the motion are stabilized.

Precautions
• Prevent wrist flexion.
• Allow the three motions of flexion, abduction, and medial rotation at the first carpometacarpal joint.

Figure 6–20. Measuring opposition with a ruler or measuring tape.

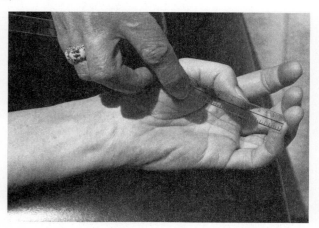

Figure 6–21. Alternate end position for measuring opposition.

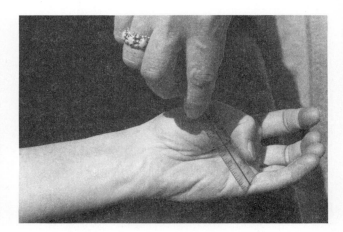

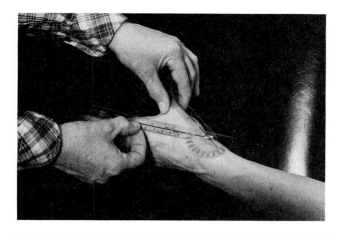

Figure 6–22. End position for carpometacarpal joint abduction.

Thumb Carpometacarpal Joint Abduction (Palmar Abduction)

In the anatomical position, thumb carpometacarpal joint abduction occurs in the sagittal plane. In the test position, the motion occurs in the transverse plane. The thumb moves at right angles to the palm of the hand. The first metacarpal abducts on the trapezium bone, and its base glides dorsally on the trapezium bone.

Motion. 0 to 60 degrees of abduction at the first carpometacarpal joint.

Position. Subject sits with the elbow flexed and the forearm in midposition between supination and pronation. The hand is supported and resting on the ulnar border. The wrist and fingers are in the anatomical position.

Goniometric Alignment (Fig. 6–22)

Axis. Placed between the first and second carpometacarpal joints on the dorsal surface.

Stationary Arm. Placed on the lateral midline of the second metacarpal bone.

Moving Arm. Placed on the midline of the dorsal surface of the first metacarpal bone.

Stabilization. The carpal and second metacarpal are stabilized.

Precautions
- Prevent medial rotation of the thumb.
- Observe web space for skin tightness.
- Prevent flexion or extension of the thumb.
- Avoid wrist joint motions.

Thumb Carpometacarpal Joint Adduction

Adduction of the carpometacarpal joint of the first digit is the return from carpometacarpal joint abduction. It is also the anatomical position for the first carpometacarpal joint. As the first metacarpal moves toward adduction, its base glides anteriorly in the opposite direction over the trapezium.

Motion. 60 to 0 degrees of adduction at the first carpometacarpal joint into the anatomical position.

Position. Subject sits with elbow flexed and forearm supported in mid-position between supination and pronation. The wrist, finger, and thumb joints assume the anatomical position.

Goniometric Alignment (Fig. 6–23)

Axis. Placed between the first and second metacarpal joints.

Stationary Arm. Placed on the midline of the lateral surface of the second metacarpal.

Moving Arm. Placed on the midline of the dorsal surface of the first metacarpal bone.

Stabilization. The carpal and second metacarpal bones are stabilized.

Figure 6–23. End position for carpometacarpal joint adduction.

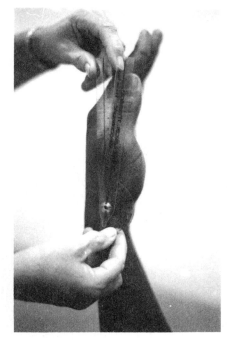

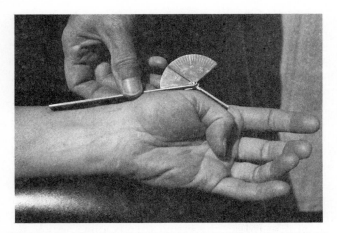

Figure 6–24. End position for metacarpophalangeal joint flexion.

Precautions
- Prevent medial rotation of the thumb.
- Prevent carpometacarpal joint flexion and extension.
- Prevent wrist joint motions.

Thumb Metacarpophalangeal Joint Flexion

In the anatomical position, flexion of the thumb metacarpophalangeal joint occurs in the coronal plane. In the test position the motion occurs in the transverse plane. The proximal phalanx flexes on the first metacarpal as the base glides in an anterior direction on the head of the first metacarpal.

Motion. 0 to 50 degrees of flexion, maintaining the interphalangeal joint in extension.

Position. Subject sits with elbow flexed and forearm and hand supported in a supinated position. The wrist, thumb, and finger joints are in the anatomical position.

Goniometric Alignment (Fig. 6–24)

Axis. Placed over the dorsal aspect of the metacarpophalangeal joint.

Stationary Arm. Placed over the dorsal midline shaft of the first metacarpal bone.

Moving Arm. Placed over the dorsal midline shaft of the proximal phalanx.

Stabilization. The metacarpal bones are stabilized.

Precautions
- Prevent wrist joint motion.
- Avoid carpometacarpal joint flexion and opposition.

Thumb Metacarpophalangeal Joint Extension and Hyperextension

Metacarpophalangeal joint extension is the return from metacarpophalangeal joint flexion to the anatomical position and beyond into hyperextension. The motion occurs in the transverse plane in the test position and in the coronal plane in the anatomical position. During the motion of extension and hyperextension, the first metacarpal bone glides posteriorly on the trapezium.

Motion. 50 to 0 degrees for extension, and 0 to 10 degrees for hyperextension. The interphalangeal joint remains extended.

Position. Subject sits with elbow flexed and forearm supinated and supported. The wrist, fingers, and first carpometacarpal joint assume a neutral position.

Goniometric Alignment (Fig. 6–25)

Axis. Placed over the dorsal aspect of the metacarpophalangeal joint. For hyperextension, the axis is placed over the palmar aspect of the metacarpophalangeal joint.

Stationary Arm. Placed along the dorsal surface of the shaft of the first metacarpal bone. For hyperextension, the stationary arm is aligned with the shaft of the first metacarpal on the palmar side.

Moving Arm. Placed along the dorsal midline of the proximal phalanx of the thumb and the palmar surface for the motion of hyperextension.

Stabilization. The first metacarpal is stabilized.

Precautions
- Prevent wrist motions.
- Avoid carpometacarpal joint motions.

Figure 6–25. End position for metacarpophalangeal joint extension and hyperextension.

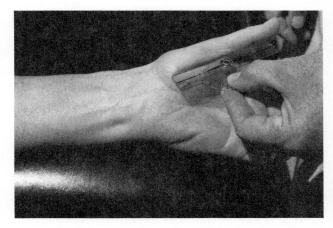

Thumb Interphalangeal Joint Flexion

Interphalangeal joint flexion of the first digit occurs in the transverse plane. As the base of the distal phalanx flexes on the head of the proximal phalanx, it glides in an anterior direction.

Motion.   0 to 80 or 90 degrees of flexion at the interphalangeal joint of the thumb.

Position.   Subject sits with elbow flexed and forearm supinated and supported. The wrist, fingers, and thumb are in the anatomical position.

Goniometric Alignment (Fig. 6–26)

Axis.   Placed over the dorsal surface of the interphalangeal joint.

Stationary Arm.   Placed along the dorsal midline surface of the proximal phalanx.

Moving Arm.   Placed along the dorsal midline surface of the distal phalanx.

Stabilization.   The proximal phalanx is stabilized.

Precautions
- Prevent wrist motions.
- Prevent metacarpophalangeal joint flexion or extension.

Thumb Interphalangeal Joint Extension and Hyperextension

Interphalangeal joint extension occurs in the transverse plane in the test position and is the return from flexion. The base of the distal phalanx of the thumb glides posteriorly on the head of the proximal phalanx during the

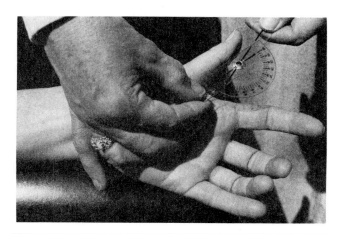

Figure 6–27.   End position for first digit interphalangeal joint extension and hyperextension.

extension and hyperextension motion. The range of motion varies from person to person.

Motion.   90 to 0 degrees for extension, and 0 to 90 degrees for hyperextension.

Position.   Subject sits with elbow flexed and forearm supinated and supported. The wrist, fingers, and thumb are in the anatomical position.

Goniometric Alignment (Fig. 6–27)

Axis.   Placed over the dorsal aspect of the interphalangeal joint. For the motion of hyperextension, the axis is over the interphalangeal joint on the palmar surface.

Stationary Arm.   Placed along the dorsal midline surface of the proximal phalanx. For hyperextension motion, the stationary arm is along the midline palmar surface of the proximal phalanx.

Moving Arm.   Placed along the midline dorsal surface of the distal phalanx. For hyperextension, the moving arm is placed on the palmar midline surface of the distal phalanx.

Stabilization.   The proximal phalanx is stabilized.

Precautions
- Prevent wrist movements.
- Prevent metacarpophalangeal and carpometacarpal joint motion.

Functional Muscle Testing
Wrist

The wrist, a distal joint of the upper limb, allows the hand to assume various positions. Changes in the position of the elbow affect the length of the forearm muscles

Figure 6–26.   End position for first digit interphalangeal joint flexion.

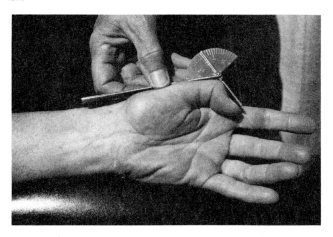

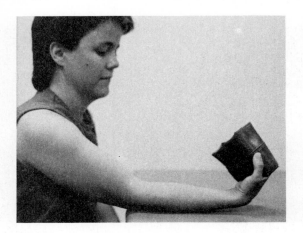

Figure 6–28.   Resisted wrist joint flexion.

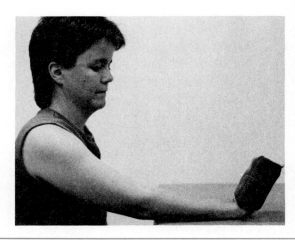

Figure 6–29.   Resisted wrist joint extension and hyperextension.

and the function of the muscles of the wrist and hand. The position of the wrist is a determining factor in the strength of the hand muscles. Its major contribution to upper limb function is to provide a stable base for hand function.

Wrist Flexion

The wrist flexor muscles lie anterior to the axis of motion; therefore they produce motion in the sagittal plane. The flexor muscles of the wrist act synergistically with finger extension.

Position.   Subject sits with forearm supinated and resting on a table.

Activity.   Subject lifts a weight or object placed in the hand (Fig. 6–28).

Muscles.   Flexor carpi radialis, palmaris longus, flexor carpi ulnaris.

Types of Contraction
· Concentric: Lifting the weight.
· Eccentric: Lowering the weight back to the table.

Resistance
· The weight offers the resistance.
· Functional: 5-pound weight.
· Functionally Fair: 3- to 4-pound weight.
· Functionally Poor: 1- to 2-pound weight.
· Nonfunctional: 0 weight.

Wrist Extension

Functional wrist extensor muscles are most important in maintaining the length–tension relationship for grippng objects. They act synergistically with the finger flexors. The functional position of the wrist is approximately 45

degrees of extension, the hand position best adapted for prehension.

Position.   Subject sits with the forearm supported in pronation.

Activity.   Subject is asked to grasp and lift a small object that can be held in the palm of the hand (Fig. 6–29).

Muscles.   Extensor carpi radialis longus, extensor carpi radialis brevis, extensor carpi ulnaris.

Types of Contraction
· Concentric: Lifting and grasping the weight.
· Eccentric: Lowering and releasing the weight.
· Isometric: Holding the wrist extended.

Resistance
· Functional: 5 repetitions.
· Functionally Fair: 3 to 4 repetitions.
· Functionally Poor: 1 to 2 repetitions.
· Nonfunctional: 0 repetitions.

Wrist Radial Deviation

The muscles that flex and extend the wrist also produce deviation; if they lie on the radial side of the midline of the wrist they radially deviate or abduct.

Postion.   Subject sits with the forearm in a position between supination and pronation.

Activity.   Subject holds a weight in the hand and lifts and lowers it to the table (Fig. 6–30).

Muscles.   Extensor carpi radialis longus, flexor carpi radialis, extensor pollicis longus, extensor pollicis brevis, and abductor pollicis longus.

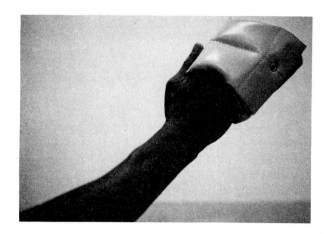

Figure 6–30. Resisted radial deviation at the wrist joint.

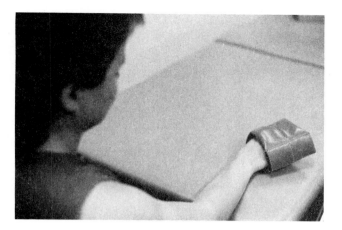

Figure 6–31. Resisted ulnar deviation at the wrist joint.

Types of Contraction
• Concentric: Lifting the weight from the table.

Resistance
• The weight offers the resistance.
• Functional: 5 repetitions.
• Functionally Fair: 3 to 4 repetitions.
• Functionally Poor: 1 to 2 repetitions.
• Nonfunctional: 0 repetitions.

Wrist Ulnar Deviation

The muscles that flex and extend the wrist also produce ulnar deviation when they lie medial to the axis for motion. A common activity that requires ulnar deviation of the wrist is writing.

Position. Subject sits with forearm pronated.

Activity. Subject holds a weight in the hand and moves it across the table (Fig. 6–31).

Muscles. Extensor carpi ulnaris, flexor carpi ulnaris, extensor digiti minimi.

Types of Contraction
• Concentric: Pushing the weight ulnarly.

Resistance
• The weight offers the resistance.
• Functional: 5 repetitions.
• Functionally Fair: 3 to 4 repetitions.
• Functionally Poor: 1 to 2 repetitions.
• Nonfunctional: 0 repetitions.

Hand

The versatility of the hand is improved by the kinematic chain of the upper limb. The hand is a mechanism for expression of our thoughts; it also enables us to feel our environment and to perform skilled activities. The thumb gives the hand prehensile ability.

Thumb

The thumb has both intrinsic and extrinsic muscles. The extrinsic muscles provide for the length–tension needed by the thumb by extending the wrist. The intrinsic or thenar muscles are active in most grasping activities, regardless of the precision needed. The thumb is not always involved in prehension.

Thumb Flexion

For flexion of the interphalangeal joint to occur alone, the extensor pollicis brevis muscle must contract to prevent flexion of the metacarpophalangeal joint. Prehension by terminal opposition is the finest and most precise form of prehension; it allows one to hold a thin object or pick up a very fine object like a pin or a toothpick. The long thumb flexor stabilizes the distal phalanx. Subterminal opposition is the most common type of prehension. It allows one to hold a relatively large object like a pencil or a piece of paper. The interphalangeal joint is usually extended and the metacarpophalangeal joint is usually flexed.

Position. Subject sits with the forearm supported and in a position midway between supination and pronation.

Activity. Subject is asked to flex the thumbs against the tension of a rubber band (Fig. 6–32).

Muscles. Flexor pollicis longus, flexor pollicis brevis.

Types of Contraction
• Concentric: Pulling against a rubber band.

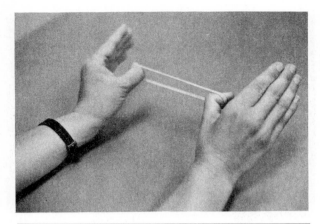

Figure 6–32. Resisted thumb flexion.

Resistance
- Slight; function is based on dexterity.
- Functional: 5 repetitions.
- Functionally Fair: 3 or 4 repetitions.
- Functionally Poor: 1 or 2 repetitions.
- Nonfunctional: 0 repetitions.

Thumb Extension

For extension of the thumb to occur, the wrist joint must be stabilized by the synergistic contraction of the flexor and extensor carpi ulnaris muscles; otherwise the wrist will abduct. The extensor pollicis longus is positioned to adduct the first metacarpal joint.

Position. Subject sits with forearm resting on a table. A rubber band is placed around the distal phalanx of the thumb and the proximal phalanx of the index or middle finger.

Activity. Subject moves the thumb away from the palm against the tension of the rubber band (Fig. 6–33).

Muscles. Extensor pollicis longus, extensor pollicis brevis.

Types of Contraction
- Concentric: Moving the thumb away from the palm.
- Eccentric: Allowing the thumb to return to the starting position.

Resistance
- The rubber band offers the resistance.
- Functional: 5 repetitions.
- Functionally Fair: 3 or 4 repetitions.
- Functionally Poor: 1 or 2 repetitions.
- Nonfunctional: 0 repetitions.

Thumb Abduction

Abduction of the thumb is an important factor in performing thumb opposition, as the thumb must be raised from the palm. The thumb must move away from the palm to perform precision grasp and many of the power grips.

Position. Subject sits with forearm resting on a table. A rubber band is placed around the distal end of the thumb and the proximal phalanx of another digit.

Activity. Subject moves the thumb at a 90-degree angle from the palm against the tension of the rubber band (Fig. 6–34).

Muscles. Abductor pollicis longus, abductor pollicis brevis.

Types of Contraction
- Concentric: Moving away from the palm at a 90-degree angle.

Resistance
- The tension in the rubber band offers the resistance.
- Functional: 5 repetitions.

Figure 6–33. Resisted thumb extension.

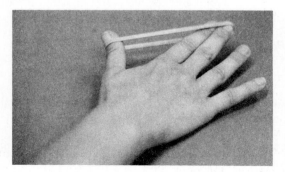

Figure 6–34. Resisted thumb abduction.

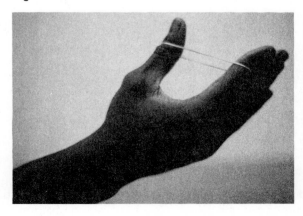

- Functionally Fair: 3 or 4 repetitions.
- Functionally Poor: 1 or 2 repetitions.
- Nonfunctional: 0 repetitions.

Thumb Adduction

When the thumb is moved away from the palm to grasp an object, it must adduct to maintain the grasp. Power grips such as cylindrical, spherical, and lateral prehension require adduction of the thumb.

Position. Subject sits with forearm resting on a table and thumb positioned next to the index finger.

Activity. Subject holds a piece of paper, in a lateral prehension position, against the pull from the examiner (Fig. 6–35).

Muscle. Adductor pollicis.

Types of Contraction
- Isometric: Holding against the pull from the examiner.

Resistance
- The examiner pulling on the paper offers the resistance.
- Functional: 5 seconds.
- Functionally Fair: 3 to 4 seconds.
- Functionally Poor: 1 to 2 seconds.
- Nonfunctional: 0 seconds.

Thumb Opposition

Bringing the distal pad of the thumb in contact with the pad of any other digit is an essential function of the hand. Loss of this function makes the hand virtually useless. Opposition of the thumb (tip to tip) is required in precision prehension, as in holding a pin or a very small object. Pad-to-pad prehension, as in holding a coin, requires opposition of the thumb also.

Position. Subject sits with forearm resting on a table. Subject holds a piece of paper between the pads of the thumb and the index finger.

Activity. Subject holds the paper against the resistance of the examiner pulling on it (Fig. 6–36).

Muscles. Opponens pollicis.

Types of Contraction
- Isometric: Holding the paper against the pull by the examiner.

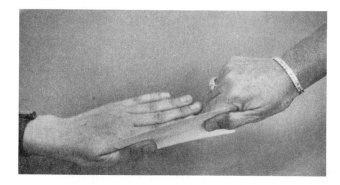

Figure 6–35. Resisted thumb adduction.

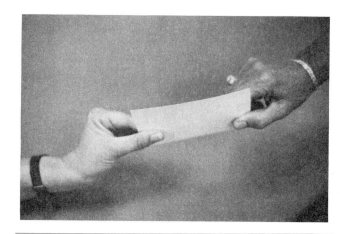

Figure 6–36. Resisted thumb opposition.

Resistance
- The examiner pulling on the paper offers the resistance.
- Functional: 5 seconds.
- Functionally Fair: 3 to 4 seconds.
- Functionally Poor: 1 to 2 seconds.
- Nonfunctional: 0 seconds.

Fingers

To maintain optimal length and tension for the function of the fingers, the wrist musculature must contract synergistically to counterbalance the force exerted by the finger muscles. If this counterbalance is not developed, the finger flexors lose their tension and power.

Finger Flexion

The flexor digitorum profundus is generally more active than the flexor digitorum superficialis. Its attachment on the distal phalanx allows the muscle to flex all joints of the digits. The flexor digitorum superficialis functions only when there is no need for distal interphalangeal flexion or during power-resistive activities.

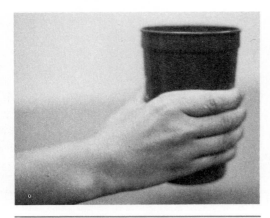

Figure 6–37.   Resisted finger flexion.

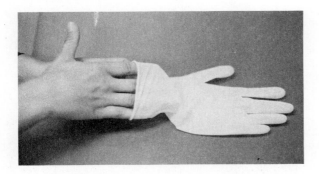

Figure 6–38.   Resisted finger extension.

Position.   Subject sits with forearm resting on a table, midway between supination and pronation.

Activity.   Subject grasps, picks up, and releases a mug, glass, or any object that requires a cylindrical grip (Fig. 6–37).

Muscles.   Flexor digitorum profundus, flexor digitorum superficialis.

Types of Contraction
· Concentric: Grasping the glass.

Resistance
· The glass offers the resistance.
· Functional: 5 repetitions.
· Functionally Fair: 3 to 4 repetitions.
· Functionally Poor: 1 to 2 repetitions.
· Nonfunctional: 0 repetitions.

Finger Extension

Extension is accomplished by both the extrinsic and intrinsic extensor musculature. The extrinsic muscles ex-tend the metacarpophalangeal joints and the intrinsic muscles extend the interphalangeal joints. The fingers move together in extension, but may move singly, as in playing the piano. The power with which these muscles contract depends on the position of the wrist joint. Writing with a pencil alternately uses the finger flexors and extensors at the interphalangeal and metacarpophalangeal joints.

Position.   Subject sits with forearm resting on a table, midway between supination and pronation.

Activity.   Subject places the hand into a glove (Fig. 6–38).

Muscles.   Extensor digitorum, extensor digiti minimi, extensor indicis, lumbricals, and dorsal and palmar interossei.

Types of Contraction
· Isometric: Keeping fingers straight to fit into appropriate finger slot.

Resistance
· The friction of the glove offers the resistance.
· Functional: 2 seconds.
· Functionally Fair: 4 to 5 seconds.
· Functionally Poor: 10 to 20 seconds.
· Nonfunctional: 21+ seconds.

Finger Abduction

The dorsal interossei have twice the muscle mass of the palmar interossei and, therefore, are stronger.

Position.   Subject sits with forearms resting on a table.

Activity.   Subject pulls against the tension of a rubber band, or the examiner may offer resistance to the motion (Fig. 6–39).

Types of Contraction
· Concentric: Pulling into abduction of the fingers.
· Isometric: Holding against the tension of the rubber band or manual resistance.

Resistance
· The rubber band offers the resistance.
· Functional: 5 seconds.
· Functionally Fair: 3 to 4 seconds.
· Functionally Poor: 1 to 2 seconds.
· Nonfunctional: 0 seconds.

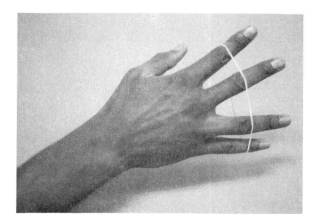

Figure 6–39. Resisted finger abduction.

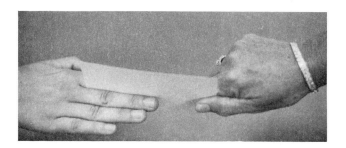

Figure 6–40. Resisted finger adduction.

Finger Adduction

The palmar interossei are responsible for adducting the index, ring, and little fingers. Both the dorsal and palmar interossei may be tested by having the subject hold a piece of paper between the fingers.

Position. Subject sits with forearm resting on a table.

Activity. Subject holds a piece of paper between the fingers (Fig. 6–40).

Muscles. Palmar interossei.

Types of Contraction
- Isometric: Holding the paper against the resistance of the tester pulling on the paper.

Resistance
- Holding the paper against a pull from the examiner.
- Functional: 5 seconds.
- Functionally Fair: 3 to 4 seconds.
- Functionally Poor: 1 to 2 seconds.
- Nonfunctional: 0 seconds.

Manual Muscle Testing

Wrist

Flexor Carpi Radialis Muscle

The flexor carpi radialis muscle produces the motion of wrist flexion from a starting position of extension. All grades are tested with the subject in the sitting or supine position with the forearm resting on a table. The fingers should remain relaxed.

Palpation. The tendon is superficial at the level of the carpal creases. It is palpated slightly lateral to the midline of the wrist (Fig. 6–41).

Position
- AG: The dorsal surface of the hand rests on the table with the fingers in slight flexion (Fig. 6–42).
- GM: Subject is positioned with the ulnar border of the hand resting on the table. Fingers are relaxed in flexion (Fig. 6–43).

Movement. Flexion of the wrist with radial deviation.

Resistance. Applied to palm of the hand into extension and ulnar deviation.

Stabilization. Forearm is stabilized.

Substitutions
- Subject may hyperextend the wrist, then relax, giving the appearance of flexion.

Figure 6–41. Palpation for flexor carpi radialis muscle.

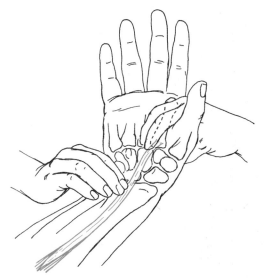

Attachments of Flexor Carpi Radialis Muscle

Muscle	Proximal	Distal	Innervation
Flexor carpi radialis	Common flexor tendon from medial epicondyle of humerus	Base of second and third metacarpal palmar surface	Median C7 (C6)

Attachments of Flexor Carpi Ulnaris Muscle

Muscle	Proximal	Distal	Innervation
Flexor carpi ulnaris	Common flexor tendon from humeral medial epicondyle, medial aspect of olecranon, and proximal border of ulna	Pisiform bone, hamate, and base of fifth metacarpal	Ulnar C8 (C7)

· Keep fingers relaxed to prevent substitution by finger flexors.
· Palpate to determine the functions of each muscle.

Flexor Carpi Ulnaris Muscle

The flexor carpi ulnaris muscle produces the motions of wrist flexion and adduction, or ulnar deviation. The test motion is wrist flexion to 90 degrees with accompanying ulnar deviation from the anatomical starting position.

Palpation. Flexor carpi ulnaris tendon is superficial and palpable immediately proximal to the pisiform (Fig. 6–44).

Position
· AG: Subject sits or lies supine with the forearm supinated and the dorsal surface of the hand resting on a table, with the fingers in slight flexion.
· GM: Subject is positioned as above but with the ulnar border of the hand resting on the table. The fingers are relaxed in slight flexion (see Figs. 6–42 and 6–43).

Movement. Flexion of the wrist joint through the test range accompanied by ulnar deviation.

Resistance. Applied to the palm of the hand into extension and radial deviation.

Stabilization. The forearm is stabilized.

Figure 6–42. Testing the flexor carpi radialis muscle in the AG position.

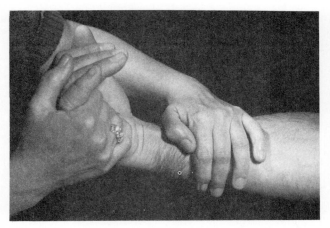

Figure 6–43. Testing the flexor carpi radialis muscle in the GM position.

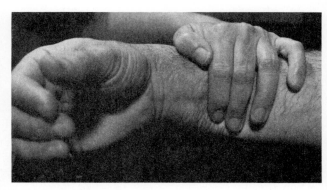

Attachments of Palmaris Longus Muscle

Muscle	Proximal	Distal	Innervation
Palmaris longus	Common flexor tendon from medial epicondyle	Palmar fascia	Median C8 (C7)

Substitutions
- Subject may hyperextend the wrist then relax, giving the appearance of flexion. Keep the fingers relaxed to prevent substitution by the finger flexors.
- Palpate to determine the function of ulnar deviation.

Palmaris Longus Muscle

The palmaris longus muscle may or may not be present. It is absent in 15 to 20 percent of the population. When present, it is located in the midline of the wrist and performs wrist flexion without deviations into abduction or adduction. It does not have a bony attachment distally but rather pulls on the palmar fascia during wrist flexion.

Palpation. If present, the tendon is superficial at the level of the carpal creases in the midline of the wrist. The tendon is more prominent if the hand is cupped during the motion of wrist flexion (Fig. 6–45).

Position
- AG: Subject sits with the dorsal surface of the hand resting on the table and the fingers relaxed.
- GM: Subject sits with the hand resting on the ulnar border and the fingers relaxed (see Figs. 6–42 and 6–43).

Movement. Flexion of the wrist.

Resistance. Applied to the palm of the hand into extension.

Stabilization. The forearm is stabilized.

Substitutions
- The superficial finger flexors may be palpated instead of the palmaris longus.
- Hyperextension of the wrist may give the appearance of wrist joint flexion.
- Prevent substitution by finger flexors by keeping them relaxed.

Extensor Carpi Radialis Longus Muscle

The extensor carpi radialis longus muscle produces the movement of wrist hyperextension and radial deviation from a starting position of flexion. For all grades of testing, the subject is either sitting or supine. The fingers must be relaxed.

Palpation. With the forearm pronated, the examiner palpates on the radiodorsal aspect of the wrist proximal to the second metacarpal (Fig. 6–46).

Position
- AG: The hand rests on the palmar surface on the table with the fingers relaxed in flexion (Fig. 6–47).

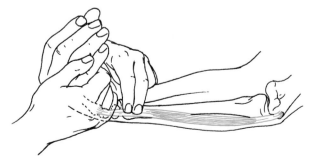

Figure 6–44. Palpation for the flexor carpi ulnaris muscle.

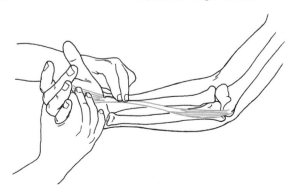

Figure 6–45. Palpation for the palmaris longus muscle.

Attachments of Extensor Carpi Radialis Longus Muscle

Muscle	Proximal	Distal	Innervation
Extensor carpi radialis longus	Distal third of lateral supracondylar ridge of humerus	Base of second metacarpal, dorsal surface	Radial C6 and C7

- GM: The hand rests on the ulnar border and the table with the fingers relaxed (Fig. 6–48).

Movement. Extend the wrist, with radial deviation.

Resistance. Applied to the dorsum of the hand into flexion and ulnar deviation.

Stabilization. Forearm is stabilized.

Substitutions
- The subject may flex the wrist, then relax.
- Keep the fingers relaxed in flexion to prevent substitution by extensor digitorum.

Figure 6–46. Palpation for the extensor carpi radialis longus muscle.

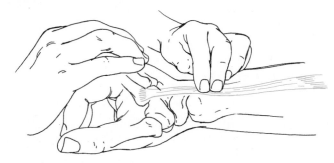

Figure 6–47. Testing the extensor carpi radialis longus muscle in the AG position.

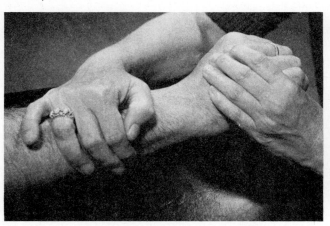

Extensor Carpi Radialis Brevis Muscle

The extensor carpi radialis brevis tendon is located over the axis for the wrist joint; it participates in the extension of the wrist joint, with no deviation.

Palpation. The extensor carpi radialis brevis is somewhat difficult to palpate. With the subject's forearm pronated and the hand off the table, the examiner places a finger in the depression over the capitate bone. The subject is asked to abduct the thumb in the sagittal plane. The extensor carpi radialis brevis contracts as a synergist to stabilize the wrist (Fig. 6–49).

Position
- AG: Subject sits with the palmar surface of the hand resting on a table, keeping the fingers relaxed in flexion.
- GM: Subject's hand rests on the ulnar border, with the fingers relaxed in flexion (see Figs. 6–47 and 6–48).

Movement. Extend the wrist.

Resistance. Applied to the dorsum of the hand into flexion.

Stabilization. The forearm is stabilized.

Figure 6–48. Testing the extensor carpi radialis longus muscle in the GM position.

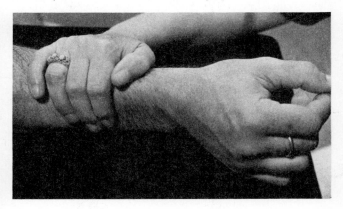

Attachments of Extensor Carpi Radialis Brevis Muscle

Muscle	Proximal	Distal	Innervation
Extensor carpi radialis brevis	Common extensor tendon from lateral epicondyle and radial collateral ligament	Base of third metacarpal	Radial C7 and C8

Attachments of Extensor Carpi Ulnaris Muscle

Muscle	Proximal	Distal	Innervation
Extensor carpi ulnaris	Common extensor tendon from lateral epicondyle of humerus and posterior aspect of ulna	Base of fifth metacarpal, medial side	Radial C8 (C7)

Substitutions
- Subject may flex the wrist, then relax.
- Keep the fingers relaxed in flexion.

Extensor Carpi Ulnaris Muscle

The extensor carpi ulnaris muscle produces the movements of wrist hyperextension and ulnar deviation. The muscle is tested as a wrist extensor muscle working in synergy with the extensor carpi radialis longus and brevis muscles.

Palpation. The extensor carpi ulnaris is palpated between the head of the ulna and the tubercle of the fifth metacarpal (Fig. 6–50).

Position
- AG: Subject sits with the hand on its palmar surface and the fingers relaxed.
- GM: Subject sits with the hand resting on its ul-

nar border, with the fingers relaxed (see Figs. 6–47 and 6–48).

Movement. Extend and deviate the wrist toward the ulna.

Resistance. Applied to the dorsum of the hand into flexion and radial deviation.

Stabilization. The forearm is stabilized.

Substitutions
- Subject may flex the wrist, then relax.
- Keep the fingers relaxed.

Fingers

Each finger is tested separately. Gravity has little effect on the fingers or thumb, therefore the test position may be any comfortable position, usually sitting or supine.

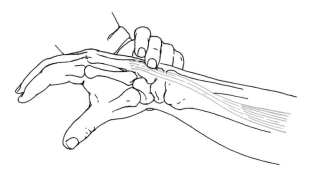

Figure 6–49. Palpation for the extensor carpi radialis brevis muscle.

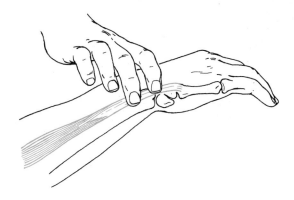

Figure 6–50. Palpation for the extensor carpi ulnaris muscle.

Attachments of Flexor Digitorum Superficialis Muscle

Muscle	Proximal	Distal	Innervation
Flexor digitorum superficialis	Common flexor tendon from medial epicondyle of humerus, ulnar collateral ligament, coronoid process of ulna, and oblique line on radius	Four tendon slips to each side of middle phalanx of medial four fingers	Median C8 (C7 and T1)

The grading key differs for the fingers and thumb (see Chap. 2). No half grades are given.

Flexor Digitorum Superficialis Muscle

The flexor digitorum superficialis muscle is a flexor of the proximal interphalangeal joints of the second through the fifth digits. The muscle assists in wrist and metacarpophalangeal joint flexion. The movement is 120 degrees of flexion of the proximal interphalangeal joints

Figure 6–51. Palpation for the flexor digitorum superficialis muscle.

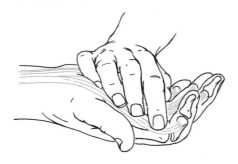

Figure 6–52. Testing position for the flexor digitorum superficialis muscle.

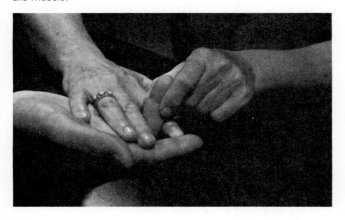

with the metacarpophalangeal joints in extension. All grades are determined with the forearm in supination; each finger is evaluated independently.

Palpation.   The flexor digitorum superficialis muscle or tendon is palpated where it crosses the palmar surface of each proximal phalanx (Fig. 6–51).

Position.   The hand rests on a table on its dorsal surface. Both the wrist and metacarpal joints are in a neutral position (Fig. 6–52).

Movement.   Flexion of the proximal interphalangeal joint without flexion of the distal interphalangeal joint. To test the flexor digitorum superficialis, the distal joint must remain inactive.

Resistance.   Applied to the palmar surface of the middle phalanx.

Stabilization.   Proximal phalanx and palm of the hand are stabilized; tips of the fingers are relaxed.

Substitutions
- Subject may quickly extend the proximal interphalangeal joint.
- The flexor digitorum profundus can cause substitute motion, flexing the distal interphalangeal joints.

Flexor Digitorum Profundus Muscle

The movement produced by the flexor digitorum profundus muscle is flexion of the distal interphalangeal joints of the second through the fifth digits, with the other finger joints remaining in extension. The muscle may assist in proximal interphalangeal joint and metacarpophalangeal joint flexion. The flexor digitorum profundus muscle is the only muscle that flexes the distal interphalangeal joint. All grades are determined with the

Attachments of Flexor Digitorum Profundus Muscle

Muscle	Proximal	Distal	Innervation
Flexor digitorum profundus	Anterior and medial surfaces of proximal three quarters of ulna	Four tendon slips to base of each distal phalanx of the medial four fingers	Radial two—medial; ulnar two—ulnar C8 (T1)

forearm in supination; each finger is evaluated independently.

Palpation.   Palpate each tendon where it crosses the palmar surface of each middle phalanx of the medial four digits (Fig. 6–53).

Position.   The hand rests on its dorsal surface on a table. Both the wrist and metacarpal joints are in a neutral position (Fig. 6–54).

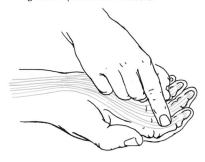

Figure 6–53.   Palpation for the flexor digitorum profundus muscle.

Figure 6–54.   Testing position for the flexor digitorum profundus muscle.

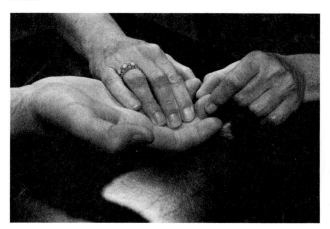

Movement.   Flexion of the distal interphalangeal joints; fingers not being tested are allowed to flex.

Resistance.   Applied to the palmar surface of the distal phalanx.

Stabilization.   The middle phalanx and proximal interphalangeal joint are stabilized.

Substitutions
- Subject may quickly extend the distal interphalangeal joint, then relax.

Extensor Digitorum, Extensor Indicis, Extensor Digiti Minimi Muscles

The test movement for the extensor digitorum, extensor indicis, and extensor digiti minimi is extension at the metacarpophalangeal joints from a starting position of flexion. Motion occurs at each of the medial metacarpophalangeal joints simultaneously. The upper limb rests on the table with the forearm pronated. All grades are tested in the sitting position.

Palpation

Extensor Digitorum.   Palpate each tendon where it crosses the dorsal aspect of the palm (Fig. 6–55).

Extensor indicis.   Palpate over the dorsal aspect of the second metacarpal, close to the head. It is the tendon closer to the ulna (Fig. 6–56).

Extensor Digiti Minimi.   Palpate over the dorsal aspect of the fifth metacarpal, close to the head of the ulna (Fig. 6–57).

Position.   The hand rests on its palmar surface on a table with the wrist in a neutral position. The metacarpophalangeal joints are flexed 90 degrees off the edge of the table (Fig. 6–58).

Movement.   Extension of the metacarpal joints, with interphalangeal joints flexed.

Attachments of Extensor Digitorum, Extensor Indicis, and Extensor Digiti Minimi Muscles

Muscle	Proximal	Distal	Innervation
Extensor digitorum	Common extensor tendon on lateral epicondyle of humerus	Four tendons, from second to fifth digit through extensor hood to base of distal phalanx	Radial C7 (C8)
Extensor indicis	Distal posterior surface of ulna	Into extensor hood of index finger with extensor digitorum	Radial C8 (C7)
Extensor digiti minimi	Common extensor tendon of lateral epicondyle of humerus	Into extensor hood of fifth finger with extensor digitorum	Radial C7 (C8)

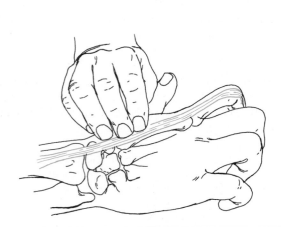

Figure 6–55. Palpation for the extensor digitorum muscle.

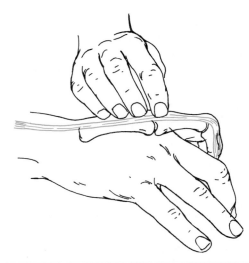

Figure 6–56. Palpation for the extensor indicis muscle.

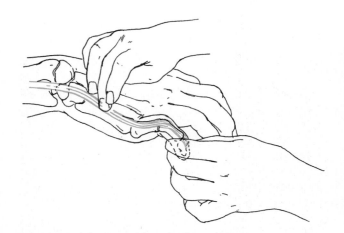

Figure 6–57. Palpation for the extensor digiti minimi muscle.

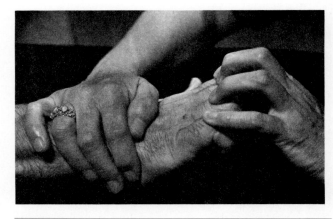

Figure 6–58. Testing position for the extensor digitorum, extensor indicis, and extensor digiti minimi muscles.

Attachments of Lumbrical Muscles

Muscle	Proximal	Distal	Innervation
First and second lumbricals	Radial side of flexor digitorum profundus tendon to index and middle fingers	Radial side of extensor expansion of the medial four fingers	Median T1 (C8)
Third and fourth lumbricals	Adjacent sides of flexor digitorum tendon to ring and little fingers		Ulnar T1 (C8)

Resistance. Applied to the distal end of the proximal phalanx on the dorsal aspect.

Stabilization. Stabilize the hand and wrist.

Substitutions
- Subject may quickly flex the metacarpophalangeal joints, then relax.
- Wrist flexion puts tension on the extensor tendons.
- Lumbricals can cause extension of the interphalangeal joints.

Lumbrical Muscles

The lumbrical muscles perform the motion of interphalangeal joint extension with the metacarpophalangeal joints held in extension. The forearm is pronated and the wrist extended. Other authors state that the lumbrical muscles produce metacarpophalangeal joint flexion simultaneously with interphalangeal joint extension.

Palpation. Because of their size and position, the lumbricals usually cannot be palpated. Therefore a "1" or "T" grade cannot be given.

Position
- Preferred: The hand rests on its palmar surface with the middle and distal phalanges flexed over the edge of the table. The metacarpophalangeal joints are supported in extension by the table. (Fig. 6–59).
- Alternate: Hand rests on palmar surface with the proximal, middle, and distal phalanges extended off the table.

Movement
- Preferred: Extension of the proximal and distal interphalangeal joints.

- Alternate: Flexion of the metacarpophalangeal joint with the proximal and distal interphalangeal joints maintained in extension.

Resistance
- Preferred: Applied to the dorsal surface of the middle and distal phalanges. The medial four fingers may be resisted simultaneously or separately.
- Alternate: Apply resistance to the palmar surface of the proximal phalanx.

Stabilization. Stabilize under the proximal phalanx of the fingers being tested. With the other hand, stabilize the wrist and metacarpophalangeal joint in the neutral position.

Substitions
- Extensor digitorum can cause hyperextension of the metacarpophalangeal joints.
- Flexion of the interphalangeal joints followed by relaxation can substitute.
- Maintain the metacarpophalangeal joints in extension.

Figure 6–59. Testing position for the lumbrical muscles.

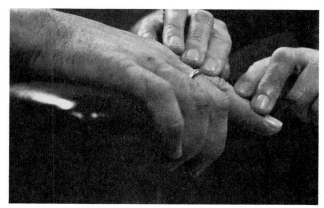

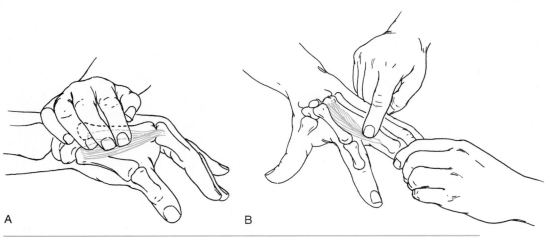

Figure 6–60.   (A) Palpation for the first dorsal interosseous muscle. (B) Palpation for the second dorsal interosseous muscle.

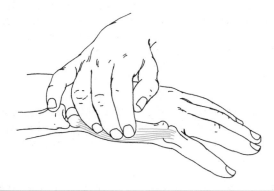

Figure 6–61.   Palpation for the abductor digiti minimi muscle.

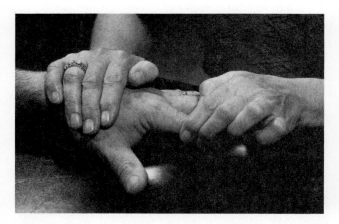

Figure 6–62.   Testing position for the first dorsal interosseous muscle.

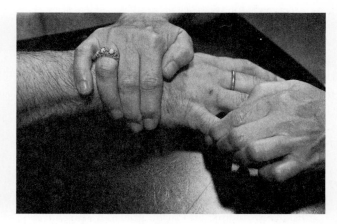

Figure 6–63.   Testing position for the abductor digiti minimi muscle.

Attachments of Dorsal Interossei and Abductor Digiti Minimi Muscles

Muscle	Proximal	Distal	Innervation
Dorsal interossei:	Between each metacarpal on adjacent sides		Ulnar T1 (C8)
First and second		Radial side of extensor expansion of index and middle fingers	
Third and fourth		Ulnar side of extensor expansion of midde and ring fingers	
Abductor digiti minimi	Pisiform bone and tendon of flexor carpi ulnaris muscle	Base of proximal phalanx of fifth finger and ulnar aspect of extensor expansion	Ulnar T1 (C8)

Dorsal Interossei, Abductor Digiti Minimi Muscles

The dorsal interossei and the abductor digiti minimi muscles produce the test motion of abduction, with the fingers in extension. The forearm is pronated and the wrist extended.

Palpations

Dorsal Interossei. Palpate the first dorsal interossei on the radial side of the second metacarpal; palpate the tendon of the second on the radial side of the proximal phalanx of the middle finger; palpate the tendon of the third on the ulnar side of the proximal phalanx of the middle finger; palpate the tendon of the fourth on the ulnar side of the proximal phalanx of the ring finger (Fig. 6–60).

Abductor Digiti Minimi. Palpate along the ulnar border of the fifth metacarpal (Fig. 6–61).

Position. The hand rests on its palmar surface on a table, with the wrist in a neutral position and the fingers extended (Figs. 6–62 and 6–63).

Movement. Move the index, ring, and little fingers away from the middle finger; the middle finger moves toward the index and ring fingers.

Resistance. Applied to the side of the distal end of the proximal phalanx of each of the four fingers.

Stabilization. Hand and fingers not being tested are stabilized.

Substitutions
- When the metacarpophalangeal joints hyperextend, they also abduct.

- Wrist flexors put extensor tendons on a stretch, which produces abduction by tendon action. Do not allow subject to push down onto the table.
- Lumbricals may assist in abduction.

Palmar Interossei Muscles

The palmar interossei muscles produce the motion of adduction of the fingers from a starting position of abduction. The forearm is pronated and the wrist and fingers are extended.

Palpation. The three tendons cross the metacarpophalangeal joints (Fig. 6–64). Palpate the first interosseous on the ulnar side of the proximal phalanx of the index finger. Palpate the second interosseous on the radial side of the proximal phalanx of the ring finger. Palpate the third interosseous on the radial side of the proximal phalanx of the little finger.

Figure 6–64. Palpation for the first palmar interosseous muscle.

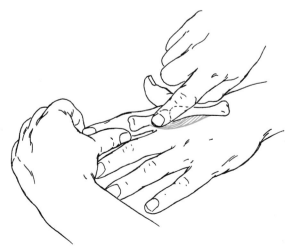

Attachments of Palmar Interossei Muscles

Muscle	Proximal	Distal	Innervation
Palmar interossei: First	Length of ulnar side of second metacarpal	Ulnar side of extensor expansion and proximal phalanx of index finger	Ulnar T1 (C8)
Second	Length of radial side of fourth metacarpal	Radial side of extensor expansion and proximal phalanx of ring finger	
Third	Length of radial side of fifth metacarpal	Radial side of extensor expansion and proximal phalanx of little finger	

Position. The hand rests on its palmar surface, with the wrist and fingers in an extended position (Fig. 6–65).

Movement. Move index, ring, and little fingers toward the middle finger from the starting position of abduction.

Resistance. Applied to the side of the distal end of the proximal phalanx.

Stabilization. The hand and fingers that are not being tested are stabilized.

Substitutions
· Finger flexors will cause the metacarpophalangeal joints to flex. Do not let the fingers press down onto table.
· If the wrist is allowed to extend, the metacarpophalangeal joints will passively flex and adduct.
· Extensor digitorum and extensor indicis may cause adduction of the index finger.
· The lumbricals may assist in adduction.

Figure 6–65. Testing position for the first palmar interosseous muscle.

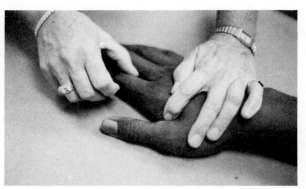

Flexor Pollicis Longus, Flexor Pollicis Brevis Muscles

The flexor pollicis longus and the flexor pollicis brevis muscles produce the flexion motion at the metacarpophalangeal and interphalangeal joints. During the test, the forearm is placed in supination and is supported by the table.

Palpation
· Palpate the tendon of the flexor pollicis longus where it crosses the palmar surface of the proximal phalanx of the thumb (Fig. 6–66).
· Palpate the muscle belly of the flexor pollicis brevis on the ulnar side of the first metacarpal (Fig. 6–67).

Position. The hand is resting on its dorsal surface on a table; the wrist is in a neutral position, and the thumb is adducted (Figs. 6–68 and 6–69).

Movement. Flexion of the metacarpophalangeal and interphalangeal joints in the coronal plane.

Resistance. Applied to the proximal phalanx for the flexor pollicis brevis and the distal phalanx for the flexor pollicis longus.

Stabilization. The first metacarpal is stabilized for the flexor pollicis brevis and the proximal phalanx for the flexor pollicis longus.

Substitutions
· The flexor pollicis longus instead of the brevis flexes the interphalangeal joint.
· The abductor pollicis brevis and adductor pollicis together may flex the metacarpophalangeal joint.
· Quick extension and relaxation of the interphalangeal joint may give the appearance of interphalangeal flexion.

Attachments of Flexor Pollicis Longus and Flexor Pollicis Brevis Muscles

Muscle	Proximal	Distal	Innervation
Flexor pollicis longus	Anterior shaft of radius, interosseous membrane, and coronoid process of ulna	Base of distal phalanx of thumb, palmar surface	Median C8 (T1)
Flexor pollicis brevis	Trapezium bone, trapezoid, and capitate, and flexor retinaculum	Base of proximal phalanx of thumb on radial side	Median and ulnar C8 (T1)

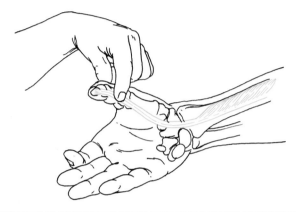

Figure 6–66. Palpation for the flexor pollicis longus muscle.

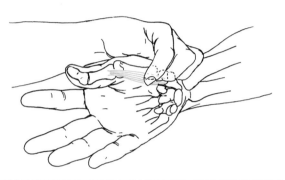

Figure 6–67. Palpation for the flexor pollicis brevis muscle.

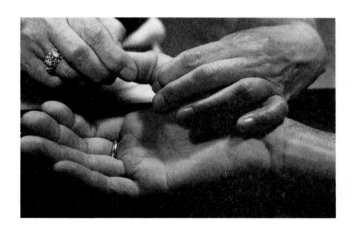

Figure 6–68. Testing position for the flexor pollicis longus muscle.

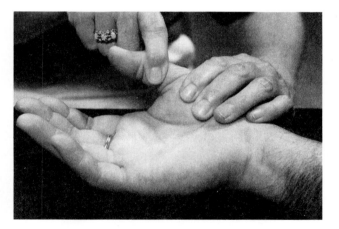

Figure 6–69. Testing position for the flexor pollicis brevis muscle.

Extensor Pollicis Longus, Extensor Pollicis Brevis Muscles

The extensor pollicis longus and brevis muscles produce the motion of extension at the metacarpophalangeal and interphalangeal joints from a starting position of complete flexion.

Palpation

- Palpate the tendon of the extensor pollicis longus where it crosses the dorsal aspect at the base of the first metacarpophalangeal joint directed toward the distal phalanx (Fig. 6–70).
- Palpate the tendon of the extensor pollicis brevis where it crosses the lateral aspect of the base of the first metacarpophalangeal joint directed toward the proximal phalanx (Fig. 6–71).

Position. The hand rests with the ulnar border on the table. With the extensor pollicis brevis, the metacarpophalangeal joint is flexed and abducted. With the extensor pollicis longus, the metacarpophalangeal joint is abducted and the interphalangeal joint flexed (Figs. 6–72 and 6–73).

Movement. Extension of the metacarpophalangeal and interphalangeal joints individually.

Resistance. Applied to the dorsal surface of the proximal phalanx for the extensor pollicis brevis and to the dorsal surface of the distal phalanx for the extensor pollicis longus.

Stabilization. The first metacarpal is stabilized for the brevis muscle and the proximal phalanx and metacarpal for the longus muscle.

Figure 6–70. Palpation for the extensor pollicis longus muscle.

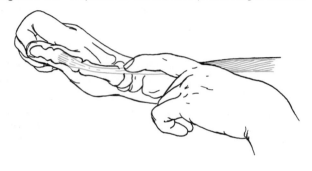

Figure 6–71. Palpation for the extensor pollicis brevis muscle.

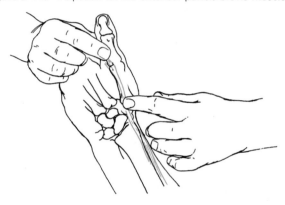

Figure 6–72. Testing position for the extensor pollicis longus muscle.

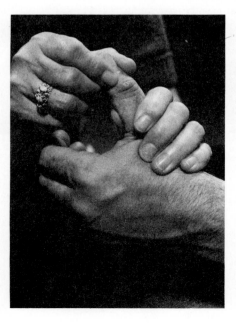

Figure 6–73. Testing position for the extensor pollicis brevis muscle.

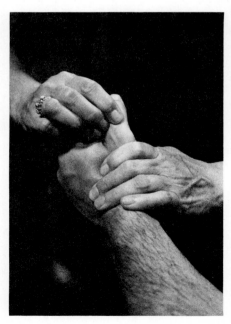

Attachments of Extensor Pollicis Longus and Extensor Pollicis Brevis Muscles

Muscles	Proximal	Distal	Innervation
Extensor pollicis longus	Middle third posterior aspect of ulna	Base of interphalangeal joint of thumb	Radial C8 (C7)
Extensor pollicis brevis	Posterior surface distally on radius	Base of proximal phalanx of thumb	Radial C8 (C7)

Attachments of Abductor Pollicis Longus and Abductor Pollicis Brevis Muscles

Muscle	Proximal	Distal	Innervation
Abductor pollicis longus	Posterior aspect of shaft of distal ulna and mid radius	Base of first metacarpal, radial side	Radial C8 (C7)
Abductor pollicis brevis	Anterior aspect of scaphoid, trapezium bones, and flexor retinaculum	Base of proximal phalanx, radial side	Median C8 (T1)

Substitutions

- The extensor pollicis longus may extend the metacarpophalangeal joint.
- Quick flexion and relaxation of the metacarpophalangeal joint may substitute.
- Quick flexion and relaxation of the interphalangeal joint may substitute.

Abductor Pollicis Longus, Abductor Pollicis Brevis Muscles

The abductor pollicis longus and brevis muscles produce the movement of abduction at the carpometacarpal joint. The test movements occur in the sagittal plane through a range of 75 degrees for the abductor pollicis brevis muscle, and in the frontal plane for the abductor pollicis

longus muscle. The metacarpophalangeal and the interphalangeal joints should remain flexed when one examines the abductor pollicis longus muscle, to lessen the effect of the thumb extensors. The forearm is positioned midway between supination and pronation or is completely supinated.

Palpation

Abductor Pollicis Longus. Palpate its tendon immediately proximal to the first carpometacarpal joint. It is the most anterior of the three tendons at the base of the carpometacarpal joint (Fig. 6–74).

Abductor Pollicis Brevis. Palpate along the anterior surface of the shaft of the first metacarpal (Fig. 6–75).

Figure 6–74. Palpation for the abductor pollicis longus muscle.

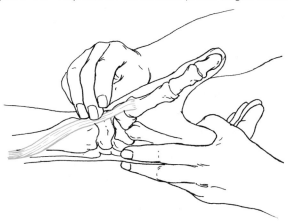

Figure 6–75. Palpation for the abductor pollicis brevis muscle.

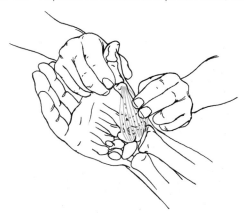

Attachments of Adductor Pollicis Muscle

Muscle	Proximal	Distal	Innervation
Adductor pollicis	Capitate and base of second and third metacarpal bones; also palmar surface of shaft of third metacarpal	Base of proximal phalanx of thumb	Ulnar T1 (C8)

Position.   The hand rests on the ulnar border, or the forearm is in supination with the wrist in a neutral position and the thumb adducted (Figs. 6–76 and 6–77).

Movement

Abductor Pollicis Longus.   The thumb abducts in the plane of the palm in the frontal plane.

Abductor Pollicis Brevis.   The thumb abducts at a right angle from the palm in the sagittal plane.

Resistance.   Applied into adduction to the distal end of the first metacarpal to test the abductor pollicis longus and on the proximal phalanx for the abductor pollicis brevis.

Stabilization.   The palm of the hand is stabilized.

Substitutions
- Lift the metacarpal toward the midline of the hand for the abductor pollicis brevis only to prevent substitution.
- The extensor pollicis longus and brevis may extend and also contribute to abduction of the first metacarpal.
- The abductor pollicis longus abducts the thumb to the radial side of the hand.

- The opponens pollicis tends to rotate thumb.
- The flexor pollicis brevis and longus are accessory muscles to the motion of abduction.

Adductor Pollicis Muscle

The adductor pollicis muscle produces the motion of adduction of the thumb from a starting position of radial abduction in the coronal plane through a range of 75 degrees. The forearm may be supinated, the hand resting on its ulnar border or pronated. The thumb remains in the plane of the palm.

Palpation.   Palpate in the first web space; push the finger and thumb deep to the first dorsal interossei (Fig. 6–78).

Position.   The hand rests on a table with the thumb abducted from the palm in the coronal plane (Fig. 6–79).

Movement.   Adduction of the first carpometacarpal joint.

Resistance.   Apply resistance to the proximal phalanx into radial abduction.

Figure 6–76.   Testing position for the abductor pollicis longus muscle.

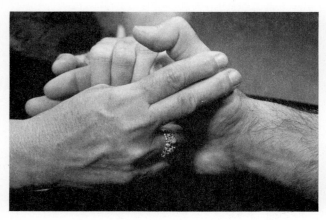

Figure 6–77.   Testing position for the abductor pollicis brevis muscle.

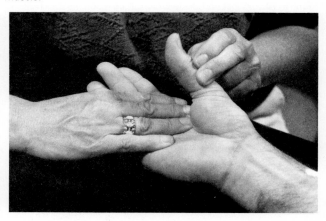

Stabilization. Stabilize the palm of the hand.

Substitutions
- The metacarpophalangeal joint flexes the flexor pollicis brevis.
- The interphalangeal joint flexes the flexor pollicis longus.

Opponens Pollicis Muscle

The opponens pollicis muscle produces the motion of opposition of the thumb at the first carpometacarpal joint. The movement is complex, initiated by palmar abduction at the first carpometacarpal joint followed by ulnar adduction, which continues to the final position with slight flexion and rotation of the carpometacarpal joint.

Palpation. Palpate along the lateral shaft of the first metacarpal. Push the abductor pollicis brevis toward the ulna and palpate deep to it (Fig. 6–80).

Position. The hand rests on its dorsal surface with the forearm supinated (Fig. 6–81).

Movement. Roll the head of the first metacarpal toward the ulnar side of the hand while keeping the tip of the thumb against the pad of the tip or base of the fifth finger.

Figure 6–78. Palpation for the adductor pollicis muscle.

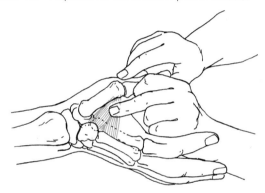

Figure 6–79. Testing position for the adductor pollicis muscle.

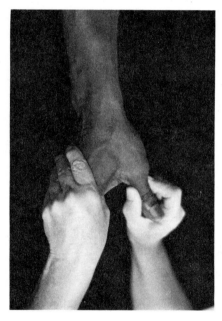

Figure 6–80. Palpation for the opponens pollicis muscle.

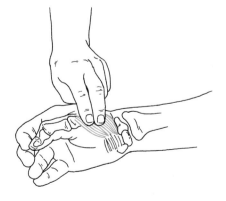

Figure 6–81. Testing for the opponens pollicis muscle.

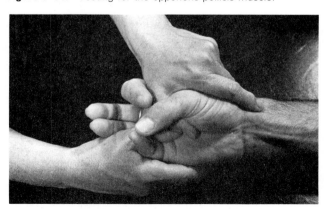

Attachments of Opponens Pollicis Muscle

Muscle	Proximal	Distal	Innervation
Opponens pollicis	Trapezium and flexor retinaculum	Entire lateral shaft of first metacarpal	Median C8 (T1)

Attachments of Opponens Digiti Minimi Muscle

Muscle	Proximal	Distal	Innervation
Opponens digiti minimi	Hook of hamate and flexor retinaculum	Entire shaft of fifth metacarpal	Ulnar T1 (C8)

Resistance. Applied to distal end of first and fifth metacarpals into derotation.

Stabilization. First and fifth metacarpals and palm of hand are stabilized.

Substitutions
· The abductor pollicis brevis can abduct the thumb without rotation.
· Motion should only occur at the carpometacarpal joints.

Opponens Digiti Minimi Muscle

The opponens digiti minimi muscle produces its action at the fifth carpometacarpal joint. The movement is rotation followed by flexion. It helps to cup the palm.

Palpation. Palpate along the shaft of the fifth metacarpal deep to the abductor digiti minimi (Fig. 6–82).

Position. The hand rests on the dorsal surface with the forearm supinated (Fig. 6–83).

Movement. Roll the fifth metacarpal toward the radial side of the hand, attempting to touch the pad of the thumb.

Resistance. Applied to the distal end of the fifth metacarpal into derotation.

Stabilization. Stabilize the palm of the hand.

Substitutions
· For the little finger flexors, motion should occur only at the carpometacarpal joint.

Figure 6–82. Palpation for the opponens digiti minimi muscle.

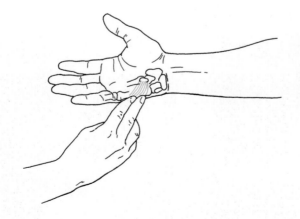

Figure 6–83. Testing position for the opponens digiti minimi muscle.

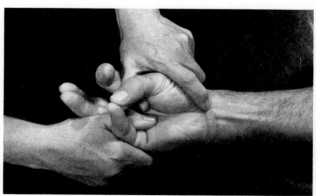

Attachments of Flexor Digiti Minimi Muscle

Muscle	Proximal	Distal	Innervation
Flexor digiti minimi	Hook of hamate, flexor retinaculum	Proximal phalanx of fifth digit	Ulnar T1 (C8)

- The abductor digiti minimi can abduct the little finger without rotation.

Flexor Digiti Minimi Muscle

The flexor digiti minimi muscle performs the motion of metacarpophalangeal joint flexion for the fifth digit and assists in opposition.

Palpation.   Palpate laterally along the shaft of the fifth metacarpal (Fig. 6–84).

Position.   The hand rests on its dorsal surface, with the forearm supinated (Fig. 6–85).

Movement.   Flexion of the fifth metacarpophalangeal joint with the interphalangeal joints remaining extended.

Resistance.   Applied to the palmar surface of the proximal phalanx.

Stabilization.   The fifth metacarpal and the palm are stabilized.

Substitutions
- The opponens digiti minimi may rotate the fifth metacarpal.
- The flexor digitorum superficialis and profundus to the fifth finger can cause flexion of the interphalangeal joints.

Clinical Tests

Palpation

The structures and landmarks of the wrist and hand that should be palpated or observed as part of the examination process include:

1. Individual carpal bones.
2. Radial styloid process.
3. Anatomical snuffbox boundaries and radial artery within.
4. Ulnar styloid process.
5. Ulnar artery at wrist.
6. Radial artery at wrist.
7. Flexor tendons where they cross the wrist.
8. Hook of the hamate where the flexor carpi ulnaris muscle inserts.
9. Carpal tunnel and components.
10. Thenar eminence.
11. Hypothenar eminence.
12. Metacarpophalangeal and interphalangeal joints.

Active and Passive Movements

The motions to be assessed during active and passive testing of the wrist and hand include:

1. Wrist flexion.
2. Wrist extension.

Figure 6–84.   Palpation for the flexor digiti minimi muscle.

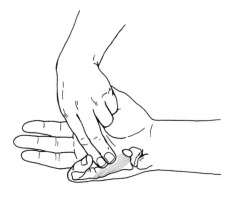

Figure 6–85.   Testing position for the flexor digiti minimi muscle.

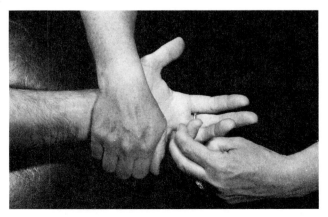

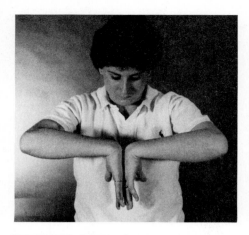

Figure 6–86. Phalen's test.

3. Wrist radial deviation.
4. Wrist ulnar deviation.
5. Metacarpophalangeal flexion of digits 1 to 5.
6. Metacarpophalangeal extension of digits 1 to 5.
7. Interphalangeal flexion of digits 1 to 5.
8. Interphalangeal extension of digits 1 to 5.
9. Abduction of the thumb.
10. Adduction of the thumb.
11. Opposition of the thumb and little finger.

Contractile Testing

Contractile testing of the wrist and hand should include:

1. Wrist flexion.
2. Wrist extension.
3. Wrist radial deviation.
4. Wrist ulnar deviation.
5. Metacarpophalangeal flexion of digits 1 to 5.
6. Metacarpophalangeal extension of digits 1 to 5.
7. Interphalangeal flexion of digits 1 to 5.
8. Interphalangeal extension of digits 1 to 5.
9. Abduction of the thumb.
10. Adduction of the thumb.
11. Opposition of the thumb and little finger.

Special Tests

Clinical Tests for Carpal Tunnel Syndrome

Phalen's Test

Indication. Phalen's test is utilized to aid in the diagnosis of carpal tunnel syndrome.

Method. The patient is instructed to flex both wrists maximally and simultaneously approximate the dorsal surfaces of both hands to assist in maintaining the flexed posture (Fig. 6–86). This position is held for at least 1 minute.

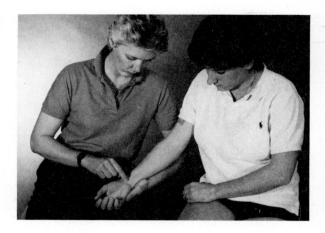

Figure 6–87. Tinel sign test for median nerve entrapment.

Results. Tingling of the palmar surface of the thumb, index, middle, and lateral half of the ring finger is a positive result.

Tinel Sign

Indication. The test for Tinel sign is an adjunct to the diagnosis of carpal tunnel syndrome for the median nerve.

Method. The subject's forearm is positioned in supination so that the examiner has easier access to the area over the carpal tunnel. The examiner taps the wrist over the carpal tunnel (Fig. 6–87).

Results. A positive test result is confirmed when the sensory changes noted above for Phalen's test occur.

Three-Jaw Chuck Test

Indication. The three-jaw chuck test is useful in assessing carpal tunnel syndrome.

Figure 6–88. Three-jaw chuck test.

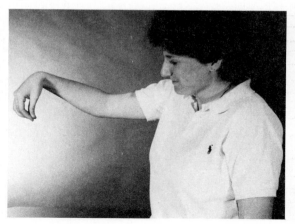

Wrist and Hand **165**

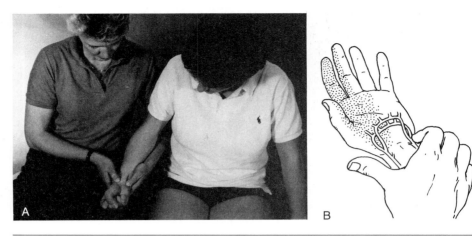

Figure 6–89. (A) In Allen's test, radial and ulnar arteries are compressed at the wrist, while the subject keeps the hand maintained in a tightly clenched fist. (B) With the hand opened, each artery is released separately. Note the flushing pattern.

Method. The subject places the hand being examined in the posture of a three-jaw chuck pinch, then flexes the wrist (Fig. 6–88). This combined posture is maintained for at least 1 minute.

Results. Reproduction of symptoms as noted in the previous two tests represents a positive result.

Other Tests

Allen's Test

Indication. Allen's test is performed to determine the integrity of the radial and ulnar arteries supplying the hand.

Method. The subject is instructed to aggressively open and close the hand several times as quickly as possible and to terminate the cycle with the hand tightly clenched into a fist. The examiner places the thumb and index finger over the radial and ulnar arteries where they cross the wrist. The examiner presses down on these two points to occlude blood flow distally (Fig. 6–89A). The subject is then asked to open the hand. The examiner releases one of the arteries and watches for flushing of the portion of the hand supplied by that particular artery (Fig. 6–89B). Finally, the remaining artery is released and again the flushing pattern is observed. This process is repeated with the opposite hand and comparisons are made.

Results. Midway through the test, when the subject opens the hand that was clenched into a fist, the hand should appear whitish or pale because of poor blood flow distal to the points of compression. Normally as each artery is released, a flushing pattern is seen as blood flow returns to the hand. If there is an absence or dim-inution of blood flow to the hand because of pathology, the hand will remain whitish, indicating a positive result.

Finkelstein's Test

Indication. An indication for Finkelstein's test would be suspected de Quervain's tenosynovitis.

Method. The subject is asked to make a fist of the test hand while enclosing the thumb within the flexed fingers. The examiner stabilizes the forearm while the wrist is passively or actively moved into ulnar deviation (Fig. 6–90).

Results. A positive result is indicated by pain laterally over the wrist. Stretching of the tendons of the abductor pollicis longus and the extensor pollicis brevis tendons where they cross the wrist is responsible for the pain. As normal persons notice some discomfort during this test, it is recommended that testing be carried out bilaterally to detect a difference.

Figure 6–90. Finkelstein's test.

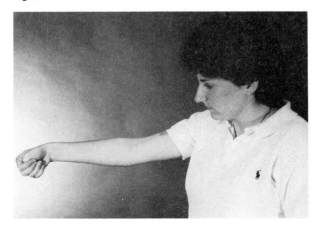

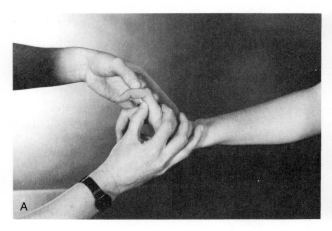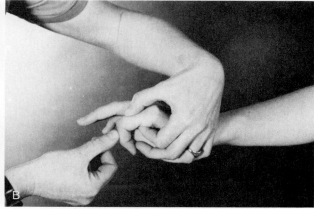

Figure 6–91. (A) In the Brunnel-Littler test, proximal interphalangeal joint flexion is assessed with the metacarpophalangeal joint maintained in extension. (B) Proximal interphalangeal joint flexion is assessed with the metacarpophalangeal joint in slight flexion.

Brunnel-Littler Test

Indication. The Brunnel-Littler test is useful in distinguishing tightness of the intrinsic hand muscles from restriction of the capsule of the metacarpophalangeal joint as the cause of loss of flexion at the metacarpophalangeal joint.

Method. The examiner stabilizes the metacarpophalangeal joint in slight extension, thereby stretching the lumbricals. While maintaining the metacarpophalangeal extension, the proximal interphalangeal joint is flexed and the quantity of motion is noted (Fig. 6–91A). Next, the metacarpophalangeal joint is slightly flexed, decreasing tension on the lumbricals. While the metacarpophalangeal joint is in flexion, the proximal interphalangeal joint is again flexed while the examiner observes the amount of flexion obtained (Fig. 6–91B).

Results. If there is restriction of proximal interphalangeal flexion while the metacarpophalangeal joint is maintained in extension, the restriction may be due to either tight intrinsics or capsular involvement at the proximal interphalangeal joint.

When proximal interphalangeal flexion is attempted while the metacarpophalangeal joint is flexed, ability to move into full flexion represents tightness of the intrinsics responsible for limitation in motion. If, during flexion of the proximal interphalangeal joint with the metacarpophalangeal joint flexed, the motion of the proximal interphalangeal joint remains incomplete, capsular restrictions must be considered as the primary cause.

Retinacular Test

Indication. This test differentiates between tightness of the retinacular ligament and restrictions in the capsule

Figure 6–92. (A) In the retinacular test, distal interphalangeal joint flexion is assessed with the proximal joint maintained in an extended position. (B) Distal interphalangeal joint flexion is assessed with the proximal joint in slight flexion.

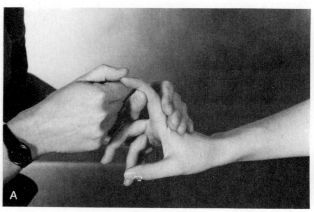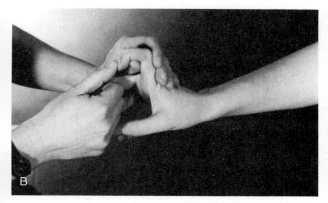

of the proximal interphalangeal joint as causes of restriction of distal interphalangeal joint flexion.

Method. The examiner positions the proximal interphalangeal joint in a neutral position while attempting to flex the distal interphalangeal joint. The degree of flexion is noted, and the process is repeated while the proximal interphalangeal joint is held in slight flexion (Fig. 6–92).

Results. The retinacular ligaments are slack when the proximal interphalangeal joint is slightly flexed. A compromise in distal interphalangeal joint flexion in that position probably is a result of capsular involvement of that joint. If the retinacular ligaments are relaxed by proximal interphalangeal flexion, thereby allowing full range of distal interphalangeal joint flexion, the initial limitation most likely was a result of retinacular ligament tightness.

Froment's Sign

Indication. The test is used to assess ulnar nerve compromise in the hand by evaluating thumb adduction.

Figure 6–93. Froment's sign.

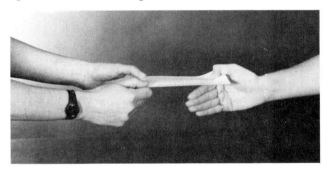

Method. A piece of paper is placed between the subject's thumb and index finger, and the subject is instructed to grip the paper as the examiner attempts to pull it from between the thumb and finger (Fig. 6–93).

Results. The test is positive if the subject tries to maintain a grip on the paper by flexing the distal interphalangeal joint of the thumb in order to compensate for thumb adductor weakness.

Joint Play (Accessory Movements)

Radiocarpal Joint

Distraction (Fig. 6–94)

Restriction. General hypomobility.

Open-Packed Position. 10 degrees of wrist flexion and slight ulnar deviation.

Positioning. Subject sits beside treatment table with forearm pronated. Stabilization may be accomplished with the use of a wedge beneath the distal radius and ulna or by stabilizing the distal forearm against the body. The stabilizing hand of the therapist holds the distal radius and ulna as close to the joint space as possible. The other hand grasps the proximal row of carpal bones.

Movement. The therapist delivers a distracting force to the proximal row of carpal bones.

Ventral Glide (Fig. 6–95)

Restriction. Wrist extension.

Positioning. Same as for distraction glide.

Figure 6–94. Distraction of the radiocarpal joint.

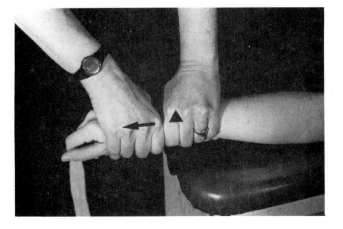

Figure 6–95. Ventral glide of the proximal carpal bones.

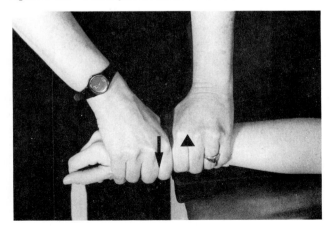

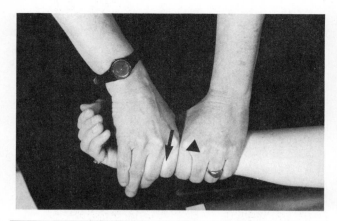

Figure 6–96. Dorsal glide of the proximal carpal bones

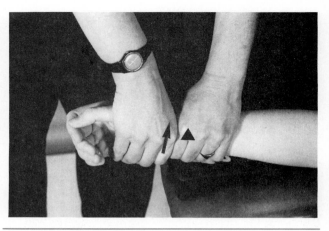

Figure 6–97. Radial glide of the proximal carpal bones.

Movement. The therapist delivers a ventral force to the proximal row of carpal bones, with the focus of the application through the radial side of the index finger, the web space, and the ulnar side of the thumb.

Dorsal Glide (Fig. 6–96)

Restriction. Wrist flexion.

Positioning. Same as for distraction glide, except that the forearm is supine.

Movement. The therapist delivers a dorsal force to the proximal row of carpal bones, with the focus of the application through the radial side of the index finger, the web space, and the ulnar side of the thumb.

Radial Glide (Fig. 6–97)

Restriction. Wrist ulnar deviation.

Positioning. Subject sits beside treatment table with forearm in the mid-position. Stabilization may be accomplished with the use of a wedge beneath the distal ulna or by stabilizing the distal forearm against the therapist's body. The stabilizing hand of the therapist holds the distal radius and ulna as close to the joint space as possible. The other hand grasps the proximal row of carpal bones.

Movement. The therapist delivers a radial force to the proximal row of carpal bones, with the focus of the application through the palmar surface of the index finger to the medial side of the ulna.

Ulnar Glide (Fig. 6–98)

Restriction. Wrist radial deviation.

Positioning. Same as for radial glide.

Movement. The therapist delivers an ulnar force to the proximal row of carpal bones, with the focus of the

application through the web space to the lateral side of the distal radius.

Second Through Fifth Carpometacarpal Joints

Distraction (Fig. 6–99)

Restriction. General hypomobility.

Open-Packed Position. Resting.

Positioning. Subject sits beside a table with the forearm pronated. The distal carpal row, which articulates with the proximal metacarpal bases, is stabilized on the wedge. One hand of the therapist provides additional stabilization by grasping the specific carpal bone with the index finger and thumb. The other hand grips the corresponding metacarpal as close to the base as possible.

Movement. The therapist creates a distraction force to the proximal metacarpal.

Figure 6–98. Ulnar glide of the proximal carpal bones.

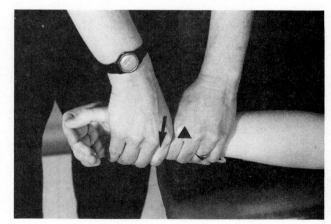

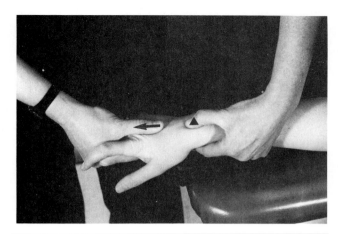

Figure 6–99. Distraction of the second to the fifth carpometacarpal joints.

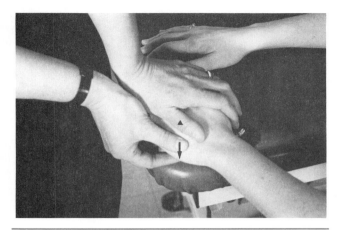

Figure 6–100. Ventral glide of the fifth metacarpal.

Ventral Glide (Fig. 6–100)

Restriction.   General hypomobility.

Positioning.   Subject sits beside a table with forearm pronated. The metacarpal adjacent to the one being mobilized is stabilized on a wedge. One hand of the therapist rests on the dorsum of the stabilized metacarpal, providing additional support. The thenar eminence of the other hand is placed on the metacarpal to be mobilized.

Movement.   Using the radial aspect of the thenar eminence the therapist imposes a ventral force to the metacarpal being mobilized. This technique applies not only to carpometacarpal joint mobilization but also to intermetacarpal mobilization.

Carpometacarpal Joint of the Thumb

Distraction (Fig. 6–101)

Restriction.   General hypomobility.

Open-Packed Position.   Midway between flexion and extension and between abduction and adduction.

Positioning.   Subject sits beside a table with forearm in mid-position. The therapist stabilizes the trapezium and trapezoid as a unit, with the thumb and index finger of one hand. The thumb and index finger of the other hand are placed on the dorsal and palmar surfaces, respectively, of the subject's first metacarpal.

Movement.   The therapist applies a distraction force to the subject's first metacarpal.

Ulnar Glide (Fig. 6–102)

Restriction.   Flexion of the thumb.

Positioning.   Subject sits beside a table with the forearm in mid-position. The therapist stabilizes the trapezium and trapezoid as a unit with the thumb and index finger of one hand. The thenar eminence of the other hand is placed on the first metacarpal of the subject's thumb, and the fingers wrap around the thumb to assist in maintaining the resting position.

Movement.   The therapist applies an ulnarly directed force through the thenar eminence to the radial aspect of the subject's metacarpal.

Radial Glide (Fig. 6–103)

Restriction.   Extension of the thumb.

Positioning.   Same as for ulnar glide.

Movement.   The therapist applies a radially directed force through the thenar eminence to the ulnar aspect of the subject's first metacarpal.

Figure 6–101. Distraction of the first carpometacarpal joint.

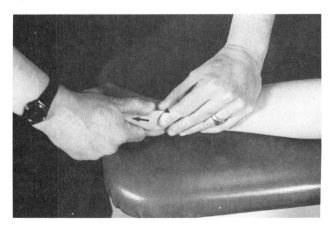

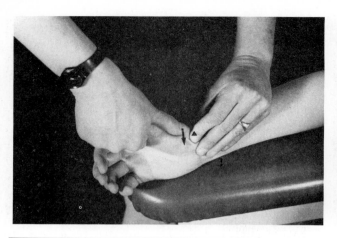

Figure 6–102. Ulnar glide of the first metacarpal.

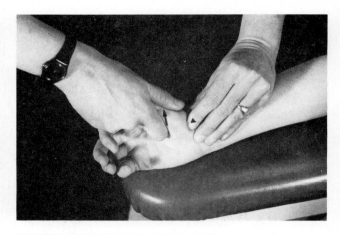

Figure 6–103. Radial glide of the first metacarpal.

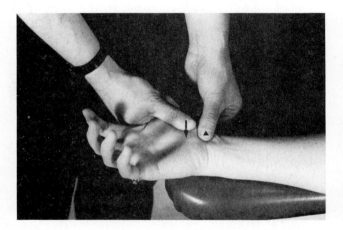

Figure 6–104. Dorsal glide of the first metacarpal.

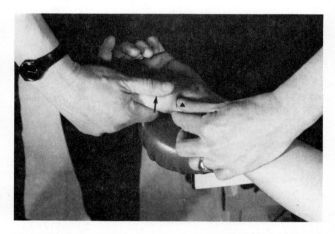

Figure 6–105. Ventral glide of the first metacarpal.

Dorsal Glide (Fig. 6–104)

Restriction. Abduction of the thumb.

Positioning. Same as for ulnar glide, except with the forearm fully supinated.

Movement. The therapist applies a dorsally directed force through the thenar eminence to the anterior aspect of the subject's first metacarpal.

Ventral Glide (Fig. 6–105)

Restriction. Adduction of the thumb.

Positioning. Same as for dorsal glide.

Movement. The therapist applies a ventrally directed force to the posterior aspect of the subject's first metacarpal.

First Through Fifth Metacarpophalangeal and Interphalangeal Joints

Distraction, Ventral, and Dorsal Glide (Fig. 6–106)

Restriction. General hypomobility, flexion, extension.

Open-Packed Position. Slight flexion.

Positioning. Subject is seated with the proximal articulating partner stabilized on the wedge. The therapist's one hand is placed on the dorsal surface of the stabilized bone to provide additional support. The thumb and index finger of the other hand are placed on the dorsal and palmar surfaces of the subject's distal articulating partner as close to the joint space as possible.

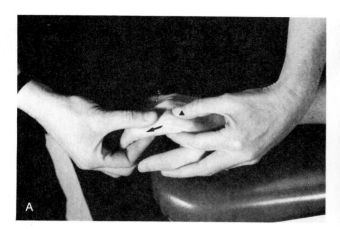

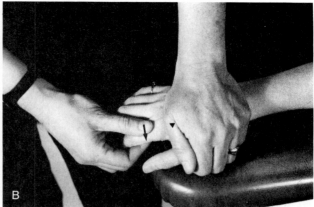

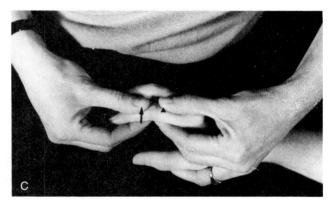

Figure 6–106. (*A*) Mobilization of metacarpophalangeal and interphalangeal joints. Distraction of the metacarpophalangeal joint (*B*) Ventral glide of the proximal phalanx. (*C*) Dorsal glide of the middle phalanx.

Movement.   The therapist applies a distraction force to the distal articulating segment for generalized hypomobility restrictions. A ventral or palmar glide is performed for restrictions in flexion, and a dorsal glide is used for limitations in extension.

Carpal Bone Mobility Testing

Kaltenborn has developed a systematic approach to examination of joint play of the individual carpal bones (Fig. 6–107). The suggested format is as follows:

1. Stabilize the capitate and move the trapezium and trapezoid as a unit.
2. Stabilize the capitate and move the scaphoid.
3. Stabilize the capitate and move the lunate.
4. Stabilize the capitate and move the hamate.
5. Stabilize the scaphoid and move the trapezium and trapezoid as a unit.
6. Stabilize the radius and move the scaphoid.
7. Stabilize the radius and move the lunate.

Figure 6–107. Anterior view of the anatomical relationship of the distal forearm and carpal bones.

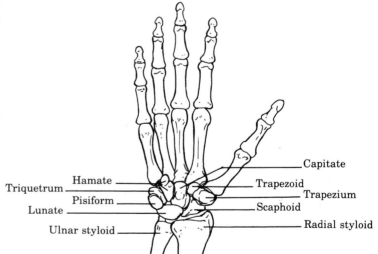

Table 6–1. Summary of Joint Play in the Wrist and Hand

GLIDE	RESTRICTION	FIXED BONE	MOVING BONE
Radiocarpal Joint			
Distraction	General hypomobility	Radius	Scaphoid/lunate/disc
Ventral	Extension	Radius	Scaphoid/lunate/disc
Dorsal	Flexion	Radius	Scaphoid/lunate/disc
Radial	Ulnar deviation	Radius	Scaphoid/lunate/disc
Ulnar	Radial deviation	Radius	Scaphoid/lunate/disc
Second Through Fifth Carpometacarpal Joints			
Distraction	General hypomobility	Carpal	Metacarpal
Dorsal	Flexion	Carpal	Metacarpal
Ventral	Extension	Carpal	Metacarpal
Carpometacarpal Joint of Thumb			
Distraction	General hypomobility	Carpal	Metacarpal
Ulnar	Flexion	Carpal	Metacarpal
Radial	Extension	Carpal	Metacarpal
Dorsal	Abduction	Carpal	Metacarpal
Ventral	Adduction	Carpal	Metacarpal
First Through Fifth Metacarpophalangeal Joints			
Distraction	General hypomobility	Metacarpal	Proximal phalanx
Ventral	Flexion	Metacarpal	Proximal phalanx
Dorsal	Extension	Metacarpal	Proximal phalanx
First Through Fifth Interphalangeal Joints			
Distraction	General hypomobility	Proximal phalanx	Distal phalanx
Ventral	Flexion	Proximal phalanx	Distal phalanx
Dorsal	Extension	Proximal phalanx	Distal phalanx

8. Stabilize the ulna with the articular disc and move the triquetrum.
9. Stabilize the triquetrum and move the hamate.
10. Stabilize the triquetrum and move the pisiform.

Table 6–1 provides a summary of joint play in the wrist and hand.

Bibliography

Backhouse KM, Hutchings RT: Color Atlas of Surface Anatomy. Baltimore, Williams & Wilkins, 1986

Daniels L, Worthingham C: Muscle Testing Techniques of Manual Examination. Philadelphia, WB Saunders, 1986

Gould A III, Davies G (eds): Orthopedic and Sports Physical Therapy. St Louis, CV Mosby, 1985

Hollinshead WH, Jenkins DB: Functional Anatomy of the Limbs and Back. Philadelphia, WB Saunders, 1981

Hoppenfeld S: Physical Examination of the Spine and Extremities. New York, Appleton-Century-Crofts, 1976

Kaltenborn M: Mobilization of the Extremity Joints. Oslo, Bygdoy Alle, 1980

Kendal FP, McCreary EK: Muscle Testing and Function. Baltimore, Williams & Wilkins, 1983

Kessler R, Hertling D: Management of Common Musculoskeletal Disorders. Philadelphia, Harper & Row, 1983

Kisner C, Colby LA: Therapeutic Exercise: Foundations and Techniques. Philadelphia, FA Davis, 1985

Magee J: Orthopedic Physical Assessment. Philadelphia, WB Saunders, 1987

Maitland GD: The Peripheral Joints: Examination and Recording Guide. Adelaide, Australia, Virgo Press, 1973

Norkin CC, White DJ: Measurement of Joint Motion: A Guide to Goniometry. Philadelphia, FA Davis, 1985

Saunders DH: Evaluation, Treatment, and Prevention of Musculoskeletal Disorders. Minneapolis, H Duane Saunders, 1985

Williams P, Warwick R (eds): Gray's Anatomy, 36th British ed. Philadelphia, WB Saunders, 1980.

Neck and
Trunk Region

Chapter 7

Jan Bühler Callahan, M. Ed., PT contributed to this chapter.

The vertebrae serve many important functions. They protect the spinal cord and assist in breathing and swallowing. They provide a base of support for the head and internal organs and indirect attachments for the limbs. They allow mobility for the trunk. The articulations for each vertebra are numerous. The bodies articulate with each other, and the articulations are cushioned by intervertebral discs. The vertebral arches articulate through the superior and inferior articulating facets. The facet joints are plane synovial joints and have three degrees of freedom of motion. The articulation with the intervertebral discs permits minimal motion and is referred to as a symphysis type of amphiarthrodial joint.

The atlanto-occipital joint has two degrees of freedom of motion—flexion and extension and lateral bending. The atlantoaxial articulation produces the primary motion of rotation. The direction of motion permitted in the remaining vertebrae depends on the direction of the facets (except for the sacrum, the segments of which are fused). The sacrum articulates with the ilium and the sacroiliac joint is capable of a limited amount of flexion and extension. The vertebrae are reinforced by intersegmental and intrasegmental ligaments and muscles.

Goniometry

Cervical Vertebrae

Cervical Flexion

Flexion in the sagittal plane occurs between all cervical vertebrae, the occipital bone, and the upper five to seven thoracic vertebrae (T5 to T7). The majority of the movement occurs between the superior and inferior facet joints followed by movement between the intervertebral discs.

Motion
- Preferred: 0 to 45 degrees of neck flexion in the sagittal plane.
- Alternate: When using a measuring tape, 0 inches.

Position. Subject sits with the trunk well supported and the neck in the anatomical position. The hands are placed in the lap and the shoulder joints are relaxed.

Goniometric Alignment (Fig. 7–1)

Axis. Placed over the external auditory meatus.

Stationary Arm. Placed parallel to the floor.

Moving Arm. Placed along a line parallel to the inferior border of the nose.

Alternates
1. A bubble or gravity-activated goniometer is fixed to the head over the ear with the base parallel to

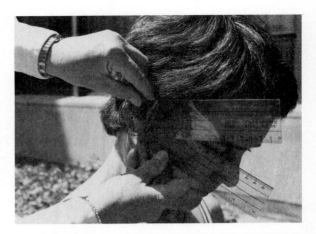

Figure 7–1. End position for cervical flexion.

the top of the ear. The goniometer is set at 0 degrees (Fig. 7–2).
2. The number of inches from the point of the chin to the midpoint of the sternal notch is measured with a tape; the subject's mouth remains closed. (Figs. 7–3 and 7–4).
3. The distance in inches from the external occipital protuberance and the spinous process of C7 is measured.

Stabilization. The trunk is stabilized.

Precautions
- Prevent trunk flexion.
- Prevent neck rotation and lateral flexion.

Cervical Extension and Hyperextension

The extension motion is the return from neck flexion. Hyperextension increases the anterior convexity of the cervical vertebrae. The motion occurs in the sagittal plane

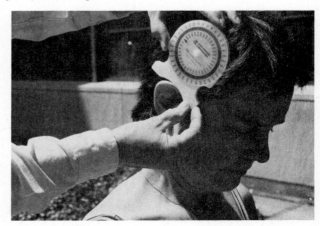

Figure 7–2. Alternate end position for cervical flexion using a gravity-activated goniometer.

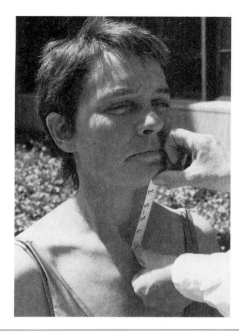

Figure 7–3. Alternate starting position for cervical flexion using a measuring tape.

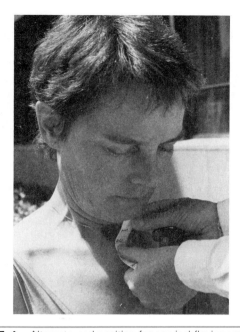

Figure 7–4. Alternate end position for cervical flexion using a measuring tape.

between the articulating facets of all the cervical vertebrae and at the atlanto-occipital joint.

Motion. 45 to 0 degrees for extension, and 0 to 45 degrees for hyperextension of the cervical vertebrae. When using a measuring tape, the distance is approximately 7 to 10 inches from complete flexion into hyperextension of the cervical vertebrae.

Position. Subject sits, the trunk supported and the neck in the anatomical position. The hands rest in the lap and the shoulder girdle joints remain relaxed.

Goniometric Alignment (Figs. 7–5 and 7–6)

Axis. Placed over the external auditory meatus.

Stationary Arm. Placed parallel to the floor.

Figure 7–5. Starting position for cervical extension and hyperextension.

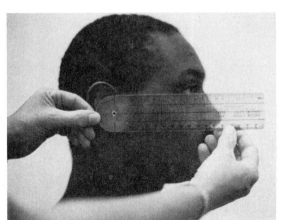

Figure 7–6. End position for cervical extension and hyperextension.

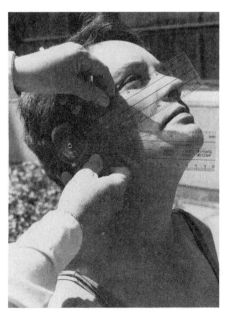

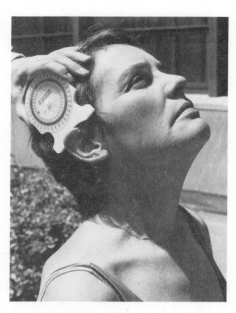

Figure 7–7. Alternate end position for cervical extension and hyperextension using a gravity-activated angle finder.

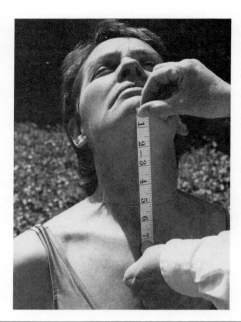

Figure 7–8. Alternate end position for cervical extension and hyperextension using a measuring tape anteriorly.

Moving Arm. Placed parallel to the inferior border of the nose.

Alternates
1. The bubble or gravity-activated goniometer is fixed to the head with the base over the top of the ear. The goniometer is set at zero (Fig. 7–7).

2. The tape measure is used to determine the distance in inches between the tip of the chin and the sternal notch (Fig. 7–8).
3. The tape measure is placed from the external occipital protuberance to the spinous process of C7. The difference between the starting and ending positions is the range of motion (Figs. 7–9 and 7–10).

Figure 7–9. Alternate starting position for cervical extension and hyperextension using a measuring tape.

Figure 7–10. End position for cervical extension and hyperextension using a measuring tape.

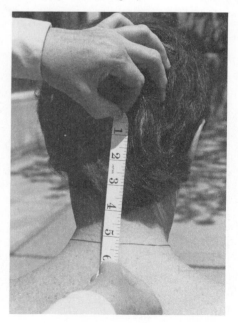

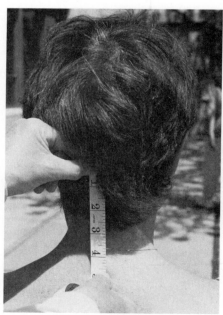

Stabilization.   The trunk and shoulder girdle are stabilized.

Precautions
- Prevent trunk flexion.
- Prevent neck lateral flexion and rotation.

Cervical Rotation

Rotation of the cervical vertebrae occurs in the transverse plane. The greatest amount of rotation occurs between the first (atlas) and the second (axis) cervical vertebrae, at the atlantoaxial joint. Rotation does occur between the articulating facets of each of the cervical vertebrae and the intervertebral discs. Cervical vertebral rotation is accompanied by lateral flexion to the same side as the rotation.

Motion.   0 to 60 to 75 degrees of cervical rotation in each direction. The distance is approximately 5 inches to each side, as measured by tape.

Position   Subject sits with the trunk supported and the neck in the anatomical position. The subject's hands are resting in the lap and the shoulder joints are relaxed.

Goniometric Alignment (Fig. 7–11)

Axis.   Placed over the center of the top of the head.

Stationary Arm.   Placed in line with the acromion process of the side being measured.

Moving Arm.   Placed in line with the tip of the nose.

Alternate.   Place the measuring tape on the midline of the chin and the acromion process. Measure the difference between the starting and ending positions. The

difference in the measurement is the amount of range of motion (Fig. 7–12).

Stabilization.   The trunk and shoulder girdle are stabilized.

Precautions
- Prevent the trunk from rotating.
- Keep the neck in the transverse plane.
- Prevent scapular elevation.

Cervical Lateral Flexion

The motion of lateral flexion occurs in the frontal plane. The lateral flexion motion is more or less equally distributed among all the joints of the cervical vertebrae. It is accompanied by rotation of the vertebrae to the same side because of the stretch of the soft tissue structures.

Motion.   0 to 45 to 60 degrees of cervical joint lateral flexion. Using a measuring tape, the distance between the starting and ending positions is approximately 5 inches to each side.

Position.   Subject sits with the trunk supported and the neck in the anatomical position. The hands lie in the lap and the shoulder girdle joints are relaxed.

Goniometric Alignment (Fig. 7–13)

Axis.   Placed over the spinous process of C7.

Stationary Arm.   Placed along the thoracic spinous processes.

Moving Arm.   Placed over the external occipital protuberance of the occipital bone.

Figure 7–11.   End position for cervical rotation.

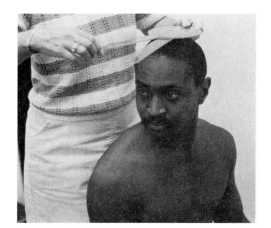

Figure 7–12.   Alternate end position for cervical rotation using a tape measure.

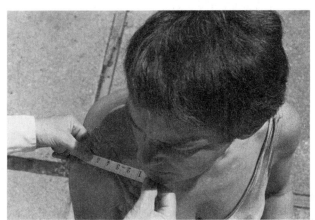

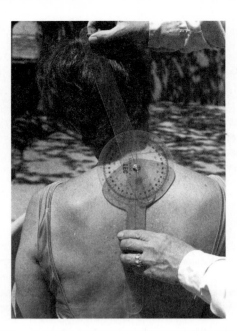

Figure 7–13. End position for cervical lateral flexion.

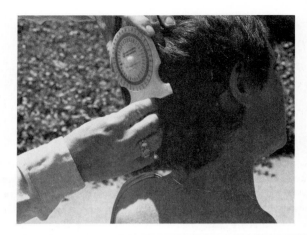

Figure 7–14. Alternate end position for cervical lateral flexion using a gravity-activated angle finder.

Alternates
1. The lower edge of a bubble goniometer is centered over the external occipital protuberance (Fig. 7–14).
2. A tape measure is used to measure the distance between the mastoid process of the temporal bone and the acromion process of the scapula. An average amount of lateral flexion motion is approximately 5 inches (Fig. 7–15).

Stabilization. The upper trunk and the shoulder girdle are stabilized.

Precautions
· Prevent shoulder elevation on the test side.
· Prevent upper trunk lateral flexion to the test side.

Thoracic and Lumbar Vertebrae

Thoracic and Lumbar Flexion

The motion of thoracic and lumbar vertebral flexion occurs in the sagittal plane. The greatest amount of motion occurs in the lumbar region, because the articular facets are positioned in the sagittal plane. The motion occurs also between the articular facets and the intervertebral discs. The discs compress anteriorly and distract posteriorly.

Motion. There is approximately a 4-inch difference between the starting and ending positions. The range of motion in the lumbar region amounts to a straightening

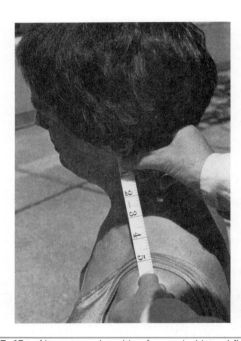

Figure 7–15. Alternate end position for cervical lateral flexion using a tape measure.

of the lordotic curve, with little or no reversal of the lumbar lordosis.

Position
· Preferred: Subject sits with the knee joints flexed.
· Alternate: Subject stands with the trunk erect.

Measuring Tape

Starting. The tape is placed proximally on the spinous process of C7 and distally to S1. *32*

Ending. Following flexion of the vertebrae, using the same bony landmarks, calculate the difference in distance between the starting and ending positions (Fig. 7–16).

Stabilization. The pelvis and hip joints are stabilized.

Precautions
- Prevent increased hip joint flexion.
- Prevent anterior tilt of the pelvis
- Allow for cervical vertebral flexion.

Thoracic and Lumbar Extension and Hyperextension

The motion of vertebral extension occurs in the sagittal plane. The majority occurs between the lumbar articular facets, because they are oriented in the sagittal plane. Extension also occurs between the intervertebral discs, which are compressed posteriorly and distracted anteriorly. The motion in the lumbar regions increases the normal lordosis and in the thoracic region decreases the normal kyphosis, or posterior convexity.

Motion. The extension motion is the distance between the starting and ending points when using a measuring tape. The difference is approximately 2 inches of thoracolumbar extension.

Position
- Preferred: Subject sits or stands with the feet flat on the floor and facing the back of the chair.
- Alternate: Subject stands erect.

Measuring Tape

Starting. Place the tape measure on the spinous process of C7.

Ending. Place the measuring tape on S1. Following the thoracolumbar extension, the difference in the starting and ending measurements is the amount of extension motion (Fig. 7–17).

Stabilization. The pelvis is stabilized.

Precautions
- Prevent an increase in hip joint extension.
- Prevent posterior pelvic tilt.
- Prevent trunk rotation.

Thoracic and Lumbar Lateral Flexion

The thoracolumbar motion of lateral flexion occurs in the frontal plane and is accompanied by thoracic and lumbar rotation to the opposite side. The most lateral flexion occurs between the thoracic articular facets and less between the intervertebral discs. The discs are compressed on the test side and distracted on the other side.

Motion. Subject bends to one side rotating as little as possible. The motion is determined by the difference between the starting and ending positions. Because of such variances in body proportions as arm and trunk length, the amount of motion is determined by comparing the sides.

Figure 7–16. End position for thoracic and lumbar flexion.

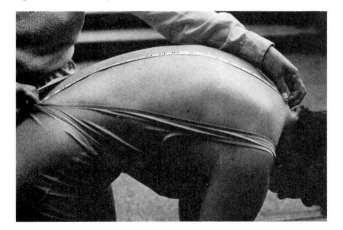

Figure 7–17. End position for thoracic and lumbar extension and hyperextension

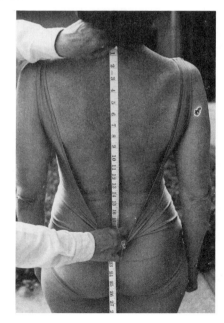

Position
- Preferred: Subject lies supine with the medial malleoli touching (Fig. 7–18).
- Alternate: Subject stands erect with the feet flat on the floor, approximately 2 inches apart (Fig. 7–19).

Measuring Tape

Starting
- Preferred: Place one end of a measuring tape on the tip of the middle finger and the other on the tip of the lateral malleolus.
- Alternate: Place one end of a measuring tape on the tip of the middle finger and the other on the floor on a point directly beneath the middle finger.

Figure 7–18. End supine position for lateral trunk flexion.

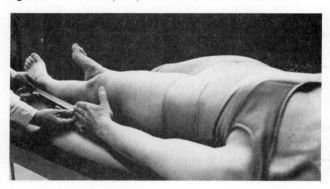

Figure 7–19. End standing position for lateral trunk flexion.

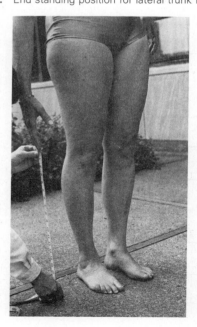

Ending. Measure the difference in inches following the lateral flexion motion.

Stabilization. The pelvis is stabilized.

Precautions
- Avoid trunk flexion, extension, and rotation.
- Prevent lateral tilting of the pelvis.

Thoracic and Lumbar Rotation

The rotation motion occurs in the transverse plane between the articular facets and the intervertebral discs. The lumbar vertebrae exhibit little or no rotation, the most occurring in the thoracic region. The motion of thoracolumbar vertebral rotation is accompanied by lateral flexion to the opposite side.

Motion. Objective measurements usually are not taken. The motion of thoracolumbar rotation is observed, and the amount of motion is compared to that on the opposite side.

Position. Subject sits erect with the feet flat on the floor in a chair without a back support or facing the back of the chair (Fig. 7–20).

Measurements. No actual measurements are taken. The motion on each side is observed.

Stabilization. The pelvis is stabilized.

Figure 7–20. End position for thoracic and lumbar rotation.

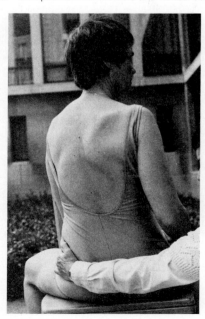

Precautions
- Prevent pelvic rotation.
- Avoid trunk flexion and extension and lateral flexion.

Functional Muscle Testing

Neck

The motions of the neck and trunk are evaluated bilaterally simultaneously.

Neck Flexion

Flexion of the head on the cervical column and flexion of the neck on the thoracic column depend on the anterior muscles of the neck. The suprahyoid and infrahyoid muscles are flexors of the head and the cervical vertebrae and support the cervical column at rest. Functionally the neck flexor muscles are weak and usually do not have to contract against gravity. They are type II phasic muscles, which fatigue more quickly than their counterparts, the neck extensor muscles. Concentrically the flexor muscles rotate the neck with synergistic action from the neck extensor muscles.

Position. Subject lies supine with the head in the anatomical position.

Activity. Subject lifts the head off the treatment table, keeping the chin tucked (Fig. 7–21).

Muscles. Sternocleidomastoids, prevertebral muscles: longus cervicis; rectus capitis anterior; rectus capitis lateralis; intertransverse; scalenus anterior, middle, posterior; suprahyoids and infrahyoids.

Types of Contraction
- Concentric: Lifting head against gravity.
- Eccentric: Lowering head.

Resistance
- The weight of the head offers the resistance.
- Functional: 5 repetitions.
- Functionally Fair: 3 to 4 repetitions.
- Functionally Poor: 1 to 2 repetitions.
- Nonfunctional: 0 repetitions.

Neck Extension

The neck extensor muscles contract continuously, holding the head up against gravity. They have a greater number of type I muscle fibers, which are fatigue resistant. The muscle group contracts eccentrically, allowing the neck to flex when the subject is in an upright or prone position. Many of the extensor muscles contract synergistically with the neck flexor muscles during the concentric contraction of neck rotation.

Position. Subject lies prone with the head in the anatomical position.

Activity. Subject lifts the head off the treatment table and holds it against gravity (Fig. 7–22).

Muscles. Upper trapezius, splenius capitis and cervicis, erector spinae group, and the transversospinalis group.

Types of Contraction
- Concentric: Lifting the head against gravity.
- Isometric: Holding the head and neck in an extended position.

Figure 7–21. Cervical flexion.

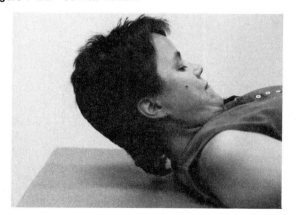

Figure 7–22. Cervical extension and hyperextension.

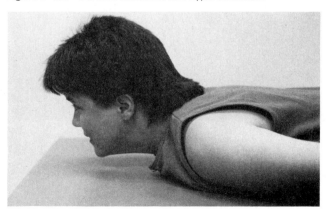

Resistance
- The weight of the head offers the resistance.
- Functional: 20 seconds.
- Functionally Fair: 10 to 19 seconds.
- Functionally Poor: 1 to 9 seconds.
- Nonfunctional: 0 seconds.

Trunk

Trunk Flexion

The trunk flexor muscles usually are not active during normal erect standing as are their counterparts, the trunk extensor muscles; however, they are essential for keeping the pelvis in its normal position. The muscles act indirectly on the vertebral column by exerting a pull on the ribs, sternum, and pelvis. The trunk flexor muscles contract strongly during strenuous activities to stabilize the trunk as a rigid support for the upper or lower limbs. The trunk flexor muscles reduce the lordotic curves of the vertebrae.

Position
- Preferred: Subject lies supine with hips and knees flexed, feet flat on the table, and shoulder joints flexed to 90 degrees (Fig. 7–23).
- Alternate: Subject stands (Fig. 7–24).

Activity
1. Subject assumes a sitting position without using the upper limbs.
2. Standing subject performs and holds a posterior pelvic tilt.

Muscles. Rectus abdominis, pyramidalis, transversus abdominis, and internal and external abdominal obliques.

Types of Contraction
1. Concentric: Coming to the sitting position.
   Eccentric: Lowering trunk to the supine position.
2. Concentric: Assuming a posterior pelvic tilt.
   Isometric: Holding the pelvic tilt.

Resistance
- The body weight provides the resistance.
- Functional: 1 repetition.
- Functionally Fair: half to three-quarter sit-up.
- Functionally Poor: initiation to half sit-up.
- Nonfunctional: 0 initiation.

Time
- Functional: 10 seconds.
- Functionally Fair: 5 to 9 seconds.
- Functionally Poor: 1 to 4 seconds.
- Nonfunctional: 0 seconds.

Trunk Extension

The trunk extensor muscles are located posterior to the axis in the sagittal plane. These muscles are thick and powerful. They contract during static erect standing and during the phases of gait. The extensor muscles are classified as fatigue-resistant, or type I, static muscles. The trunk extensors control forward trunk flexion in the standing position. The extensor muscles increase the lordotic curves of the vertebrae.

Figure 7–23. Trunk flexion.

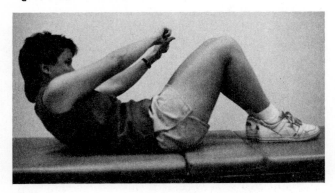

Figure 7–24. Posterior pelvic tilt for trunk flexion.

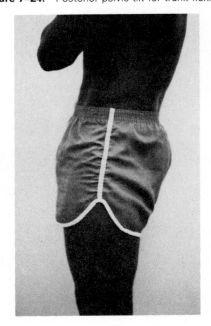

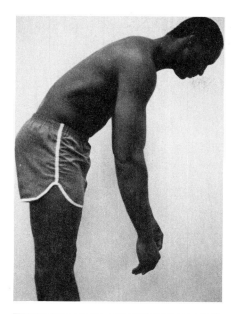

Figure 7-25. Thoracic and lumbar extension from a position of flexion.

Position. Subject stands, the upper limbs by the sides of the trunk.

Activity. Subject leans forward toward the floor and returns to the upright position (Fig. 7–25).

Muscles. Erector spinae, transversospinalis, and the interspinales.

Types of Contraction
- Eccentric: Lowering the trunk toward the floor.
- Concentric: Raising the trunk to the upright position.

Resistance
- The body weight offers the resistance.
- Functional: 5 repetitions.
- Functionally Fair: 3 to 4 repetitions.
- Functionally Poor: 1 to 2 repetitions.
- Nonfunctional: 0 repetitions.

Trunk Rotation With Flexion

Rotation of the trunk requires simultaneous contraction of the muscles from each side. These muscles make up the external and intermediate layer of abdominal muscle and run an oblique course. They form a girdle around the abdomen forming the "waist."

Position. Subject lies supine, with the hips and knees flexed.

Activity. Subject performs a sit-up on the diagonal. The activity is performed first to one side, then to the other (Fig. 7–26).

Muscles. Internal and external abdominal obliques.

Types of Contraction
- Concentric: Coming to the sitting position.
- Eccentric: Lowering trunk to the supine position.

Resistance
- The weight of the trunk offers the resistance.
- Functional: 1 sit-up to each side.
- Functionally Fair: half to three-quarter sit-up.
- Functionally Poor: initiation to half sit-up.
- Nonfunctional: 0 initiation.

Trunk Lateral Flexion

The muscles that perform lateral trunk flexion are located lateral to the axis of motion on one side of the trunk both anteriorly and posteriorly. For lateral flexion of the trunk to occur, the pelvis and lower limbs are fixed. Laterally flexing the trunk from an erect posture causes the opposite trunk muscles to contract eccentrically.

Position. Subject either sits or stands.

Activity. Subject slowly leans to one side, then to the other (Fig. 7–27).

Muscles. Erector spinae and abdominals on the same side.

Types of Contraction
- Eccentric: Leaning to one side.
- Concentric: Returning to the erect position.

Figure 7–26. Thoracic and lumbar rotation.

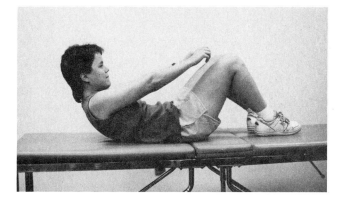

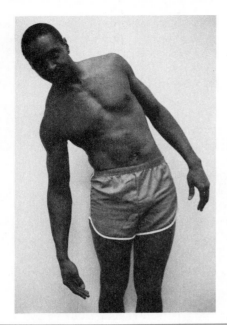

Figure 7–27. Lateral thoracic and lumbar flexion.

Resistance
· The weight of the trunk offers the resistance.
· Functional: 5 repetitions.
· Functionally Fair: 3 to 4 repetitions.
· Functionally Poor: 1 to 2 repetitions.
· Nonfunctional: 0 repetitions.

Manual Muscle Testing

Sternocleidomastoid Muscles

The sternocleidomastoid muscles produce the basic motion of flexion of the neck in the sagittal plane through a test range of 45 degrees, or just beyond the straightening of the lordosis. Usually both sides are tested si-

multaneously, but they may be tested unilaterally by having the patient rotate to the opposite side.

Palpation. Superficially on the anterolateral aspect of the neck (Fig. 7–28).

Position
· AG: Subject lies supine (Fig. 7–29).
· GM: Subject is in sidelying position with the head supported on a surface that allows easy motion (Fig. 7–30).

Movement. Flexion of the neck in the sagittal plane.

Resistance. Applied to the anterior forehead into extension.

Stabilization. The thorax is stabilized.

Substitutions
· Palpate each muscle to be sure that both sternocleidomastoid muscles are functioning.
· Rectus capitis anterior and the rectus capitis lateralis muscles are accessory neck flexors.
· Suprahyoid, infrahyoid, and platysma are also accessory muscles for the motion of neck flexion.
· Scalene muscles and the longus colli and capitis flex the neck.

Anterior, Middle, and Posterior Scalene Muscles; Longus Colli Muscle; Longus Capitis Muscle

The scalene muscles flex the neck when both sides contract simultaneously. Unilaterally, the muscles flex laterally and rotate the neck to the same side. The longus colli and capitis muscles produce neck flexion in the sagittal plane. The starting position is with the neck in extension.

Figure 7–28. (A) Palpation for the sternocleidomastoid muscle in neck flexion. (B) Palpation for the sternocleidomastoid muscle during neck flexion with rotation to the opposite side.

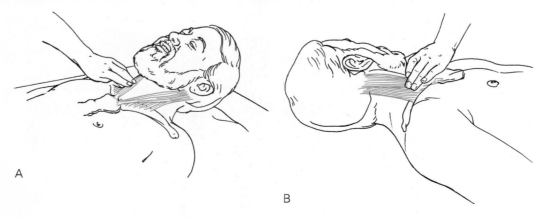

A

B

Attachments of Sternocleidomastoid (Sternal and Clavicular) Muscles

Muscle	Proximal	Distal	Innervation
Sternocleidomastoid (sternal) (clavicular)	Superior aspect of manubrium sterni medial third of clavicle	Mastoid process	Spinal accessory CN IX

Palpation

Scalene Muscles. Place the fingertips above the clavicle in the triangle formed by the sternocleidomastoid and trapezius muscles. Have the subject force inspiration (Fig. 7–31).

Longus Colli and Longus Capitis. The longus colli and longus capitis muscles are too deep to palpate.

Position
· AG: Subject lies supine.
· GM: Subject is in sidelying position with the head supported on a surface that allows easy motion.

Movement. Flexion of the neck in the sagittal plane.

Figure 7–29. Testing the sternocleidomastoid muscle in the AG supine position.

Figure 7–30. Testing the sternocleidomastoid muscle in the GM sidelying position.

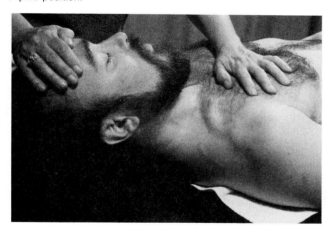

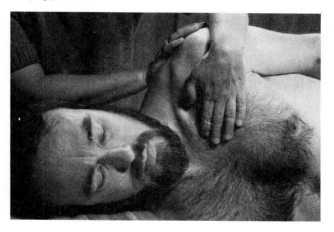

Figure 7–31. (*A*) Palpation for the anterior, middle, and posterior scalene muscles. (*B*) Location of the scalene muscles.

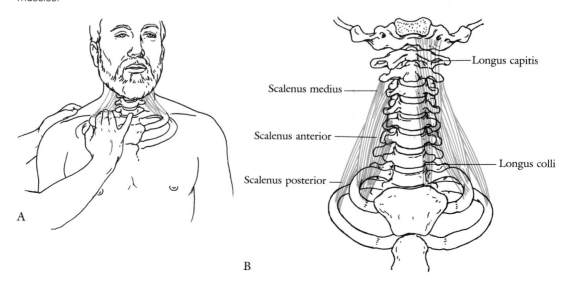

Attachments of Scalene, Longus Colli, and Longus Capitis Muscles

Muscle	Proximal	Distal	Innervation
Scalenus Anterior	Anterior tubercles of C3–6	Superior crest of first rib	Ventral primary rami of cervical spinal nerves
Middle	Posterior tubercles of C2–7	Superior crest of first rib	
Posterior	Posterior tubercles of C5–7	Outer surface of second rib	
Longus colli	Anterior tubercles of C3–5, anterior surface of C5–7, T1–3	Tubercle of the atlas, anterior tubercles of C5 and C6, anterior surface of C2–4	Ventral primary rami of cervical spinal nerves
Longus capitis	Anterior tubercles of C3–6	Inferior occipital bone, basilar portion	Ventral primary rami of cervical spinal nerves

Resistance. Applied to the anterior forehead into extension.

Stabilization. The thorax is stabilized.

Substitutions
· Sternocleidomastoid muscle is a neck flexor.
· Rectus capitis anterior, rectus capitis lateralis, suprahyoid and infrahyoid, and platysma muscles also flex the neck.

Splenius Capitis and Cervicis Muscles

The splenius capitis and cervicis muscles produce the motion of extension of the neck through a range of 90 degrees, or 10 inches from a starting position of 45 degrees of flexion. Usually both sides are tested simultaneously, although they may be tested separately.

Palpation. The splenius capitis and cervicis muscles lie deep to the upper trapezius muscles. Place the fingertips under the lateral border of the upper trapezius muscle. The fibers are directed toward the mastoid process (Fig. 7–32).

Position
· AG: Subject lies prone with a pillow under the thorax or with the head over the edge of the treatment table (Fig. 7–33).
· GM: Subject is in sidelying position with the head supported on a low-friction surface (Fig. 7–34).

Movement. Extension of the head and neck.

Resistance. Applied to the occiput in a downward and forward direction.

Stabilization. Upper posterior thorax is stabilized.

Figure 7–32. Palpation for the splenius capitis and cervicis muscles.

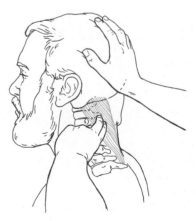

Figure 7–33. AG prone position for testing the splenius capitis and cervicis muscles.

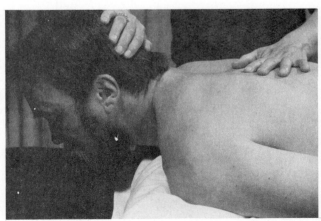

Attachments of Splenius Capitis and Cervicis Muscles

Muscles	Proximal	Distal	Innervation
Splenius capitis	Inferior ligamentum nuchae, spinous process of C7 and T1–4 vertebrae	Mastoid process, occipital bone, and lateral third of superior nuchal line	Cervical spinal nerve and ventral primary rami of the cervical spinal nerves
Splenius cervicis	Spinous processes of T3–6 vertebrae	Posterior tubercles of C1–3	

Attachments of Rectus Abdominis Muscle

Muscle	Proximal	Distal	Innervation
Rectus abdominis, upper	Pubic crest and symphysis	Costal cartilages of 5th to 7th ribs and xiphoid process	Ventral primary rami T5–10
Lower			T10–L1

Substitutions
- Deviations to the left or right indicate that one side is stronger than the other.
- Upper trapezius, erector spinae, and intertransversarii muscles extend the neck.

Upper Rectus Abdominis Muscle

The upper portion of the rectus abdominis muscle is tested for flexion of the upper trunk in the sagittal plane, through a range such that the inferior angles of the scapulae clear the table. The subject should curl up slowly.

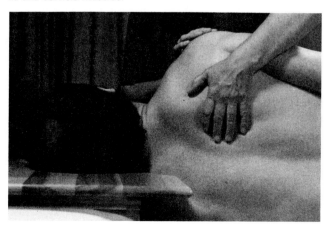

Figure 7–34. GM sidelying position for testing the splenius capitis and cervicis muscles.

Palpation. Palpate the rectus abdominis on both sides of the midline between the umbilicus and the xiphoid process (Fig. 7–35).

Position. Subject lies supine.

Movement
- For 0 to P or 0 to 2 grades: Depression of the lower portion of the thorax (Figs. 7–36 and 7–37).
- For P+ to N or 2+ to 5 grades: Partial sit-up (Figs. 7–38 to 7–42).

Resistance. No external resistance is given; resistance is determined by position of the upper limbs.

Stabilization. Pelvis and lower limbs are stabilized.

Grades
0: No contraction is palpated.
T or 1: Contraction without depression of the thorax.
P−: Contraction with partial depression of the thorax.
P or 2: Contraction with full depression of the thorax.
P+: Upper limbs at side of trunk; trunk begins motion against gravity.
F: Upper limbs at side of trunk; spines of scapulae clear the table.
F or 3: Upper limbs at side of trunk; inferior angles of the scapulae clear the table.

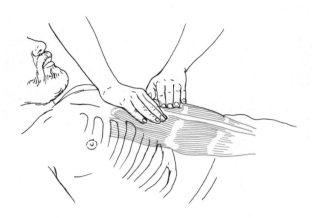

Figure 7–35. Palpation for the upper rectus abdominis muscle.

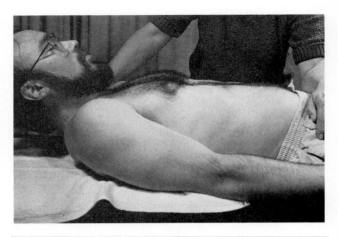

Figure 7–36. Appearance of "poor minus" performance of the rectus abdominis muscle.

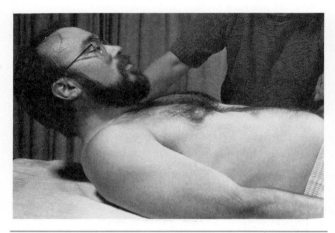

Figure 7–37. Appearance of "poor" performance of the rectus abdominis muscle.

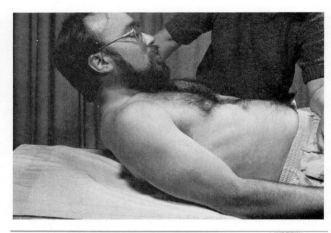

Figure 7–38. Appearance of "poor plus" performance of the rectus abdominis muscle.

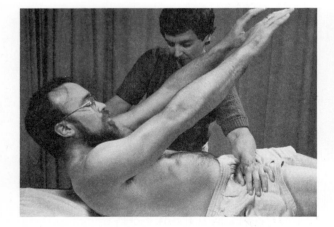

Figure 7–39. Appearance of "fair plus" performance of the rectus abdominis muscle.

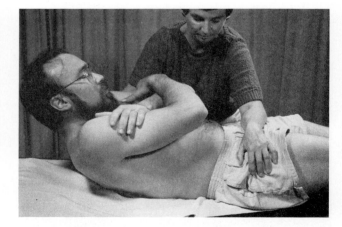

Figure 7–40. Appearance of "good" performance of the rectus abdominis muscle.

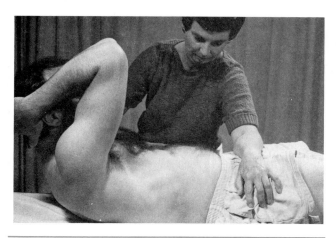

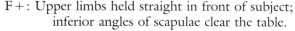

Figure 7–41. Appearance of "good plus" performance of the rectus abdominis muscle.

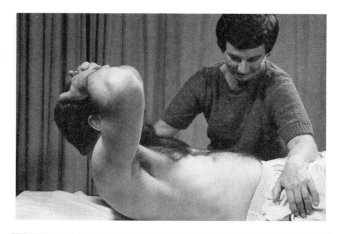

Figure 7–42. Appearance of "normal" performance of the rectus abdominis muscle.

F + : Upper limbs held straight in front of subject; inferior angles of scapulae clear the table.

G or 4: Upper limbs across chest; inferior angles of scapulae clear the table.

G + : Hands placed behind the head with elbows pointing forward; inferior angles clear the table.

N or 5: Hands on top of head with the shoulder horizontally abducted; inferior angles clear the table.

Substitutions

- Patient may jerk up using momentum; the sit-up should be performed slowly.
- For grades of P + to F or 2 + to 3, patient may push up with the upper limbs.
- For grades of T to P or 1 to 2, the patient may breathe deeply, causing depression of the lower portion of the thorax.
- The internal and external abdominal obliques of each side contracting together can produce trunk flexion in the sagittal plane.
- Deviation of the umbilicus to one side indicates greater strength of that side.

Lower Rectus Abdominis Muscle

The lower portion of the rectus abdominis muscle is tested during the motion of flexion of the lower trunk until the sacrum clears the treatment table.

Palpation. Palpate the rectus abdominis on both sides of the midline between the umbilicus and the symphysis pubis (Fig. 7–43).

Position. The subject lies supine, with the hips and knees flexed and the feet flat on the table; the upper limbs are crossed over the chest (Figs. 7–44 and 7–45).

Movement. Posterior pelvic tilt, the sacrum is lifted from the table.

Resistance. No external resistance is applied. Weight of the lower limbs and the number of repetitions provide the resistance.

Stabilization. No stabilization is necessary.

Grades

0: No contraction.

T or 1: Contraction felt but no movement.

P − : Partial pelvic tilt.

P or 2: Complete pelvic tilt.

P + : Initiates lifting of sacrum.

F − : Lifts sacrum through half the range.

F or 3: Lifts sacrum through full range 1 time.

Figure 7–43. Palpation for the lower rectus abdominis muscle.

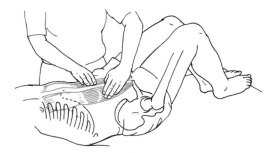

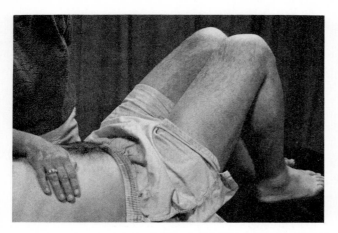

Figure 7–44. "Poor minus" performance for the lower portion of the rectus abdominis.

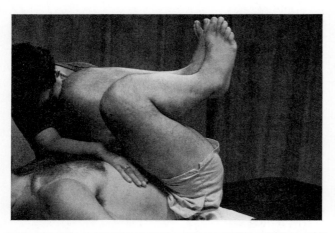

Figure 7–45. "Fair" performance for the lower portion of the rectus abdominis.

F+: Lifts sacrum through full range 2 to 3 times.
G or 4: Lifts sacrum through full range 4 to 6 times.
G+: Lifts sacrum through full range 7 to 9 times.
N or 5: Lifts sacrum through full range 10 times.
P+ to N or 2+ to 5: Subject brings knees to chest, then lifts sacrum off the table.

Substitutions
- For grades of P− and P or 2, subject may breathe deeply, causing the abdomen to depress, thus giving the appearance of posterior pelvic tilt.
- For grades of P+ to N or 2+ to 5, subject may push with the upper limbs or jerk up. Be sure subject comes up slowly and keeps the upper limbs relaxed.
- The umbilicus may deviate toward the strong side.

Attachments. See attachments for upper rectus abdominis muscle.

External and Internal Abdominal Oblique Muscles

The external and internal abdominal oblique muscles are tested against gravity during trunk flexion and rotation or a diagonal sit-up. In the gravity-minimized (GM) position, the motion is rotation only. The end point of the test range is when both scapulae clear the table. Both rotation and flexion occur at the same time, and the trunk must roll up evenly without extension in the lumbar area. The movement takes place at the same speed over the full range, without a jerk at the beginning of motion. The external abdominal oblique muscle contracts when the subject rotates to the opposite side, and the internal abdominal oblique muscle contracts when the subject rotates to the same side. If the trunk is rotating toward the left, the right external abdominal oblique and the left internal abdominal oblique contract to perform the diagonal sit-up.

Palpation

External Abdominal Oblique. Palpate below the ribs and costal cartilages of the lowest ribs in the midclavicular line.

Internal Abdominal Oblique. Palpate immediately medial to the anterior superior iliac spine in the midclavicular line (Fig. 7–46).

Position
- AG: Subject lies supine with the lower limbs extended (Figs. 7–47 to 7–50).
- GM: Subject sits with the upper limbs at the sides of the trunk. If the patient is unable to sit, an alternate position is used: subject lies supine with the hips and knees flexed, feet flat on the table. In this position, however, the subject may depress the lower thorax and elevate the pelvis when performing the rotation.

Figure 7–46. Palpation for the external and internal oblique abdominal muscles.

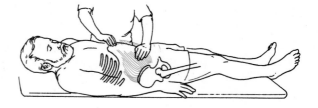

Attachments of External and Internal Abdominal Oblique Muscles

Muscle	Proximal	Distal	Innervation
External abdominal oblique	Lateral surface of caudad 8 pairs of ribs	Linea alba, inguinal ligament, anterior superior iliac spine, pubic tubercle, and anterior half of iliac crest	Ventral primary rami of T5–L1
Internal abdominal oblique	Inguinal ligament, iliac crest, and thoracolumbar fascia	Pubic crest, linea alba, and 10th–12th ribs	Ventral primary rami of T7–L1

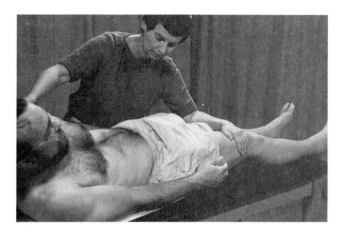

Figure 7–47. "Poor plus" performance for the external and internal oblique abdominal muscles.

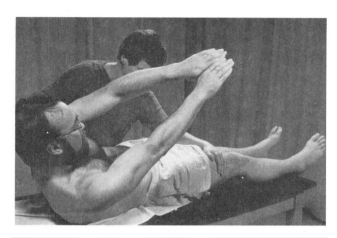

Figure 7–48. "Fair plus" performance for the external and internal oblique abdominal muscles.

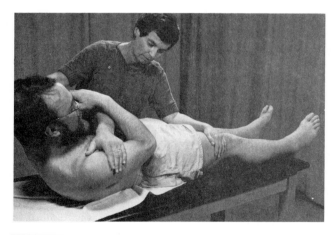

Figure 7–49. "Good" performance for the external and internal oblique abdominal muscles.

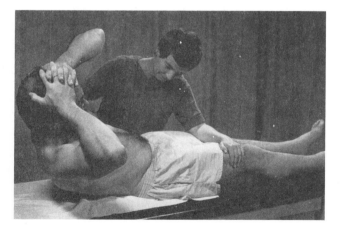

Figure 7–50. "Normal" performance for the external and internal oblique abdominal muscles.

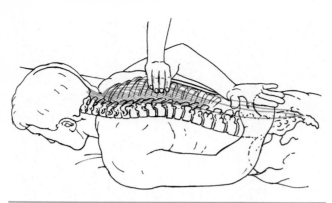

Figure 7–51. Palpation for the thoracic erector spinae muscles.

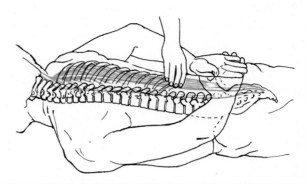

Figure 7–52. Palpation for the lumbar erector spinae muscles.

Movement. Subject attempts to perform a diagonal sit-up.

Resistance. No external resistance is applied; it is determined by the position of the upper limbs.

Stabilization. Pelvis and lower limbs are stabilized.

Grades

0: No contraction palpated.
T or 1: Contraction felt, but no rotation.
P−: Partial rotation.
P or 2: Full rotation.
P+: Beginning elevation of the opposite scapula, upper limbs relaxed.
F−: Elevation of half of the opposite scapula, upper limbs relaxed.
F or 3: Inferior angle of the opposite scapula clears the table, upper limbs relaxed.
F+: Upper limbs straight in front of subject. The opposite scapula clears the table, and part of the scapula on the side toward which the person is reaching comes off the table.
G or 4: Upper limbs cross the chest. Opposite scapula clears the table and part of the scapula on the side toward which the person is reaching comes off the table.
G+: Upper limbs behind the neck with the elbows directed forward. Both scapulae clear the table.
N or 5: Upper limbs on top of head with the shoulders abducted. Both scapulae clear the table.

Substitutions

- In the gravity-minimized position, the deep rotators of the back may rotate the trunk.

- In the against-gravity (AG) position, subject may jerk up. Motion shoud be performed slowly and evenly.
- Rectus abdominis and the short rotators of the back assist in the motion of trunk flexion with rotation.

Erector Spinae, Transversospinalis, Interspinales, and Cervical, Thoracic, and Lumbar Intertransversarii Muscles

The intrinsic back muscles are tested in the motion of cervical, thoracic, and lumbar vertebral extension from a starting position of slight flexion. The motion is tested through a range of minimal extension.

Palpation. Palpate the erector spinae on either side of the midline in the thoracic and lumbar vertebral region. These muscles are too deep to palpate in the cervical region (Figs. 7–51 and 7–52).

Position

- AG: For the thoracic muscles, subject lies prone with pillows under the abdomen and the upper limbs resting on the buttocks (Fig. 7–53). For the lumbar muscles, subject lies prone with pillows under the hips and the hands resting on the buttocks (Fig. 7–54).
- GM: For the thoracic muscles, subject sits backward in a chair with the back slightly rounded and relaxed and the hands on the back of the chair (Fig. 7–55). For the lumbar muscles, subject sits with the lower back arched, increased lumbar lordosis, and the pelvis tilted anteriorly (Fig. 7–56). Alternatively, subject lies supine and the back is arched in both the thoracic and lumbar region.

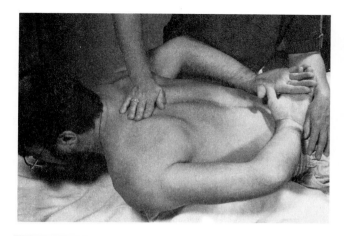

Figure 7–53.   AG prone position for the thoracic erector spinae muscles.

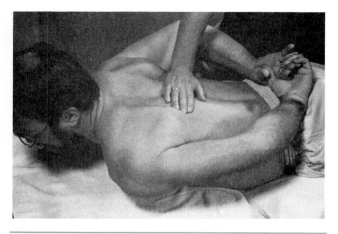

Figure 7–54.   AG prone position for the lumbar erector spinae muscles.

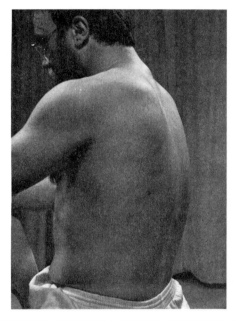

Figure 7–55.   GM sitting position for the thoracic erector spinae muscles.

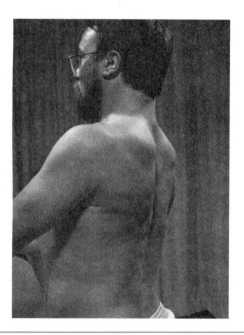

Figure 7–56.   GM sitting position for the lumbar erector spinae muscles.

Movement.   Subject extends the upper and lower portions of the trunk.

Resistance.   Applied to the upper portion of the thoracic spine for the thoracic portion, and to the lower portion of the thoracic spine for the lumbar portion.

Stabilization

Thoracic.   Pelvis and lumbar vertebrae are stabilized.

Lumbar.   Pelvis and hips are stabilized.

Substitutions

- Observe the motion of intrinsic extensors in adjacent areas in the specific test area.
- The subject may push off from the table with an anterior thrust of the shoulders. Keep scapulae adducted.
- To ensure contraction of the trunk extensors, have the subject relax the shoulders at the completion of the test range.
- Observe lumbar vertebrae motion during hip extension.

Attachments of Intrinsic Back Muscles

Muscle	Proximal	Distal	Innervation
Cervical Spine			
Suboccipital muscles	Atlas and axis	Transverse processes of atlas and occipital bone	Dorsal primary rami of the cervical spinal nerves
Iliocostalis cervicis	3rd–6th rib angles	Posterior tubercles of C4–6	
Longissimus cervicis	Transverse processes of T1–4 or T5	Posterior tubercles of C2–6	
Longissimus capitis	Transverse processes of T1–4 or T5 and C4 or 5–7	Mastoid process	
Spinalis cervicis	Ligamentum nuchae, spinous process of C7	Spinous processes of axis and C3 and C4	
Spinalis capitis	Transverse processes of upper thoracic and lower cervical vertebrae	Occipital bone between superior and inferior nuchal lines	
Semispinalis cervicis	Transverse processes of T1–6	Spinous processes of C2–5	
Semispinalis capitis	Transverse processes of T1–6 and C4–7	Between superior and inferior nuchal lines	
Multifidi	Transverse processes of cervical vertebrae	Cervical vertebra's spinous process of each two vertebrae immediately superior	
Rotatores	Transverse process of cervical vertebrae	Lamina of immediately superior cervical vertebra	
Interspinalis	Between spinous processes six pairs of cervical vertebrae		
Intertransversarii	Between transverse processes six pairs of cervical vertebrae	Posterior: dorsal and ventral primary rami Anterior: ventral primary rami of spinal nerves	
Thoracic Spine			
Iliocostalis thoracis	Angles of the lower 6 ribs	Angle of upper 6 ribs and transverse process of C7	Dorsal primary rami of the thoracic spinal nerves
Longissimus thoracis	Lumbar transverse processes Thoracolumbar fascia	Transverse processes of all thoracic vertebrae and lower nine pairs of ribs between the angle and tubercle	
Semispinalis thoracis	Transverse processes of thoracic vertebrae	Spinous process of C6 and C7 and T1–4	
Multifidi	Transverse processes of thoracic vertebrae	Spinous process of 2 to 4 immediately superior vertebrae	
Rotatores	Transverse processes of thoracic vertebrae	Lamina of vertebra immediately superior	
Intertransversarii	11 pairs between thoracic transverse processes		
Interspinales	Two to three pairs between 1st and 2nd and 11th and 12th spinous processes		

Attachments of Intrinsic Back Muscles (continued)

Muscle	Proximal	Distal	Innervation
Lumbar Spine			
Iliocostalis lumborum	Spinous processes of lumbar vertebrae and T11 and T12 Posterior iliac crest and supraspinous ligament Crest of the sacrum	Inferior border of the angles of the lower 6 or 7 ribs	
Multifidis	Sacrum Posterior superior iliac spine Sacroiliac ligaments Transverse processes of lumbar vertebrae	Spinous process of 2 to 4 immediately superior vertebrae	Dorsal primary rami of the lumbar spinal nerves
Rotatores	Transverse processes of lumbar vertebrae	Lamina of immediately superior vertebra	
Interspinalis	Four pairs between lumbar spinous processes		
Intertransversarii	Four pairs between lumbar transverse processes	Dorsal and ventral primary rami of lumbar spinal nerves	

Quadratus Lumborum Muscle

The quadratus lumborum muscle is tested in the motion of hip hiking, moving the pelvis in the coronal plane unilaterally. The iliac crest approximates the 12th rib. The test range is 25 to 30 degrees, or 3 inches.

Palpation. Palpate the quadratus lumborum with subject either supine or standing. The lateral trunk flexors must be relaxed in order that the examiner can place the fingers deep under the erector spinae muscles. Have the subject bend the trunk laterally, then relax. The fingers are placed over the posterior iliac crest and below the 12th rib directed toward the vertebrae (Fig. 7–57).

Position
- AG: Subject stands on a block or stool holding onto the examiner lightly to maintain balance, with the test leg hanging free (Fig. 7–58).
- GM: Subject is either supine or prone, with test leg abducted 15 degrees and the pelvis laterally tilted (Fig. 7–59).

Movement. Subject hikes the hip by elevating the pelvis on the test side.

Resistance. Applied to the iliac crest in the direction of lateral tilt of the pelvis.

Stabilization. Trunk is stabilized on the opposite side.

Substitutions. Flexion of the trunk to the opposite side may give the appearance of hip hiking.

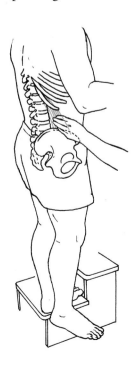

Figure 7–57. Palpation for the quadratus lumborum muscle.

Attachments of Quadratus Lumborum Muscle

Muscle	Proximal	Distal	Innervation
Quadratus lumborum	Iliolumbar ligaments Iliac crest Transverse processes of lower lumbar vertebrae	Inferior border of 12th rib Transverse processes of L1–4	Ventral primary rami of L1–3

Cervical Spine

Clinical Tests

The examiner should clear associated areas for dysfunction: the shoulder girdle, thoracic region (including the thoracic outlet), and temporomandibular joint.

Palpation

The following structures and landmarks should be palpated or observed during cervical spine evaluation. Areas of pain, tenderness, muscle guarding, atrophy, swelling, or congestion should be noted.

1. Spinous processes of C2 through T3.*
2. Transverse processes of C1.

Note: To differentiate between C6, C7, and T1, find the first prominent spinous process at the cervicothoracic junction. Palpate the spinous process of the superior vertebra and the interspinous space. Bend the head and neck backward while continuing palpation. If the superior spinous process seems to "disappear" in the backward bent position, the C6–7 interspace has been identified. If both spinous processes remain palpable, the C7–T1 interspace has been identified.

3. Mastoid process.
4. Angles of the mandible.
5. External occipital protuberance.
6. Articular pillars.
7. Zygapophyseal joints (facet articulations).
8. Carotid (Chassaignac's) tubercle of C6.
9. First rib, anterior and posterior attachments.
10. Hyoid bone.
11. Thyroid cartilage.
12. Sternal notch.
13. Sternoclavicular articulations.
14. Boundaries of anterior and posterior triangles.
15. Carotid arteries.
16. Trunks of the brachial plexus.
17. Scapula.
    Superior angle.
    Medial (vertebral) border.
    Spine.
    Acromion process.
18. Muscles and their attachment sites.
    Trapezius.
    Sternocleidomastoid.

Figure 7–58.   Testing the quadratus lumborum muscle in the AG standing position.

Figure 7–59.   Testing the quadratus lumborum muscle in the GM supine position.

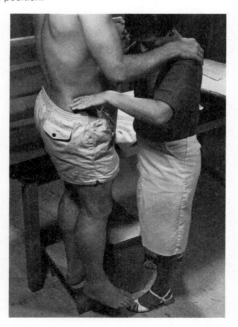

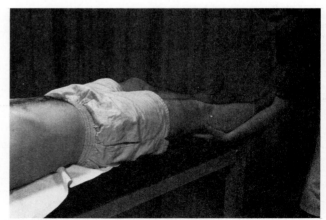

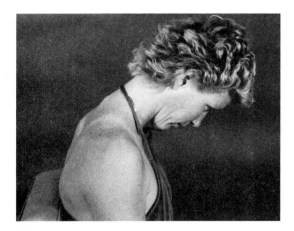

Figure 7–60. Forward bending.

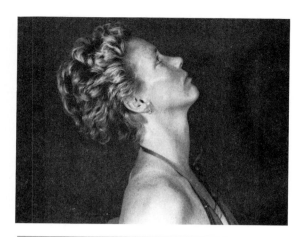

Figure 7–61. Backward bending.

Levator scapulae.
Scalenes.
Rhomboids.
Posterior suboccipital muscles.

Gross Active and Passive Movement

The motions to be assessed for the active and passive range include:

1. Forward bend (Fig. 7–60).
2. Backward bend (Fig. 7–61).
3. Right and left rotation in neutral and forward bent positions (Fig. 7–62).
4. Right and left sidebending with rotation to the same and opposite sides (Fig. 7–63). (*Note:* In true sidebending, the head naturally rotates to the same side. If the subject artificially keeps the head facing forward during sidebending, as is commonly done, rotation in the opposite direction must occur at the atlantoaxial articulation.)

End feel is assessed by gentle overpressure at the end of painless range. Sustained positioning assesses for the onset of latent paresthesia.

Contractile Testing

Contractile testing of the cervical spine should include:

1. Forward bending.
2. Backward bending.
3. Right and left sidebending.
4. Right and left rotation.

Special Tests
Vertebral Artery

Indication. The following three tests all assess vertebrobasilar artery insufficiency. Tests should be performed bilaterally, starting with the side on which no symptoms are expected. A test is terminated *immediately* with the onset of signs or symptoms, which typically

Figure 7–62. (*A*) Rotation in neutral position. (*B*) Rotation in forward bent position.

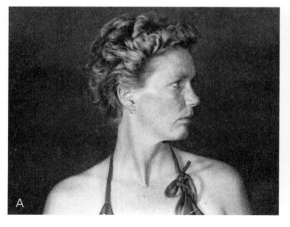

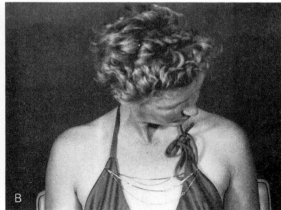

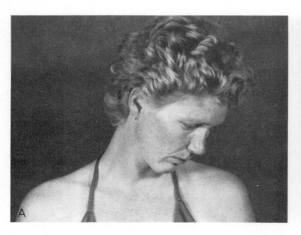
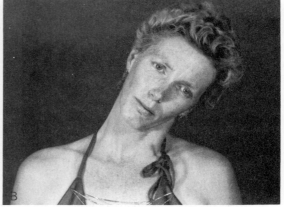

Figure 7–63. (A) Rotation with sidebend to the same side. (B) Rotation with sidebend to the opposite side.

abate when the head is returned to the neutral position. These symptoms include faintness, dizziness, nystagmus, and personality changes. It is suggested that no thrust manipulations be performed if there is a positive result. Also, the vertebral artery should be retested after each manual therapy procedure, since an increase in cervical range of motion may produce a positive result in the new range.

Quadrant Test

Method.   Subject lies supine with a pillow beneath the upper and middle thoracic spine. The head is supportd by the therapist in a neutral position. The head is brought into sidebending with rotation to the same side, and the subject is observed for 8 to 12 seconds for signs or symptoms. If there are none, the head is moved into backward bending and again observed for signs or symptoms (Fig. 7–64). The test is terminated immediately if signs or symptoms develop.

Backward Bending Test

Method.   With subject and examiner positioned as in the quadrant test, the subject's head is brought into full backward bending, without sidebending or rotation. The subject is observed for signs or symptoms for 8 to 12 seconds (Fig. 7–65).

Maigne's Test

Method.   With the subject supine, the examiner brings the head into a position of full backward bending and rotation or into the set-up position for the intended manipulation. The subject holds the position for as long as 30 seconds, while the examiner observes and questions the subject for signs and symptoms (Fig. 7–66).

Results.   The results of these tests are positive if the subject experiences or demonstrates signs of vertigo, nystagmus, slurred speech, tinnitus, nausea, vomiting, syncope, or visual disturbance. The subject's eyes should be

Figure 7–64.   Quadrant test.

Figure 7–65.   Backward bending test.

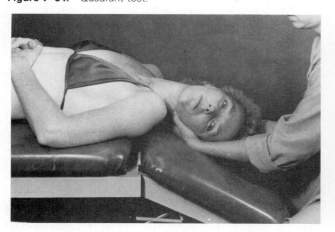
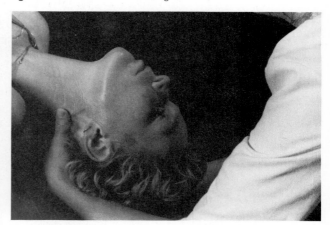

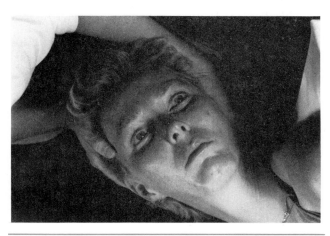

Figure 7–66.   Maigne's test.

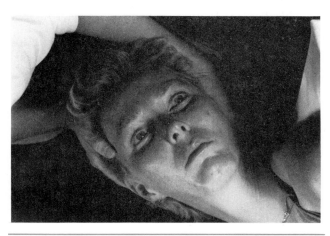

Additional Notes on Vertebral Artery.   Inner ear involvement can produce signs and symptoms like those of a positive vertebral artery test. For this reason, the subject may also be tested sitting or standing and should rotate the trunk while maintaining the head orientation. If this rotation of the cervical spine also causes signs and symptoms, the vertebral artery is still suspected of compromise. If negative, an inner ear problem is a potential source of symptoms.

Alar Ligament Test

Indication.   The alar ligament test reveals rupture of the alar ligament or fracture of the odontoid process of C2.

Method.   Subject lies supine. The therapist supports the head beneath the occipital region while palpating the C2 spinous process. A gentle force is given to produce suboccipital sidebending of the atlanto-occipital articulation, first to one side then to the other (Fig. 7–68). The spinous process is palpated during this movement to assess concurrent C2 rotation (the spinous process of C2 is palpated rotating in the opposite direction).

Results.   C2 rotation to the same side must be immediate. If there is a lag or no concurrent movement, the result is positive. This is a *life-threatening* situation.

Compression and Distraction Test

Indication.   The compression and distraction test is used to assess disc protrusion or intervertebral foramen compromise.

open and the subject should be speaking to be properly assessed. Again, the test is terminated immediately if symptoms are observed.

Hautant's Test

Indication.   Hautant's test is for vertebrobasilar artery insufficiency.

Method.   Subject is seated with the arms outstretched, forearms supinated (Fig. 7–67A). Subject is instructed to close the eyes and bring the head into full backward bending and rotation (Fig. 7–67B).

Results.   Observe the subject for signs and symptoms. A positive test result is indicated if one hand sinks and pronates on the side of compromise.

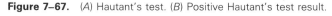

Figure 7–67.   (*A*) Hautant's test. (*B*) Positive Hautant's test result.

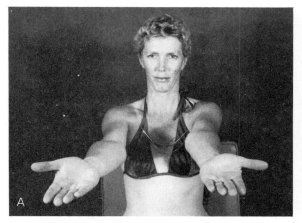

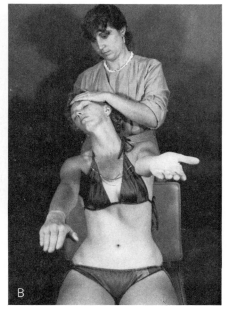

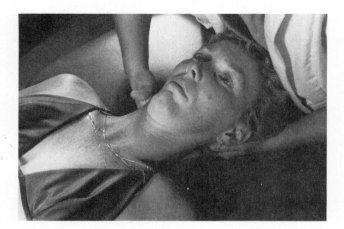

Figure 7–68.   Alar ligament test.

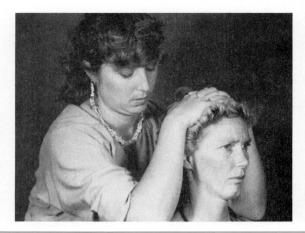

Figure 7–69.   Compression test.

Method 1, Compression.   Subject is seated, with the head and neck in a neutral position. The examiner, with fingers interlocked and placed on top of the subject's head, provides gentle downward force (Fig. 7–69). Take care not to cause forward, backward, or sideways bending of the cervical spine.

Method 2, Distraction.   The examiner contacts the mastoid processes with the base of the palms. A gentle, even force lifts the weight of the subject's head straight upward (Fig. 7–70).

Results.   In the presence of a disc protrusion or compromised intervertebral foramen, compression of the spine tends to aggravate symptoms while distraction (decompression) tends to relieve them.

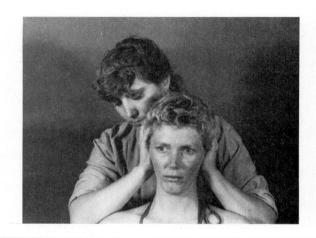

Figure 7–70.   Distraction test.

Joint Play: Passive Intervertebral Movement (PIVM)

Palpation of PIVM During Assessment of Gross Range of Motion

Segmental movement is assessed at the interspinous space. Forward and backward bending movements (Figs. 7–71 and 7–72) are palpated by contacting the spinous processes with opposite sides of one digit and guiding the head through these motions. The spinous processes will be felt to approach each other in backward bending and to separate in forward bending. To assess sidebending and rotation movements, the spine should first be bent forward to the level of testing for localization. Sidebend (Fig. 7–73) and rotation (Fig. 7–74) are assessed with contact on the lateral aspect of the spinous processes and the interspinous space. The contact will be on the side toward which the upper spinous process is expected

to move (e.g., *right* rotation of C5 on C6 will cause the spinous process of C5 to move to the *left*. The examiner, therefore, palpates on the *left*).

Suboccipital Forward Bending

Method.   Subject lies supine. The examiner stabilizes the axis with a contact over the articular pillars (Fig. 7–75A). With the opposite palm on the forehead, the examiner attempts to bend the head forward as if the subject were nodding. Centrally applied pressure produces bilateral movement (Fig. 7–75B), while more lateral pressure tends to localize testing to the same side (Fig. 7–75C).

Results.   Suboccipital forward bending assesses backward glide of the atlantooccipital articulation and forward glide of the atlantoaxial joint.

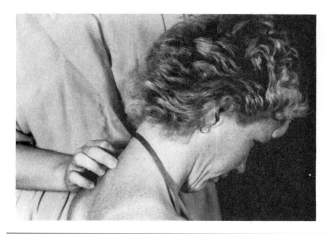

Figure 7–71. Forward bending of cervical spine.

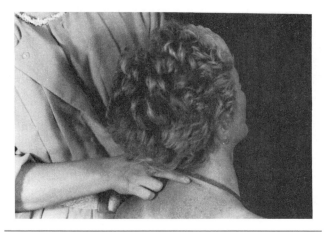

Figure 7–72. Backward bending of cervical spine.

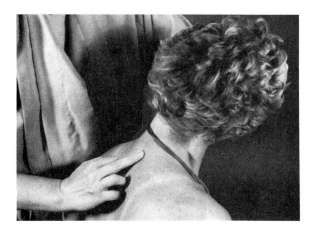

Figure 7–73. Sidebending of cervical spine.

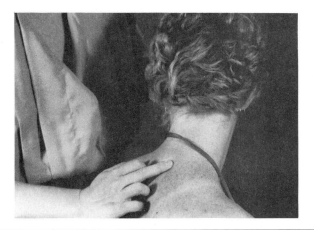

Figure 7–74. Rotation of cervical spine.

Suboccipital Backward Bending

Method. The subject lies supine. The examiner supports the head under the occiput with the second digits at the level of the atlas. The examiner can now use these digits as a fulcrum to bend the head backward at the suboccipital level. The examiner can assess one or both sides.

Results. Suboccipital backward bending assesses forward glide of the occipital condyles on the atlas and backward glide and tilt of the atlas on the axis.

Suboccipital Sidebending

Method. Subject lies supine. The examiner supports the head at the occiput, with the second digit metacarpophalangeal joint of each hand lying just distal to the mastoid process but not contacting the transverse process of C1. Gentle sidebending is produced by the hands

acting as a force couple, localizing movement to the occipitoatloid level, which causes rotation of the axis to the same side via the alar ligaments.

Results. Suboccipital sidebending assesses lateral glide of the atlantooccipital joint in the opposite direction, forward glide of the same side of the atlantoaxial joint, and backward glide of the atlantoaxial joint to the opposite side.

Suboccipital Rotation

The subject must pass the vertebral artery test before this test is performed.

Method. With the subject supine, the neck is brought into very slight foward bending and is then passively bent and rotated to one side. This action will cause facet locking on the side of the bend or rotation. The head is then rotated toward the opposite side, with the apposed

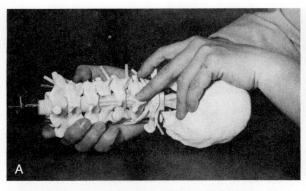

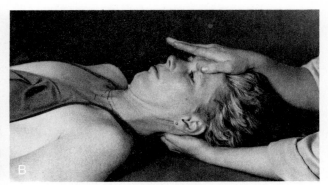

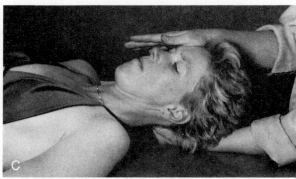

Figure 7–75. (*A*) Hand contact for suboccipital forward bending. (*B*) Central pressure producing bilateral movement. (*C*) Lateral pressure testing unilateral movement.

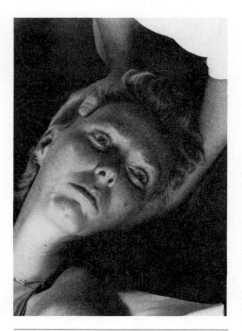

Figure 7–76. Suboccipital rotation.

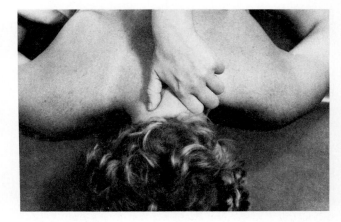

Figure 7–77. Hand contact for forward and backward glide.

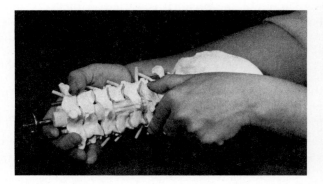

Figure 7–78. Forward and backward glide.

Table 7–1. Summary of Cervical Spine Joint Play

GLIDE	RESTRICTION	FIXED BONE	MOVING BONE
Atlanto-occipital Joint			
Anterior	Backward bend	Atlas	Occiput
Backward	Forward bend	Atlas	Occiput
Frontal plane	Side bend, same direction	Atlas	Occiput
Rotation	General hypomobility	Atlas	Occiput
Atlantoaxial Joint			
Forward	Forward bend, atlantoaxial rotation in opposite direction Atlantooccipital sidebend in opposite direction	Axis	Atlas
Backward	Backward bend, atlantoaxial rotation in same atlanto-occipital direction; sidebend in same direction	Axis	Atlas
Frontal	General hypomobility	Axis	Atlas
C2, C3–T3, T4 Joints			
Forward	Forward bend, sidebend in opposite direction, rotation in opposite direction	Inferior vertebra	Superior vertebra
Backward	Backward bend; sidebend in same direction, rotation in opposite direction	Inferior vertebra	Superior vertebra
Side	General hypomobility	Inferior vertebra	Superior vertebra

facets blocking forward gliding movement of the lower segment facet (Fig. 7–76). The test movement is then repeated in the opposite direction.

Results. Suboccipital rotation assesses backward glide of the facets on the side toward which the head is rotated and forward glide of the facets on the side of bending.

Forward and Backward Glide: C2, C3–T3, T4

Method
- *Unilateral*: The pad of the thumb is placed over the articular pillar of one side. Force is applied in a direction parallel to the joint plane to assess for end feel or provocation of symptoms (Fig. 7–77).
- *Bilateral*: Contact to bilateral articular pillars of the same vertebra is made with the pad of the thumb and the metacarpophalangeal joint of the second digit of the same hand. Force is applied parallel to the joint plane (Fig. 7–78).

Results. The forward and backward glide test assesses forward glide of the inferior motion segment and backward glide of the superior segment.

Midcervical Side Glide

Method. Subject lies supine with the neck in a neutral position. The examiner places the metacarpophalangeal joint of the second digit on the articular pillar. Using the opposite hand to support the neck, the examiner applies lateral force along the transverse plane. This force tends to "gap" the facet of the opposite side at the same level as a test of joint play.

Summary of Joint Play of the Cervical Spine

As a standard of reference, vertebral movement or position is always described by the superior vertebra with respect to the inferior vertebra, independent of which vertebra actually moves (i.e., cephalad–caudal versus caudal–cephalad sequence). Table 7–1 provides a summary of joint play of the cervical spine.

Thoracic Spine

Clinical Tests

Associated areas to be cleared for dysfunction include the cervical spine, shoulder girdle (especially for scapulothoracic dysfunction), and the lumbar spine.

Palpation

Palpation during evaluation of the thoracic spine should include:

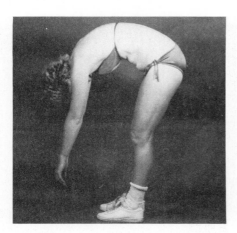

Figure 7–79. Forward bending of the trunk.

1. Spinous processes.
2. Transverse processes.
3. Ribs (including costochondral and costovertebral attachments, rib margin, and intercostal spaces; special attention should be paid to the first rib and its relationship to the clavicle anteriorly).
4. Sternum (including manubrium, body, xiphoid process, and the sternal angle).
5. Sternoclavicular joint.
6. Scapula.
7. Cervicothoracic junction.
8. Paravertebral muscles.

Gross Active Movement

The movements to be assessed for range as well as quality of movement include:

1. Forward bending (Fig. 7–79).
2. Backward bending (Fig. 7–80).
3. Sidebending (Fig. 7–81).
4. Rotation (Fig. 7–82).

Rotation is best observed by evaluating the sidebending component. The rules of sidebending and rotation change; the midthoracic levels are transitional. The lower segments follow the rule of opposite sidebending and rotation as in the lumbar spine in the erect position. The upper segments follow the rule of same sidebending and rotation as in the cervical spine.

Contractile Testing

Contractile testing should include all the motions assessed during gross active movement.

Special Tests

Positional Faults

Indication. Testing for positional faults enables the examiner to locate a possible spinal dysfunction. A finding of misalignment of the spinous processes must be correlated with the actual detection of mobility dysfunction at the same vertebral level in order to be considered valid.

Figure 7–80. Backward bending of the trunk.

Figure 7–81. Trunk sidebending.

Figure 7–82. Trunk rotation.

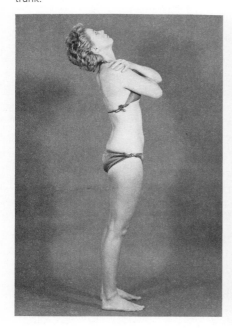

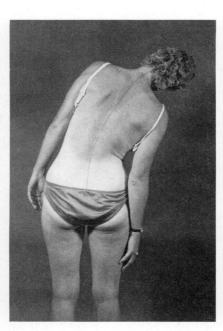

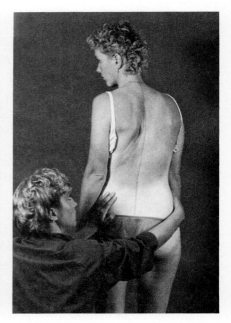

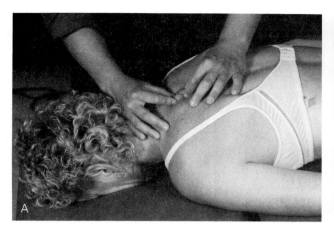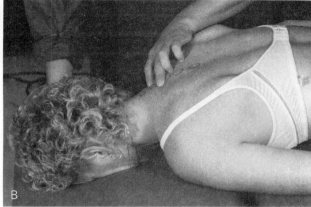

Figure 7–83. Testing for positional faults. (*A*) Palpation for rotational positional faults. (*B*) Palpation for forward and backward positional faults.

Method. The examiner pinches the spinous processes of two adjacent vertebrae between the thumb and forefinger of each hand and evaluates them for alignment along the length of the spine (Fig. 7–83*A*). The examiner then evaluates the distance between successive vertebrae (Fig. 7–83*B*).

Results. Each spinous process should be aligned between adjacent vertebrae and the interspinous distances should be similar, though it gradually changes, being narrower at both the upper and lower thoracic levels and greatest in the midthoracic region. A misaligned spinous process or an abnormal intervertebral space indicates either a potential motion segment dysfunction or a bony abnormality. If the segment moves normally upon PIVM testing, it is considered normal. If mobility is abnormal at the level of the positional fault, treatment is indicated. For example, a vertebra in an apparently forward bent position indicates restriction of forward glide of the superior motion segment or restriction of backward glide of the inferior one; this can be unilateral or bilateral. Therefore, only with motion testing can a more definitive assessment of the actual dysfunction be concluded.

Skin Rolling

Indication. Skin rolling is used to assess soft tissue mobility and to locate trigger points, areas of congestion, and temperature discrepancies.

Method. The examiner lifts an area of skin between the thumb and forefinger of each hand. The skin is "rolled" forward along the length and in the direction desired (Fig. 7–84).

Results. Ease, looseness, and lack of tenderness of the skin, although variable from person to person, are normal. Areas that feel tethered, congested, hot, or cold, or ones that are tender are usually sites of involvement that require treatment.

Joint Play: Passive Intervertebral Movement

Palpation of PIVM During Gross Range of Motion

Segmental movement is assessed at the interspinous space as in cervical spine evaluation for the upper thoracic levels. The examiner can support and guide movement of the midthoracic and lower thoracic levels by controlling the shoulders and thorax (Fig. 7–85). The spinous process is palpated during forward and backward bending, sidebending, and rotation. Assessment of sidebending and rotation is facilitated by forward bending to the level of testing. The examiner decides whether the

Figure 7–84. Skin rolling.

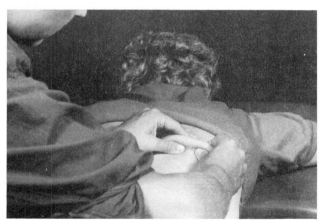

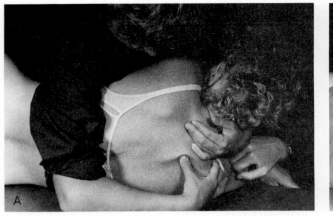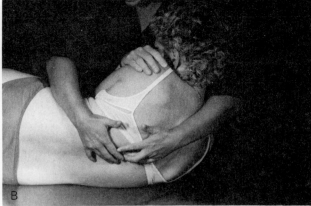

Figure 7–85. Assessment of segmental movement at the (A) midthoracic and (B) lower thoracic levels.

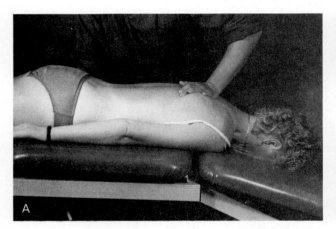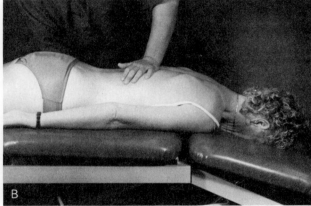

Figure 7–86. Spring testing of the (A) midthoracic and (B) lower thoracic levels.

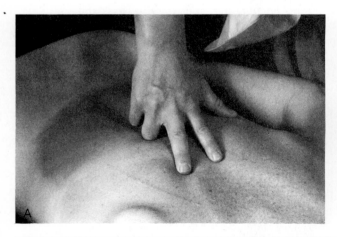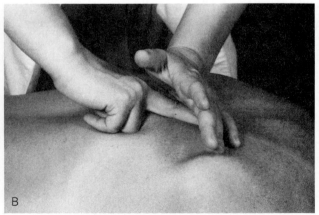

Figure 7–87. Hand positioning for posterior–anterior glide.

end feel is normal, hypermobile, or hypomobile and observes for provocaton of symptoms.

Spring Test

Method.   The examiner places the pisiform of the cephalad hand on the spinous process of each vertebra, producing a gentle springing force in a direction perpendicular to the contour of the spine (Fig. 7–86).

Results.   The spring test assesses forward bending of the superior motion segment and backward bending of the inferior segment.

Posterior and Anterior Glide

Method.   The examiner touches the transverse processes of a vertebra with the pads of the second and third digits of the caudal hand (Fig. 7–87A) and presses the hypothenar eminence of the other (mobilizing) hand over these two digits (Fig. 7–87B). Gentle force is applied in the posterocaudal–anterocephalic direction to follow the plane of the joint.

Results.   This method assesses forward bending of the inferior motion segment and backward bending of the superior segment.

Rotatory Glide

Method.   Contact is made as for posterior and anterior glide, except that the dummy hand touches two adjacent vertebrae, for example, the left transverse process of T6 and the right transverse process of T7. (The reverse set-up will also be tested.) The hypothenar eminence of the mobilizing hand produces a posterior and anterior force.

Results.   This method tests right rotation of T6 on T7 by producing forward glide of the left T6–7 articulation and backward glide of the right T6–7 articulation. This test is fairly well localized to single motion segments.

Rib (Costovertebral) Mobility

Method.   The subject lies in a prone position. The examiner uses the thumb web space along the length of the rib, including the costovertebral angle (Fig. 7–88). The examiner assesses mobility in the posterior and anterior (following the obliquity of the rib), cranial-caudal, and caudal-cranial directions.

Results.   The examiner identifies areas of normal mobility, hypermobility, and hypomobility of the costovertebral articulations.

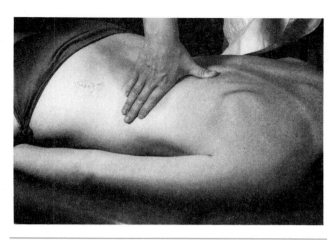

Figure 7–88.   Costovertebral mobility.

Summary of Joint Play of the Thoracic Spine

Table 7–2 provides a summary of joint play of the thoracic spine.

Lumbar Spine

Clinical Tests

Associated areas to be cleared of dysfunction include the lower thoracic spine, the sacroiliac joints, and the hips.

Palpation

The landmarks to be identified include:

1. Spinous processes.
2. Iliac crest, including anterior and posterior superior iliac spines (ASIS and PSIS).
3. The 12th rib.

Table 7–2.   Summary of Thoracic Spine Joint Play

GLIDE	RESTRICTION
Forward	Forward bend, sidebend to the opposite side, rotation to the opposite side
Backward	Backward bend, sidebend to the same side, rotation to the same side
Rotation	Rotation to the same side, backward glide of the same side, and forward glide of the opposite side facets
Spring test	General hypomobility of the costovertebral facet joints

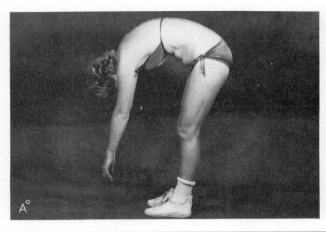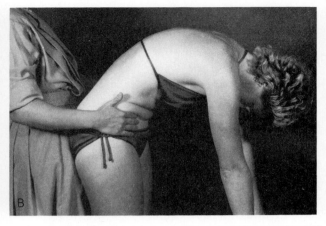

Figure 7–89. (A) Unrestricted forward bending of the lumbar spine. (B) Restricted movement of the pelvis during lumbar forward bending.

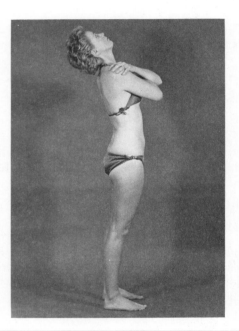

Figure 7–90. Backward bending of lumbar spine.

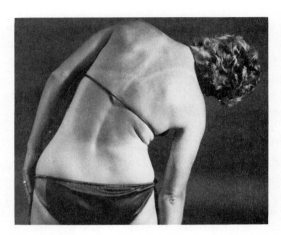

Figure 7–91. Sidebending of lumbar spine.

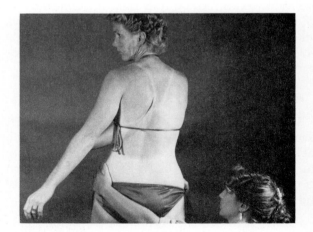

Figure 7–92. Rotation of lumbar spine.

Gross Active Movement

The motions to be assessed for active and passive range include:

1. Forward bending (Fig. 7–89).
2. Backward bending (Fig. 7–90).
3. Side bending (Fig. 7–91).
4. Rotation in erect and forward bent positions (Fig. 7–92).

Note: In the erect position, sidebending and rotation are to the same side. In forward bend, sidebending and rotation are to the opposite side.

Contractile Testing

Contractile testing of the lumbar spine should include forward, backward, and right and left sidebending and right and left rotation.

Special Tests

Tests for Dural Signs by Increased Tension on Spinal Nerve Roots

The following eight tests were designed and interpreted as tests of involvement or irritability of the lumbar spinal nerve roots by assessing reproduction of symptoms when the nerve roots are tensed. The examiner must remember that the spinal nerve roots are not the only structures provoked by these tests. In addition to the spinal nerve root, vertebral facets, and sacroiliac and hip joint structures, the hamstrings and fascial elements are also put under stress. The examiner must be aware that one of these other structures may be the source of symptoms or influence them. These elements must be properly assessed before it is possible to conclude which structure is at fault.

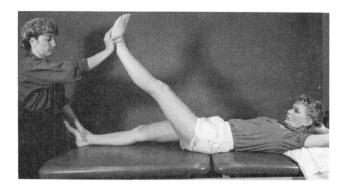

Figure 7–93.   Straight leg raise.

Straight Leg Raise (SLR) Test

Method.   The subject lies supine and raises one lower limb to 90 degrees of hip flexion. The hip is slightly adducted and internally rotated, and the knee is fully extended (Fig. 7–93). The angle between the elevated lower limb and the table at the point of onset of symptoms is noted if the test is positive.

Results.   Normal range should approach 80 to 90 degrees of hip flexion. Limitation of range accompanied by reproduction of symptoms (lower back pain, sciatic pain, or paresthesia) is a positive test result.

Laseque's Sign

Method.   The subject lies supine and flexes one lower limb at the hip to 90 degrees, with the knee and ankle in a relaxed position (Fig. 7–94A). With the ankle in a neutral position, the knee is then extended until symptoms are reproduced or a full extension position is attained (Fig. 7–94B).

Results.   The result is positive if symptoms are reproduced in the lower back or the involved limb.

Figure 7–94.   (A + B) Laseque's sign

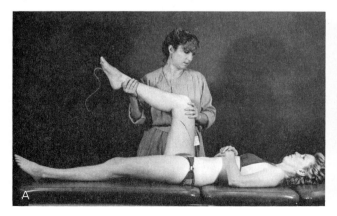

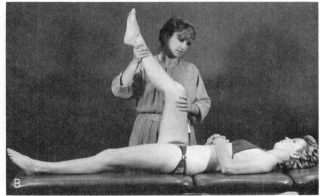

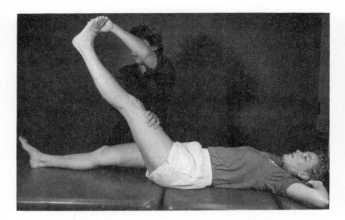

Figure 7–95. Braggard's test.

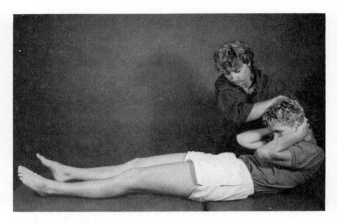

Figure 7–96. Brudzinski's test.

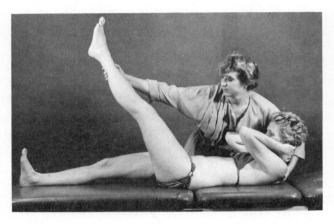

Figure 7–97. Soto-Hall test.

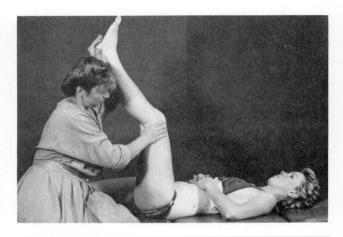

Figure 7–98. Cram's test.

Braggard's Test

Method. The subject lies supine and raises the involved lower limb to the point just short of where symptoms begin. The ankle of the limb is then passively dorsiflexed (Fig. 7–95).

Results. The result is positive if symptoms are reproduced in the lower back or the involved extremity.

Lermitte's Test (Crossed Leg–Straight Leg Raise)

Method. The subject lies supine and raises the uninvolved lower limb.

Results. The result is positive if pain is reproduced in the back or in the involved limb.

Brudzinski's Test

Method. The subject lies supine with both hands behind the neck. The examiner helps the subject flex the head and neck and upper back (Fig. 7–96).

Results. A positive result is indicated by pain in the low back, pelvic girdle, or lower limb.

Soto-Hall Test

Method. The subject lies supine. The examiner raises the involved lower limb, keeping it straight, to a point just short of the onset of pain. The subject's head and neck are then passively flexed (Fig. 7–97).

Results. Test results are positive if symptoms are reproduced.

Cram's Test (Bowstring Test, Popliteal Pressure Test)

Method. The subject lies supine. The examiner raises the involved straight leg to the point of onset of pain, then slightly flexes the knee until the pain is alleviated. The knee position is maintained; the hip is flexed further, to a point just short of the onset of pain. The examiner then presses on the posterior tibial nerve where it passes through the popliteal fossa (Fig. 7–98).

Results. Test results are positive if symptoms are reproduced.

Brechterew's Test

Method. The subject is seated and asked to extend both knees simultaneously (Fig. 7–99).

Results. Test results are positive if symptoms are reproduced in the involved limb.

Tests to Increase Intrathecal Pressure

The following three tests assess the effect of increased intrathecal pressure. A positive result suggests either intrathecal or extrathecal pathology (e.g., disc protrusion, tumor), including the meninges themselves.

Valsalva's Maneuver

Method. The subject is asked to hold a breath and then bear down, as if to have a bowel movement.

Results. Test results are positive if the subject reports reproduction or exacerbation of spinal pain or radiation into the limb.

Milgram's Test

Method. The subject lies supine. The examiner asks the subject to lift both lower limbs simultaneously 2 to 4 inches off the table while holding the position for 30 seconds (Fig. 7–100*A*).

Results. Test results are positive if the subject is unable to hold the limbs elevated for 30 seconds, or experiences reproduction of pain in the spine or radiation into the limb (Fig. 7–100*B*).

Naphziger's Test

Method. The subject lies supine. The examiner *gently* compresses the internal jugular veins bilaterally for approximately 10 seconds, then asks the patient to cough.

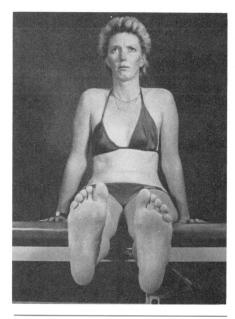

Figure 7–99. Brechterew's test.

Results. Test results are positive if the subject experiences reproduction of pain either in the spine or the limbs.

Repeated Forward and Backward Bending: Standing and Lying (McKenzie's Extension Principles)

Indication. Repeated bending is performed to differentiate between derangement of the disc and mechanical dysfunction of other spinal structures.

Method. For all of the following tests, the effect of the first movement on the subject's pain is noted. The effect is noted again after the repeated movements have been performed. Movements should be repeated as many

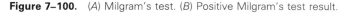

Figure 7–100. (*A*) Milgram's test. (*B*) Positive Milgram's test result.

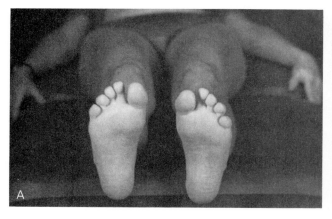

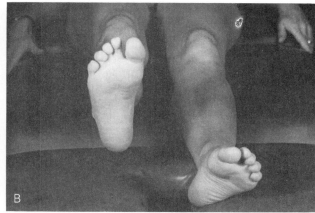

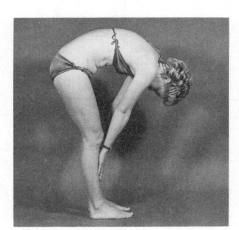

Figure 7–101. Forward bend standing.

as 10 times unless the subject reports reproduction or increased intensity or radiation of pain into the lower limb. The subject's range of motion during the repeated motions should also be observed.

Forward Bend Standing. The subject stands with the feet about 12 inches apart and is asked to run the hands down the front of the legs, as if to touch the toes, as far as can be tolerated and then to return to the upright position (Fig. 7–101).

Backward Bend Standing. The subject stands with the feet 12 inches apart and the hands placed in the small of the back. The subject bends backward over the hands, then returns to the upright position (Fig. 7–102). (*Note:*

If the subject is in a lateral shift position related to the symptoms, the examiner should attempt to correct this postural fault with a side glide technique before repeated testing of backward bending [Fig. 7–103]).

Forward Bend Supine. The subject is supine, grasping both knees with the hands. The subject bends forward, pulling the knees to the chest (Fig. 7–104). Knee flexion eliminates compression of the spine by the body weight and tension on the nerve root.

Backward Bend Prone. The subject lies prone with the hands positioned as if to do a push-up. The subject is asked to straighten the upper limbs and raise the trunk, keeping the pelvis and lower limbs in contact with the table, and then to return to the starting position (Fig. 7–105). In this position, body weight compression is diminished.

Results. The results of these tests are considered to indicate disc derangement, joint or soft tissue dysfunction, or a postural syndrome. No pain during testing indicates that pain experienced at other times by the subject is due to a postural syndrome in which time and positioning are key factors. Pain felt at the extremes of motion that does not progressively worsen with repetition and in fact is relieved with return from the end position is indicative of joint or soft tissue dysfunction. Disc derangement is indicated by progressive worsening of symptoms, especially with repeated movements, with increasingly intense pain or peripheralization of pain.

Figure 7–102. Backward bend standing.

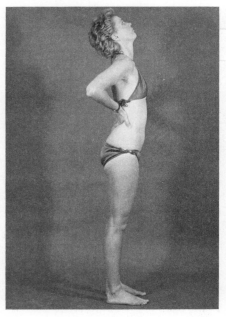

Figure 7–103. Lateral shift position.

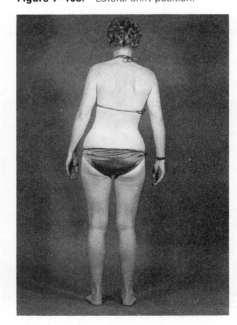

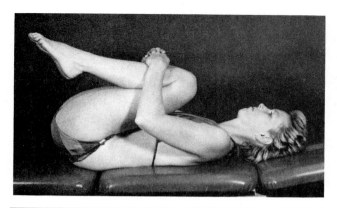

Figure 7–104. Forward bend in supine position.

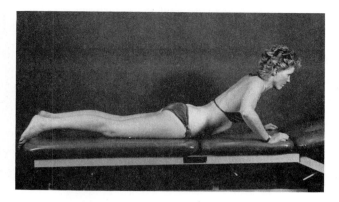

Figure 7–105. Backward bend in prone position.

Side Glide

Indication. Side glide reproduces, increases, or decreases the subject's symptoms and indicates whether a lateral shift is relevant to the symptoms.

Method. The subject stands with the examiner at one side. The examiner grasps the subject's pelvis with both hands and places a shoulder against the subject's lower thorax (Fig. 7–106). Equal and opposite forces are applied transversely by both hands.

Results. End feel and sustained positioning (10 to 15 seconds) are assessed for the effects on the subject's symptoms (increase or decrease and centralization or peripheralization of pain).

Compression and Distraction

Indication. Compression and distraction are used to assess for the presence of a bulging disc that may be compressing the spinal nerve roots.

Method
- **Compression:** The examiner stands behind the seated subject. Placing the hands on the subject's shoulders, the examiner provides moderate, even downward force through the trunk, taking care not to cause forward, backward, or sideways bending (Fig. 7–107).
- **Distraction:** The subject sits with upper limbs crossed. The examiner, standing behind, reaches around the thorax, grasping the subject's ipsilateral

Figure 7–106. Side-glide technique.

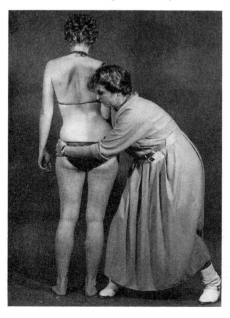

Figure 7–107. Compression test.

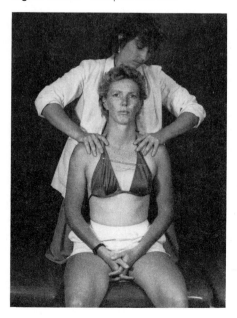

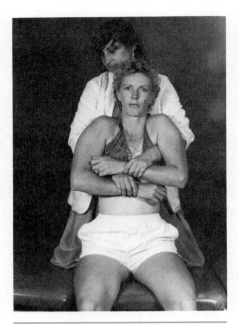

Figure 7–108. Distraction test.

forearm. By straightening up or leaning back, the examiner can distract the spine along its vertical axis (Fig. 7–108). If the subject has shoulder pathology, the examiner may put less strain on that area by just bear hugging around the thorax and distracting without applying forces to the shoulder.

Results. In the presence of a bulging disc, increased compression tends to exacerbate symptoms while distraction tends to diminish them.

Femoral Nerve Stretch

Indication. Femoral nerve stretch is used to determine whether there is any irritation of the femoral nerve or root.

Method. The subject is prone. The examiner flexes the subject's knee while supporting the thigh just proximal to the knee (Fig. 7–109). The examiner stabilizes the pelvis while extending the hip to provide a further stretch of the femoral nerve.

Results. Pain reproduced or exacerbated in the subject's back indicates a positive result for femoral nerve or nerve root irritation.

Tests To Evaluate Malingering

Flip Sign

Indication. The flip sign is used to assist in determining if the subject may be inventing symptoms.

Method. If the subject has a positive straight leg raise test when supine but the examiner suspects malingering, the subject is requested to assume a short sitting position with the legs dangling over the side of the table. Under the guise of examining for an unrelated problem (e.g., to check the knee or foot), the subject extends the knee now set up in a variant of the straight leg raise position.

Results. Reproduction of stretch of an irritated nerve root should occur in both the supine and sitting positions for this test. The subject who is malingering may fail to report symptoms in the variant position. The examiner should then be alerted to observe the subject carefully in the seated position; the subject may merely lean back or grimace rather than verbalize the complaints.

Hoover's Test

Indication. Hoover's test is used to help determine whether the subject may be malingering or withholding effort.

Method. With the subject supine, the examiner places one hand under each heel, then asks the subject to raise one lower limb. The examiner should feel an increase in pressure under the opposite heel as the subject tries to gain leverage with the effort (Fig. 7–110). The test is repeated with the opposite limb.

Results. If no increased pressure is felt from the opposite limb, the subject is probably not putting forth full effort.

Burn's Test

Method. The subject is asked to kneel on a chair and bend to touch fingers to the floor (Fig. 7–111).

Results. The subject who is unable to perform the task or overbalances the chair is likely to be malingering.

Figure 7–109. Femoral nerve stretch.

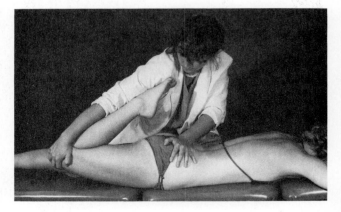

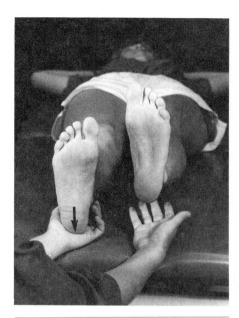

Figure 7–110.   Hoover's test.

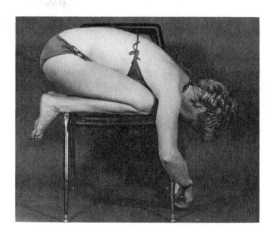

Figure 7–111.   Burn's test.

Joint Play: Passive Intervertebral Movement

Palpation and Assessment of Intersegmental Movement

All movements are described as the motion of the superior segment in relation to the inferior one.

Forward Bend

Method.   The subject is in the sidelying position. The examiner brings the uppermost limb or both limbs into hip and knee flexion (Fig. 7–112*A* and *B*). The hip must typically be flexed at least 90 degrees before lumbar movement is recruited. While using the cephalad hand

to palpate the interspinous space, the examiner brings the hip into further flexion, thereby recruiting movement at each segmental level for assessment of mobility.

Results.   This test assesses the superior glide of the facets.

Sidebending

Method 1.   The subject is in the sidelying position, with hips and knees flexed 90 degrees. The examiner uses the craniad hand to palpate at the interspinous level on the side of sidebending. The caudad hand contacts the ischial tuberosity of the upper innominate (pelvis) and rocks the pelvis superiorly (Fig. 7–113*A*). The result is sidebending of the lumbar spine in the direction of

Figure 7–112.   Forward bending. (*A*) Assessment of lumbar intersegmental forward bending by flexion of uppermost limb. (*B*) Assessment of lumbar intersegmental mobility by flexion of both lower limbs.

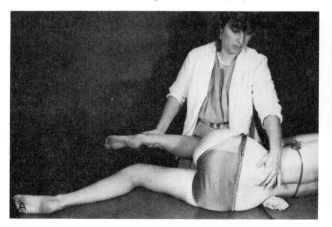

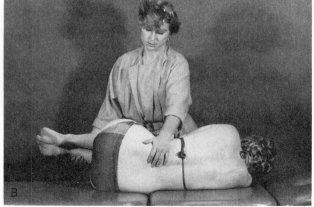

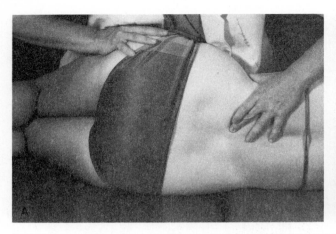
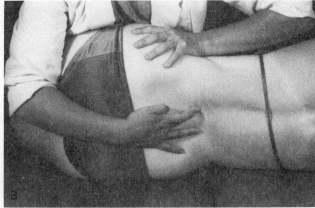

Figure 7–113. Sidebending. (*A*) Lumbar sidebending to the left. (*B*) Lumbar sidebending to the right.

the upper side. The spine is bent forward to each segmental level to localize testing. The examiner then contacts the iliac crest and pushes inferiorly to rock the pelvis and produce lumbar sidebending to the opposite direction (Fig. 7–113*B*). The examiner palpates the other side.

Method 2. The subject is in the sidelying position with the hips and knees flexed 90 degrees. The subject is moved toward the edge of the table, guarded by the examiner, so that the lower limbs may be lowered over the side of the table. The examiner, supporting at the ankles, raises the subject's limbs to rock the pelvis, in turn causing ("upward") sidebending of the lumbar spine (Fig. 7–114). The examiner palpates each segment at the interspinous space on the side toward which the subject is bent. The opposite sidebend is tested by lowering the limbs below the level of the table to rock the pelvis in the opposite direction. The palpating finger moves to the lower side in the direction of sidebending.

Results. Sidebending evaluates inferior and medial glide of the ipsilateral side and superior and lateral glide of the contralateral facet joints.

Sidebending of L5–S1

Method. The subject lies supine. The examiner "slings" the subject's knees over the examiner's shoulders so that the hips and knees are flexed 90 degrees. The examiner locks the fingers together, and with the forearm contacts the top of the subject's thighs as far proximally as possible (Fig. 7–115). Caudal distraction is produced to the side away from the examiner.

Results. Sidebending of L5–S1 assesses inferior glide of the sacrum on the L5 inferior facet of that side.

Rotation

Method 1. The subject lies prone as the examiner flexes the knees to 90 degrees to use as a lever. The spine is palpated at the interspinous space on the side toward which the limbs are rotated or the side opposite the direction of rotation. Even though rotation is being imparted from inferior to superior, the standard reference position of the superior vertebra in relation to the inferior vertebra is maintained (Fig. 7–116*A*). The examiner moves the limbs in the opposite direction to produce the

Figure 7–114. Sidebending using the lower limbs as leverage.

Figure 7–115. Sidebending of L5–S1.

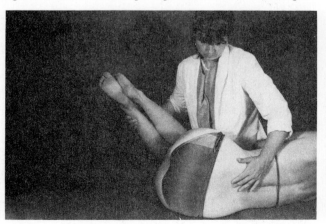
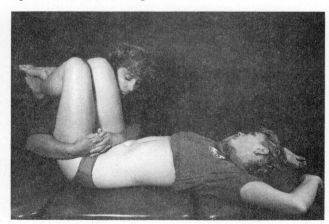

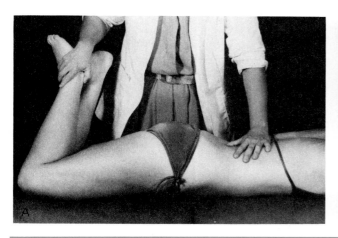 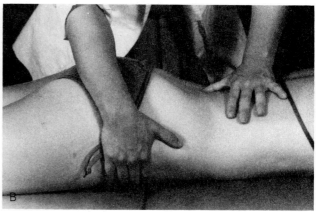

Figure 7–116.   Rotation: (A) Method 1, using lower limbs for leverage; (B) Method 2, using pelvis as leverage.

opposite rotation, changing the palpation to the appropriate side.

Method 2.   The subject lies prone. The examiner rotates the lumbar spine by lifting the ASIS of one side (Fig. 7–116B). The spine rotates toward the side opposite the side lifted. The examiner palpates at the interspinous level on the side opposite the direction of rotation. The examiner then lifts the opposite ASIS.

Method 3.   The subject is in a sidelying position facing the examiner. The examiner localizes the segment by having the subject bend forward to the level being tested. The examiner rotates the thorax to the segment being tested. Palpation will be on the lower side of the interspinous space.

Results.   Rotation evaluates lateral and superior glide of the ipsilateral facet joints and medial and inferior glide of the contralateral facet joints.

Posterior-Anterior Spring Test

Method.   The subject lies prone. The examiner presses the pisiform to the spinous process to spring the vertebra in a posterior-anterior direction. The forearm of the examiner is perpendicular to the contour of the subject's back.

Results.   The posterior-anterior spring test evaluates general hypomobility of the superior and inferior motion segments.

Rotation

Method.   The subject lies prone. The examiner palpates the 12th rib and the iliac crest (Fig. 7–117A). Pressing the pisiform over the level of the transverse process, the examiner applies downward force on one side to produce rotation of that vertebra (note that two motion segments are involved) to the opposite side (Fig. 7–117B). L2, L3, and L4 can be tested in this fashion. The examiner will have to angle the testing hand to follow the oblique angles of the 12th rib and the iliac crest to make proper contact.

Results.   The rotation spring test evaluates general mobility of the ipsilateral facet joints of the superior and inferior motion segments.

Figure 7–117.   (A) Identification of 12th rib and iliac crest. (B) Spring test for rotation of vertebrae.

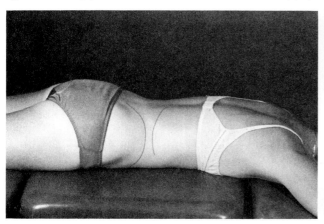 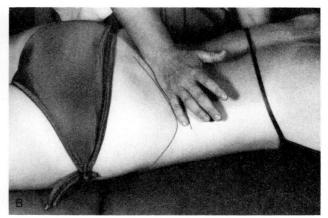

Table 7–3. Summary of Lumbar Spine Joint Play

GLIDE	RESTRICTION
Forward	Forward bend, sidebend to the opposite side, rotation to the same side
Backward	Backward bend, sidebend to the same side, rotation to the opposite side
Rotation	Rotation to the same side, sidebending to the opposite side

Summary of Joint Play of the Lumbar Spine

Table 7–3 provides a summary of lumbar joint play.

Sacroiliac Joint

The following tests permit the examiner to assess the sacroiliac joint for hypermobility or hypomobility by evaluating end feel or observing relationships of bony landmarks. Most are additionally provocation tests of joint irritability to test for reproduction of symptoms, especially those localized to the sacroiliac joint.

Palpation

The structures and landmarks that should be palpated or observed during sacroiliac joint evaluation include:

1. ASIS.
2. PSIS.
3. Iliac crests.
4. Pubic tubercle.
5. Posterior sulci.
6. S2 tubercle.
7. Sacrotuberous ligament.
8. Greater trochanters.
9. Muscles. Although many of the following muscles are primarily considered hip muscles, their attachments on the innominate bone make them susceptible to aberrant stresses and strains when there is mechanical dysfunction of the sacroiliac joint. Special attention should be paid to such things as the innominate attachments and locating trigger points and areas of congestion. Muscles to be examined are:
     Piriformis.
     Tensor fasciae latae.
     Gluteus maximus.
     Hamstrings.
     Rectus femoris.
     Sartorius.
     All adductor group muscles.
10. Iliotibial band.

Alignment of Landmarks

Indication. Inspection and palpation of pelvic landmarks help to determine the presence of sacroiliac malalignment or leg-length discrepancy. Malalignment may also be indicated by other clinical signs and symptoms.

Method. The landmarks, which should be palpated bilaterally, comparing the two sides for equal levels with the patient standing, are (*anterior*) ASIS, pubic tubercle, greater trochanter, and iliac crest, and (*posterior*) PSIS, gluteal fold, and popliteal crease.

With the subject supine, the levels of the medial malleoli are compared. If a discrepancy is found, the knees are flexed and the feet are placed flat on the table. This technique can differentiate between femoral and tibial leg-length discrepancy.

With the subject prone, the knees are first extended and then flexed 90 degrees where the levels of the heels are compared. The latter position determines whether the length discrepancy is in the femurs or the tibiae.

Results. A torsional dysfunction would be suspected if there is an opposite relationship between anterior structures and posterior structures. For example, if the right ASIS is found to be inferior to the left ASIS but the right PSIS is superior to the left, a torsional positional fault would be indicated. The direction and side of dysfunction would be determined when this is considered with other clinical evidence. Other possibilities may include an upshifted or downshifted innominate bone. Innominate irregularities might be confused with leg-length discrepancy if only the pelvic region landmarks were assessed. Evaluating more distal limb landmarks would clarify the diagnosis, as would careful consideration of the history of onset. If the history included trauma, the examiner should try to analyze the mechanical forces involved, as these will assist in determining the side and direction of sacroiliac dysfunction.

Special Tests

Supine-Sit Test

Indication. The supine-sit test evaluates sacroiliac torsion by comparing functional leg lengths. Because of the eccentric position of the acetabulum, a functional leg-length discrepancy due to sacroiliac torsion will become apparent by rotating the pelvis from the supine to the sitting position.

Method. The subject lies supine. The examiner holds both ankles and gives a slight even traction force to make sure the subject is lying straight. The lower limbs are then placed on the table. With the thumbs placed just distal to the medial malleoli of the ankles, the examiner compares leg lengths (Fig. 7–118*A* and *B*). The subject is then asked to rise into the straight leg sitting position

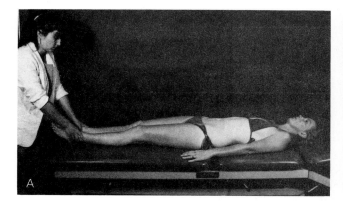

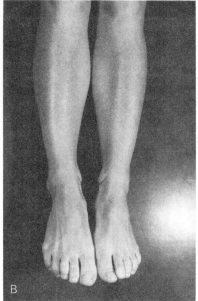

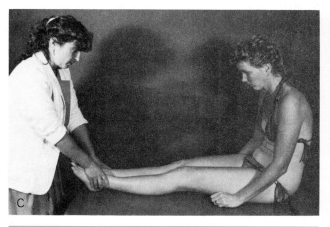

Figure 7–118. (*A*) Initial position of supine-to-sit test. (*B*) Symmetrical level of medial malleoli. (*C*) Final position for supine-to-sit test. (*D*) Asymmetrical position of medial malleoli.

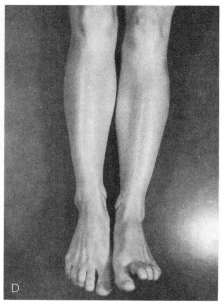

and leg lengths are again compared (Fig. 7–118*C* and *D*). The examiner must note whether the relationships remain the same or change with the change of position.

Results. A change of length between the two positions is a positive indication of sacroiliac torsion. No change in relationship suggests no torsion.

Anterior Gapping

Indication. Anterior gapping implicates the sacroiliac articulation as a source of symptoms.

Method. The subject lies supine (a pillow can be placed beneath the knees to decrease lumbar lordosis). The examiner crosses the upper limbs to contact the subject's right ASIS with the right hand and the subject's left ASIS with the left hand. A force directed laterally to each ASIS is given as though to separate them (Fig. 7–119). This force causes tension on the anterior structures of the sacroiliac joint while compressing the posterior structures. Pressure can be constant or oscillating.

Results. The result is positive if motion reproduces localized sacroiliac pain.

Posterior Gapping

Indication. Posterior gapping implicates the sacroiliac joint as a source of symptoms. This test is the complement to anterior gapping.

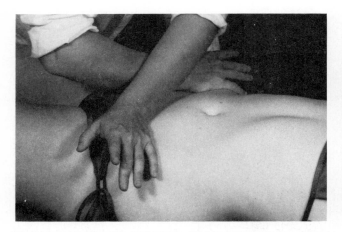

Figure 7–119. Anterior gapping of the sacroiliac joint.

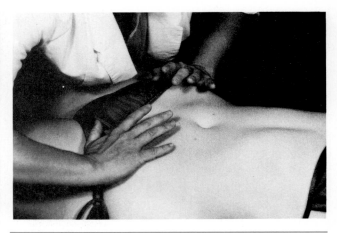

Figure 7–120. Posterior gapping of the sacroiliac joint.

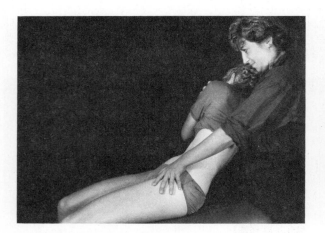

Figure 7–121. Posterior torsion test of the sacroiliac joint.

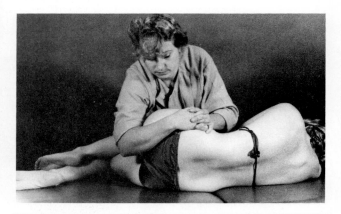

Figure 7–122. Anterior torsion test of the sacroiliac joint.

Method. The subject lies supine. The examiner contacts the lateral aspect of the ASIS bilaterally. Force is directed medially as if to approximate the ASISs, producing tension on the posterior sacroiliac structures while compressing the anterior structures (Fig. 7–120). The force can be constant or oscillating.

Results. The result is positive if pain is reproduced, localized to the sacroiliac joint.

Posterior-Anterior Spring Test

Indication. The posterior-anterior spring test implicates the sacroiliac joint as a source of pain.

Method. The subject lies prone. The innominate is stabilized by contact of the ASIS with the table (contact can be improved by placing a rolled towel beneath the ASIS bilaterally) and the hypothenar eminence of the caudal hand of the examiner contacts the PSIS on the side to be tested. The cranial hand of the examiner con-

tacts the apex of the sacrum and produces a short posterior-anterior stress to "spring" the joint. The examiner should spring test several levels of the sacrum, working toward the base.

Results. Test results are positive if pain is reproduced, especially if it is localized to the sacroiliac joint.

Torsion

Indication. Torsion testing assesses for provocation of torsional dysfunction of the sacroiliac joint.

Method

Posterior Torsion

1. The subject sits. The examiner, standing behind, supports the subject at the shoulders and leans the subject back against the trunk while stepping backward. The examiner then rotates the subject to one side while contacting the ASIS of the opposite side, blocking it from movement, thereby

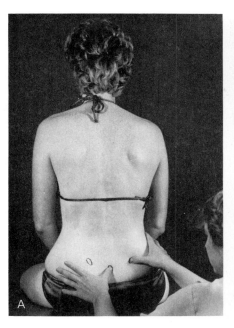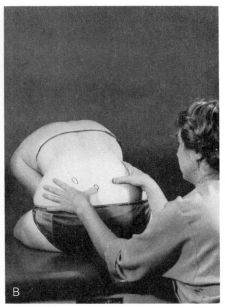

Figure 7–123.   Piedallu's sign. (*A*) Comparison of the PSIS levels and the S2 tubercle in sitting. (*B*) Comparison of the PSIS levels and the S2 tubercle in the forward bent position.

producing posterior torsion on that side (Fig. 7–121).

2. The subject is lying on the side opposite that to be tested. The examiner contacts the ASIS with the cephalad hand and the posterior aspect of the ischial tuberosity with the other. The hands are used as a force couple to produce a posterior rotation torque to the innominate along the anterolateral-posteromedial plane of the joint.

Anterior Torsion.   Hand position is changed from that for posterior torsion so that the caudal hand now contacts the ischial tuberosity for the anterior-inferior aspect, and the cephalad hand contacts the forearm along the iliac crest. Following the plane of the joint, a force couple produces an anterior rotatory torque to the innominate (Fig. 7–122). Forces can be constant or oscillating.

Results.   Test results are positive if symptoms are provoked, especially if they are localized to the sacroiliac joint.

Piedallu's Sign

Indication.   Piedallu's sign indicates restriction of sacroiliac joint mobility.

Method.   The subject is sitting on a firm surface. The examiner locates and compares the levels of the PSISs to each other and then compares each PSIS to the level of the S2 tubercle (Fig. 7–123*A*). The patient is asked to bend forward, flexing the hips and trunk. The positional relationships of the landmarks are again compared (Fig. 7–123*B*).

Results.   Frequently, sacroiliac dysfunction is indicated by the PSIS of the restricted side being inferior to that on the uninvolved side. Test results are positive if, with a finding of uneven PSISs, the relationship of PSIS to S2 reverses upon forward bending.

Test for Sacroiliac Restriction When Subject Stands

Indication.   The standing test evaluates the sacroiliac for restricted mobility.

Method.   The subject stands. The examiner stands behind the subject and locates and compares the position of one PSIS relative to the S2 tubercle (Fig. 7–124*A*). The subject is then asked to raise the knee of the side being palpated (as in marching). The examiner again compares the positional relationship of the landmarks (Fig. 7–124*B*). Comparison should also be made for the ischial tuberosity and the S2 tubercle.

Results.   With normal sacroiliac mobility the PSIS would move caudally and the ischial tuberosity would move laterally with respect to the S2 tubercle. Test results

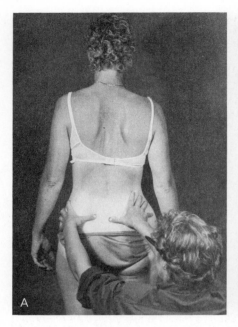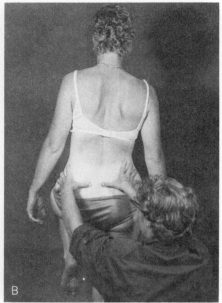

Figure 7–124A and B. Test for sacroiliac restriction standing.

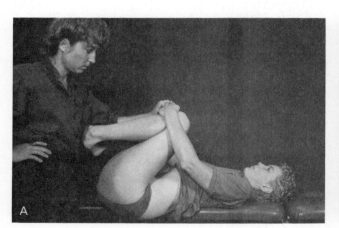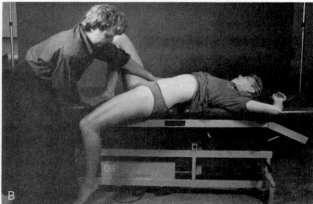

Figure 7–125. (*A*) Gaenslin's test (*B*) Lower limb of unsupported side is lowered over the side of the table.

are positive if the PSIS or the tuberosity is restricted in the cephalad direction.

Gaenslin's Test (Passive Hip Extension)

Indication. Gaenslin's test implicates the sacroiliac joint as a source of symptoms.

Method. The subject is supine, holding knees to chest. The examiner helps the subject move the lower trunk to the edge of the table, so that the near-side innominate bone has fully cleared the table and the (pad-

ded) edge of the table supports the sacrum (Fig. 7–125*A*). The lower limb of the unsupported side is then lowered over the side of the table (Fig. 7–125*B*).

Results. Test results are positive if pain is reproduced, particularly if it is localized to the sacroiliac joint.

Shear Test

Indication. The shear test implicates the sacroiliac joint as a source of symptoms, assessing the joint in the caudad and cephalad directions.

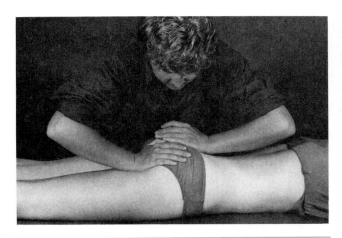

Figure 7–126. Caudal shear of the sacrum on the ilium.

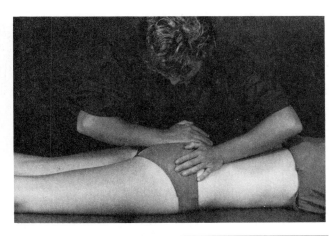

Figure 7–127. Cephalad shear of the sacrum on the ilium.

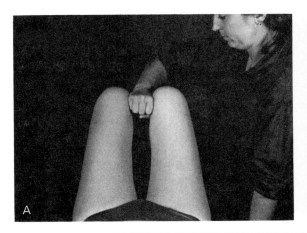

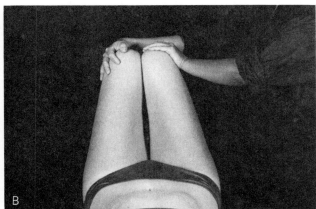

Figure 7–128. (*A*) Isometric adduction. (*B*) Isometric abduction.

Method

Caudal Shear. The subject lies prone. The examiner contacts the base of the sacrum with the cephalad hand and stabilizes the innominate bone at the ischial tuberosity. With the forearms parallel to the table, a shear force is applied to move the sacrum on the innominate in the caudad direction (Fig. 7–126).

Cephalad Shear. The caudad hand contacts the apex of the sacrum, while the cephalad hand stabilizes the innominate along the iliac crest. A shear force is given to move the sacrum on the innominate in the cephalad direction (Fig. 7–127).

Results. Results are positive if symptoms are reproduced, particularly if they are localized to the sacroiliac joint.

Isometric Adduction and Abduction

Indication. Isometric adduction and abduction implicate the sacroiliac joint as a source of symptoms by stressing the joint with resisted muscle contraction.

Method. The subject lies supine with the hips and knees flexed, feet flat on the table. The examiner isometrically resists bilateral adduction, then abduction contractions (Fig. 7–128*A* and *B*).

Results. Test results are positive if pain is reproduced and localized to the sacroiliac joint.

Bibliography

Corrigan B, Maitland GD: Practical Orthopedic Medicine. Boston, Butterworth & Co, 1983

Daniels L, Worthingham C: Muscle Testing Techniques of Manual Examination. Philadelpha, WB Saunders, 1986

Grieve GP: Common Vertebral Joint Problems. New York, Churchill Livingstone, 1981

Grieve GP: Mobilization of the Spine, 4th ed. New York, Churchill Livingstone, 1984

Grieve GP (ed): Modern Manual Therapy of the Vertebral Column. New York, Churchill Livingstone, 1986

Grimsby O: Manual Therapy of the Spine, 2nd ed. New York, Sorlandets Sysikalase Institutt A-S, 1980

Hoppenfeld S: Physical Examination of the Spine and Extremities. New York, Appleton-Century-Crofts, 1976

Kendall FP, McCreary EK: Muscle Testing and Function. Baltimore, Williams & Wilkins, 1983

Magee DJ: Orthopedic Physical Assessment. Philadelphia, WB Saunders, 1987

McKenzie RA: The Lumbar Spine. Lower Hutt, New Zealand, Spinal Publications, 1981

Maitland GD: Vertebral Manipulation, 5th ed. Boston, Butterworth & Co, 1986

Norkin CC, White DJ: Measurement of Joint Motion: A Guide to Goniometry. Philadelphia, FA Davis, 1985

Paris SV: The Spine (course notes). Atlanta, Institute Press, 1979

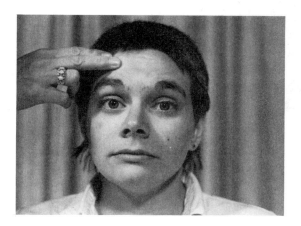

Figure 8–2. Location of the occipitofrontalis muscle.

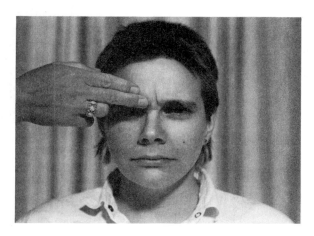

Figure 8–3. Location of the corrugator muscle.

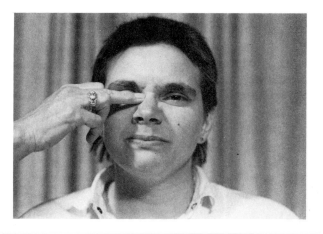

Figure 8–4. Location of the procerus muscle.

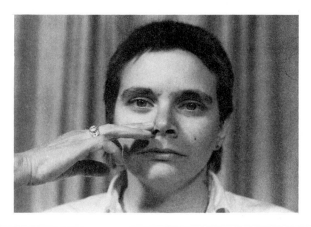

Figure 8–5. Location of the nasalis muscle.

Palpation. Palpate along the lateral portion of each side of the nose.

Movement. Draw the skin on the lateral nose upward, forming transverse wrinkles over the bridge of the nose.

Innervation. Facial nerve, buccal branches.

Nasalis (Alar and Transverse) Muscles

The nasalis muscles have an alar portion over the alar cartilage that flares the nostrils, and a depressor septi and transverse portion, horizontal fibers that compress the nostrils (Fig. 8–5).

Palpation. Palpate over the alar portion of the nose.

Movement. Dilate and compress the nostrils, changing the aperature of the nostrils.

Innervation. Facial nerve, buccal branches.

Muscles of the Eye

Orbicularis Oculi Muscle

The orbicularis oculi is an expansive sphincter muscle that encircles the eye, extending down over the cheek area. Two portions of the muscle are tested together, the orbital and palpebral parts. The starting position is with the eyes open wide. Contraction of the muscle fibers narrows the orbital opening and encourages the flow of tears by helping to empty the lacrimal gland. (Fig. 8–6).

Palpation. Palpate as close to the upper and lower eyelids as possible without interfering with the motion.

Movement. Close the eyes tightly.

Resistance. Following the movement, resistance can be applied to lift the eyelids.

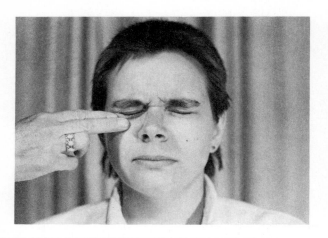

Figure 8–6. Location of the orbicularis oculi muscle.

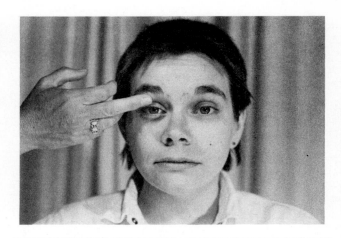

Figure 8–7. Location of the levator palpebrae muscle.

Innervation. Facial nerve, temporal and zygomatic branches.

Superior Levator Palpebrae Muscle

The levator palpebrae muscle is located deep to the skin of the upper eyelid. The starting position is with the eyes slightly open.

Palpation. Palpate the upper eyelid (Fig. 8–7).

Movement. Lift the upper eyelids.

Innervation. Oculomotor nerve.

Extrinsic Eye Muscles: Superior, Inferior, Medial, and Lateral Rectus, and Superior and Inferior Oblique

The extrinsic eye muscles are tested bilaterally and simultaneously because they usually do not function independently. All these muscles attach to the sclera of the eye from a cartilaginous ring around the optic nerve posteriorly in the orbit. The muscles are tested as the examiner is looking at the subject; the subject's left eye is to the examiner's right. The eye muscles are not palpated; instead, the movements are observed for symmetry. The six extrinsic eye muscles rotate the eyeball in the orbit about three axes (Figs. 8–8 and 8–9).

Movement. Subject moves eyes up and right; examiner observes the right superior rectus and left inferior oblique muscles (Fig. 8–10).

- Subject moves eyes up and left; examiner observes the left superior rectus and right inferior oblique muscles (Fig. 8–11).
- Subject moves eyes left; examiner observes the left lateral rectus and right medial rectus muscles (Fig. 8–12).
- Subject moves eyes right; examiner observes the right lateral rectus and left medial rectus muscles (Fig. 8–13).
- Subject moves eyes down and right; examiner observes the right inferior rectus and left superior oblique muscles (Fig. 8–14).
- Subject moves eyes down and left; examiner observes the left inferior rectus and right superior oblique muscles (Fig. 8–15).

Figure 8–8. Extrinsic muscles of the eye.

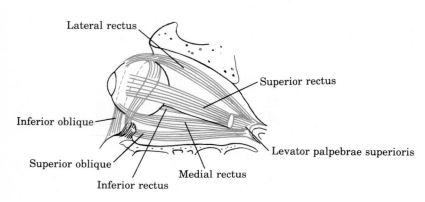

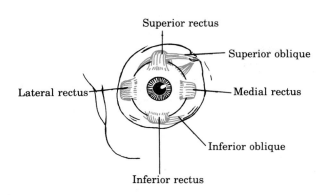

Figure 8–9. Extrinsic muscles of the eye.

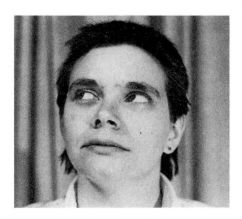

Figure 8–10. The right superior rectus and left inferior oblique muscles control this eye movement.

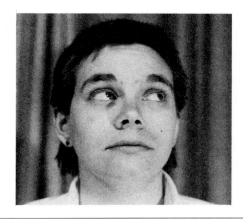

Figure 8–11. The left superior rectus and right inferior oblique muscles control this eye movement.

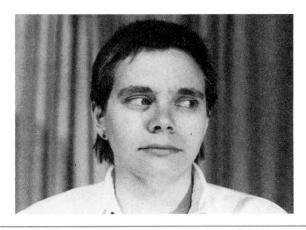

Figure 8–12. The left lateral rectus and right medial rectus muscles control this eye movement.

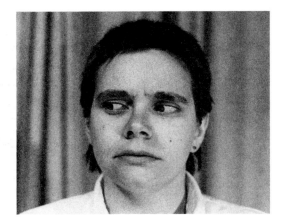

Figure 8–13. The right lateral rectus and left medial rectus muscles control this eye movement.

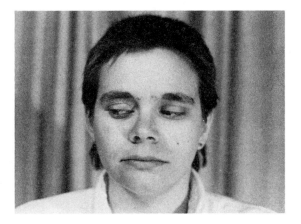

Figure 8–14. The right inferior rectus and left superior oblique muscles control this eye movement.

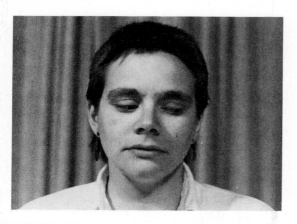

Figure 8–15. The left inferior rectus and right superior oblique muscles control this eye movement.

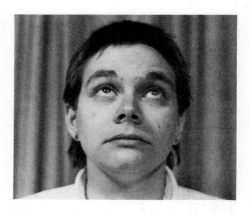

Figure 8–16. The left and right superior rectus muscles control this eye movement.

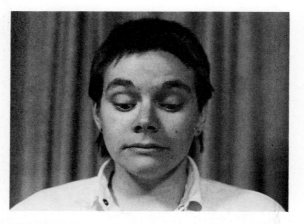

Figure 8–17. The left and right inferior rectus muscles control this eye movement.

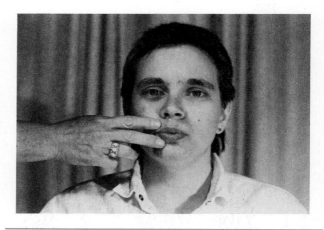

Figure 8–18. Location of the orbicularis oris muscle.

- Subject moves eyes up; examiner observes the left superior rectus and right superior rectus muscles (Fig. 8–16).
- Subject moves eyes down; examiner observes the left inferior rectus and right inferior rectus muscles (Fig. 8–17).

Innervation. Lateral rectus, abducens; superior oblique, trochlear; superior rectus, oculomotor; inferior rectus, oculomotor; medial rectus, oculomotor; inferior oblique, oculomotor.

Muscles of the Mouth

Orbicularis Oris

The orbicularis oris muscle is a sphincter with a wide distribution of muscle fibers that encircle the mouth extending onto the cheeks. The function of the muscle is to close the lips or pucker the lips as in kissing. It also helps to hold food between the teeth during mastication.

Palpation. Palpate above and below the lips (Fig. 8–18).

Movement. Close and protrude the lips.

Innervation. Facial nerve, buccal branches.

Major and Minor Zygomatic Muscles

The zygomatic muscles extend from the lateral angle of the mouth upward and laterally over the cheek.

Palpation. Palpate lateral to the angle of the mouth (Fig. 8–19).

Movement. Raise the corners of the mouth upward and laterally as in smiling.

Innervation. Facial nerve, buccal branches.

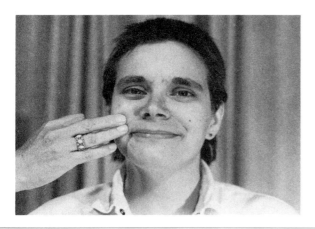

Figure 8–19. Location of the major and minor zygomatic muscles.

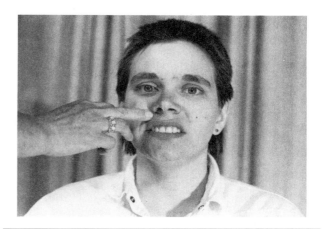

Figure 8–20. Location of the levator anguli oris muscle.

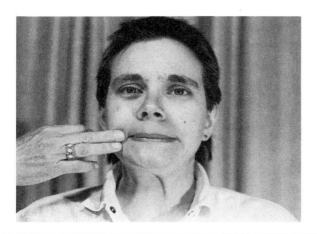

Figure 8–21. Location of the risorius muscle.

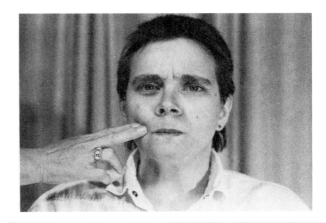

Figure 8–22. Location of the buccinator muscle.

Levator Anguli Oris Muscle

The levator anguli oris muscle is located at the angle of the mouth and extends superiorly, intermingling with other facial muscles. It lies deep to the zygomatic muscle and therefore is not easily palpated.

Palpation. Palpate on the upper lip at the angle of the mouth (Fig. 8–20).

Movement. Raise the upper border of the lip straight up as in sneering and showing the canine tooth.

Innervation. Facial nerve, buccal branches.

Risorius Muscle

The risorius muscle is extremely thin, extending laterally from the angle of the mouth. The function of the muscle is to produce the facial expression of grinning.

Palpation. Palpate the lateral angle of the mouth (Fig. 8–21).

Movement. Draw the corners of the mouth laterally.

Innervation. Facial nerve, mandibular and buccal branches.

Buccinator Muscle

The buccinator muscle lies deep in the cheek region. A thin, flat muscle, it aids in mastication by pressing the cheeks against the teeth during chewing. The buccinator is also used in sucking or blowing when the cheeks are compressed against the teeth.

Palpation. Palpate lateral to the angle of the mouth (Fig. 8–22).

Movement. Press the cheeks firmly against the teeth.

Innervation. Facial nerve, buccal branches.

Levator Labii Superioris Muscle

The levator labii superioris muscle extends from the superior border of the upper lip to the cheek lateral to the nose. It functions to raise the upper lip. A few people are able to use this muscle to evert the upper lip as chimpanzees do.

Palpation. Palpate lateral to the midline of the upper lip (Fig. 8–23).

Movement. Protrude and elevate the upper lip.

Innervation. Facial nerve, buccal branches.

Depressor Anguli Oris and Platysma Muscles

The depressor anguli oris muscle is located inferior to the angle of the mouth extending onto the chin. The platsyma muscle extends from the cheek area over the clavicle onto the anterior chest wall. These muscles function to tense the skin of the chin and neck as in shaving and draw down the corners of the mouth. The platsyma assists in depressing the mandible.

Palpation. Palpate the anterior lateral neck and inferior lateral to the lower lip (Figs. 8–24 and 8–25).

Movement. Draw the corner of the mouth downward and tense the skin over the neck.

Innervation. Facial nerve, cervical for the platysma and buccal and mandibular for the depressor anguli oris.

Figure 8–23. Location of the levator labii superioris muscle.

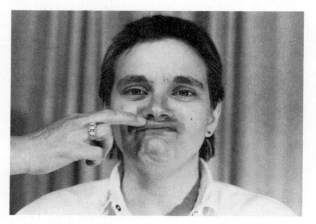

Figure 8–24. Location of the depressor anguli oris muscle.

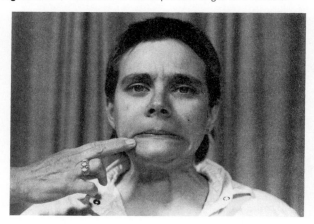

Figure 8–25. Location of the platysma muscle.

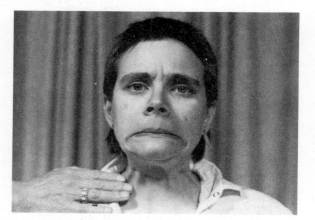

Figure 8–26. Location of the depressor labii inferioris muscle.

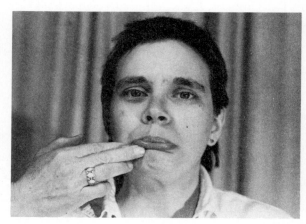

Attachments of Temporalis Muscle

Muscle	Proximal	Distal	Innervation
Temporalis	Floor of temporal fossa	Coronoid process and anterior ramus of mandible	Mandibular division of trigeminal nerve

Depressor Labii Inferioris Muscle

The depressor labii inferioris muscle protrudes the lower lip. It is located below the lower lip.

Palpation. Palpate below the lower lip and lateral to the midline (Fig. 8–26).

Movement. Protrude the lower lip, as in pouting.

Innervation. Facial nerve, buccal branches.

Mentalis Muscle

The mentalis muscle is located in the midline of the chin. It wrinkles the skin on the chin, as when a person is about to cry.

Palpation. Midline of chin (Fig. 8–27).

Movement. Raise the skin on the chin.

Innervation. Facial nerve, mandibular branches.

Muscles of Mastication

Temporalis Muscle

The temporalis muscle is thick and fan-shaped, covering the temporal region of the head. It performs the function of closing the jaw, moving the mandible to the same side as in chewing and grinding food. The starting position is with the mouth relaxed, partially open.

Palpation. Palpate the side of the head in the region over the temporal bone (Fig. 8–28).

Movement. Elevate and retract the mandible.

Resistance. Applied with a tongue depressor placed between the teeth and pulled out after the movement has occurred. Test both sides (Fig. 8–29).

Figure 8–27. Location of the mentalis muscle.

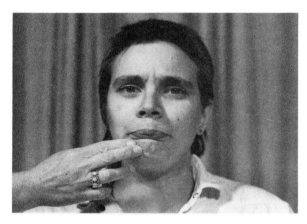

Figure 8–28. Location of the temporalis muscle.

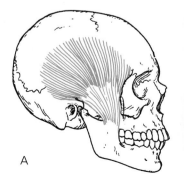

A

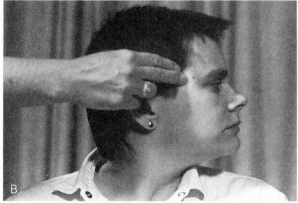

B

Attachments of Masseter Muscle

Muscle	Proximal	Distal	Innervation
Masseter	Inferior and deep surface of zygomatic arch	Lateral ramus and coronoid process of mandible	Mandibular division of trigeminal nerve

Masseter

The name of the masseter muscle comes from the Greek word meaning "masticator," or "chewer." The thick quadrate muscle is located on the side of the mandible. It elevates and helps to protract the mandible and clenches the teeth. The starting test position is with the mouth relaxed and partially open.

Figure 8–29. Resistance applied by pulling on a tongue depressor.

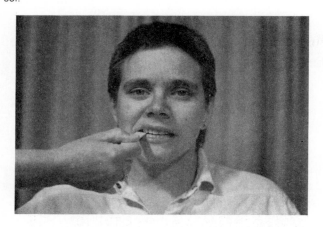

Figure 8–30. Location of the masseter muscle.

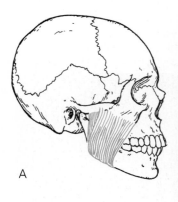
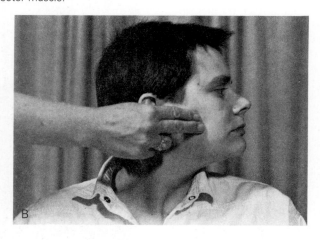

Palpation. Palpate the cheek above the angle of the mandible (Fig. 8–30).

Movement. Elevate the mandible, as in closing the jaw.

Resistance. Applied to the mandible using a tongue blade.

Lateral Pterygoid Muscle

The lateral pterygoid muscle has two short heads that have horizontal fibers. The muscle is deep. It lies on the medial side of the mandible and protracts the mandible and moves the jaw toward the opposite side, as in grinding and chewing.

Palpation. Palpate the pterygoid at its attachment to the neck of the mandible and joint capsule.

Movement. Acting together, the pterygoids protrude and depress the jaw (Figs. 8–31 to 8–33).

Resistance. Applied to the anterior surface of the chin.

Attachments of the Lateral Pterygoid Muscle

Muscle	Proximal	Distal	Innervation
Lateral pterygoid	Greater wing of sphenoid and lateral pterygoid plate	Neck of mandible and articular cartilage	Mandibular division of trigeminal nerve

Medial Pterygoid Muscle

The medial pterygoid muscle is thick and square, with two heads. The fibers run in a vertical plane. The muscle elevates the jaw.

Palpation. The medial pterygoid is too deep to palpate.

Movement. Elevate and protrude the mandible (Fig. 8–34).

Resistance. Applied to the mandible with a tongue depressor.

Suprahyoid Muscles: Mylohyoid, Geniohyoid, Stylohyoid, Digastric

The suprahyoid muscles lie superior to the hyoid bone and attach it to the skull. Their function is to elevate the hyoid bone and the larynx for swallowing and speaking.

Figure 8–31. Pterygoid muscles.

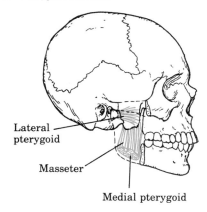

Lateral pterygoid

Masseter

Medial pterygoid

Figure 8–32. Lateral pterygoid protruding mandible—lateral view.

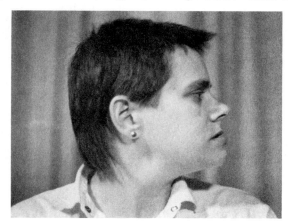

Figure 8–33. Lateral pterygoid protruding mandible—anterior view.

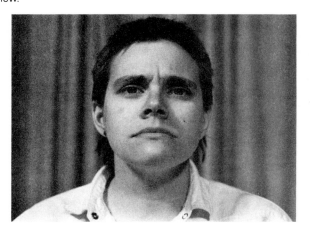

Figure 8–34. Right medial and lateral pterygoid muscles moving the mandible toward the left side.

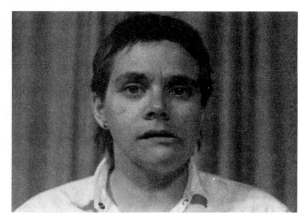

Attachments of Medial Pterygoid Muscle

Muscle	Proximal	Distal	Innervation
Medial pterygoid	Medial surface of lateral pterygoid plate and tuberosity of maxilla	Medial surface of mandible close to angle	Mandibular division of trigeminal nerve

Attachments of Suprahyoid Muscles

Muscle	Proximal	Distal	Innervation
Mylohyoid	Medial surface of mandible	Body of hyoid bone	Mylohyoid branch of trigeminal nerve, mandibular division
Geniohyoid	Mental spine of mandible	Body of hyoid bone	Ventral ramus of C1 via hypoglossal nerve
Stylohyoid	Styloid process of temporal bone	Body of hyoid bone	Facial nerve
Anterior and posterior digastric	Internal surface of mandible and mastoid process of temporal bone	By intermediate tendon to hyoid bone	Anterior, mylohyoid branch of trigeminal nerve Posterior, facial

Attachments of Infrahyoid Muscles

Muscle	Proximal	Distal	Innervation
Sternohyoid	Manubrium and medial end of clavicle	Body of hyoid bone	Ansa cervicalis
Omohyoid	Superior angle of scapula	Inferior body of hyoid bone	Ansa cervicalis
Sternothyroid	Posterior surface of manubrium	Thyroid cartilage	Ansa cervicalis
Thyrohyoid	Thyroid cartilage	Inferior body and greater horn of hyoid bone	C1 via hypoglossal

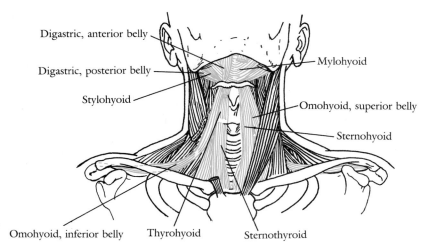

Figure 8–35. Suprahyoid and infrahyoid muscles.

Digastric, anterior belly
Digastric, posterior belly
Stylohyoid
Mylohyoid
Omohyoid, superior belly
Sternohyoid
Omohyoid, inferior belly
Thyrohyoid
Sternothyroid

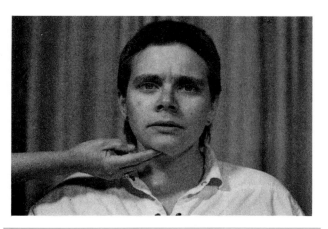

Figure 8–36. Suprahyoid muscle contraction during resisted tongue protrusion.

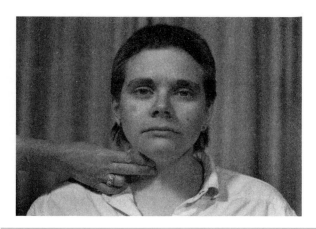

Figure 8–37. Infrahyoid muscle contraction during swallowing.

Collectively the muscles also depress the mandible (Fig. 8–35).

Palpation.   Palpate in the floor of the mouth (Fig. 8–36).

Movement.   Press the tip of the tongue against the front teeth.

Resistance.   Applied to the surface of the hyoid bone in an effort to protrude the tongue.

Infrahyoid Muscles: Sternohyoid, Thyrohyoid, Omohyoid, Sternothyroid

The infrahyoid muscles are often called strap muscles because of their thin, straplike appearance. As their name implies, they attach to the hyoid bone and stabilize it against the upward pull of the suprahyoid muscles and depress the hyoid bone and larynx during swallowing and speaking.

Palpation.   Palpate below the hyoid bone immediately lateral to the midline (Fig. 8–37).

Movement.   Depress the hyoid following swallowing or speaking.

Resistance.   None is applied; the movement of the larynx and hyoid bone are observed.

Clinical Tests of the Temporomandibular Joint

Palpation

The palpation of structures associated with the TMJ include the temporomandibular ligament, the lateral capsule, and the retrodiscal tissue in the posterolateral aspect of the joint. Palpation is performed with the subject's mouth alternately closed and open, in the following manner:

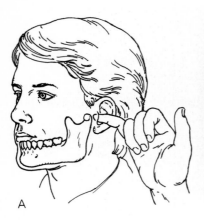
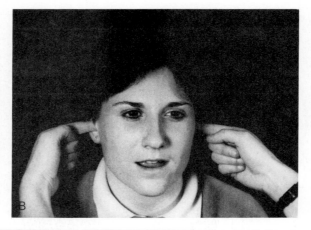

Figure 8–38. Palpation of the temporomandibular joint. (*A*) With little finger; (*B*) with index finger.

1. With the subject's mouth open, place the index or fifth fingers bilaterally into the external auditory meati with the palmar portion of the finger forward (Fig. 8–38). Instruct the subject to close the mouth. When the examiner feels the condyle against the finger, the TMJ is in its resting, or "freeway space," position, in which the space between the upper and lower front teeth should be 2 to 4 mm. Anything greater represents hypermobility of both TMJs.

2. With the subject's mouth open, palpate around the lateral pole and along the line of the temporomandibular ligament, as well as the tissues in the posterolateral portion of the joint cavity. The temporomandibular ligament originates at the inferior aspect of the zygomatic arch and travels obliquely and posteroinferiorly.

3. With the subject's mouth closed, palpate for joint effusion around the lateral pole and along the temporomandibular ligament.

Other structures that should be observed or palpated include the following:

1. Examine the teeth for abnormalities in positioning, for missing teeth, and for tenderness.
2. Examine the mandible for left-to-right symmetry. Measure the distance between the posterior aspect of the TMJ and the notch of the chin for symmetry (Fig. 8–39).
3. Palpate the hyoid bone for normal, painless movement while the subject swallows. The hyoid can be found anterior to C2,3 (Fig. 8–40).
4. The thyroid cartilage, located anterior to C4,5 can be easily palpated and moved with the neck

Figure 8–39. Measurement for symmetry of the mandible.

Figure 8–40. Palpation of the hyoid bone.

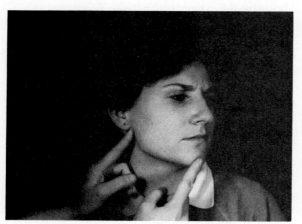
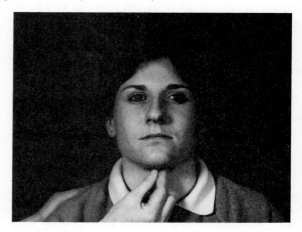

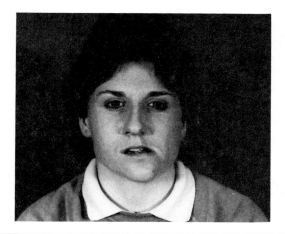

Figure 8–41. Active lateral excursion of the mandible.

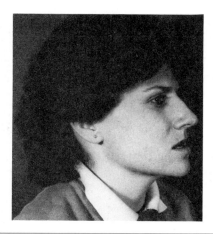

Figure 8–42. Active protrusion of the mandible.

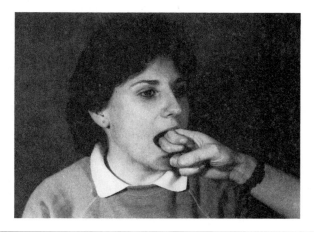

Figure 8–43. Normal range of opening of the mouth.

in a neutral position. Crepitation of this structure may be felt when the neck is in a position of backward bending and the thyroid cartilage becomes taut.

5. Palpate the mastoid processes for symmetry.
6. Palpate the bony landmarks of the cervical spine, including the spinous processes, transverse processes, and facet joints.
7. Palpate the musculature of the cervical region, including the suboccipital muscles, sternocleidomastoid, scalenes, and platysma.
8. Palpate the muscles of mastication for symmetry and function. These muscles include the lateral pterygoid, medial pterygoid, masseter, and temporalis muscles.
9. Assess the tongue for resting position, movements, frenulum length, and size. A large tongue exerts excessive pressure against the teeth and may interfere with dental occlusion. A small tongue exerts too little pressure on the teeth. A short frenulum may interfere with tongue function.

Active Movements

The active movements that should be assessed as part of the evaluation of the TMJ region include:

1. The opening and closing of the mouth.
2. Lateral excursion of the mandible (Fig. 8–41).
3. Protrusion of the mandible (Fig. 8–42).

Opening and Closing the Mouth. Normally, when a person opens and closes the mouth, the movement of the mandible is fluid and smooth because both TMJs function symmetrically. The normal mandible opens and closes in a linear manner at the midline.

The subject's ability to open the mouth should be assessed. The normal range of opening is about 35 mm. The examiner can quickly determine range by attempting to place two or three flexed interphalangeal joints into the open mouth (Fig. 8–43).

If hypomobility of one TMJ is present, the mandible will deviate in a **C** to that side of the open mouth. The subject that demonstrates an **S** movement of the jaw while opening the mouth is probably suffering from a muscle imbalance. A subject's inability to open the mouth indicates a lack of rotation of the TMJ.

With the mouth closed, the mandible should remain in the midline, and the midpoints of the upper teeth should meet those of the lower teeth (Fig. 8–44).

Lateral Excursion of the Mandible. If lateral excursion of the mandible is noted when the subject's mouth is open, the amount of excursion should be measured. The examiner takes a millimeter ruler and determines a midline reference point.

Contralateral structures that are implicated as a cause of lateral deviation include the disc, the masseter, temporalis, and lateral pterygoid muscles, and the lateral ligament.

Protrusion of the Mandible. The patient is directed to protrude the mandible, a motion that should be readily and easily performed. Abnormal protrusion to one side may also indicate involvement of the structures associated with lateral excursion (see above).

Passive Movements

The usual indication for passive motion assessment is to determine the end feel in the open and closed positions. In the closed position, there should normally be a bony end feel as a result of the teeth coming together. The end feel with the mouth open is equivalent to tissue stretch.

Figure 8–44. Correct alignment of the mandible and teeth.

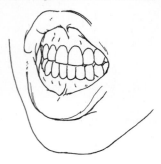

Figure 8–45. Forced biting.

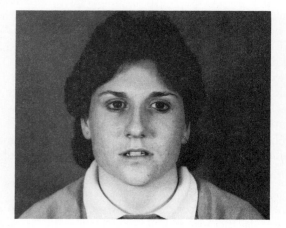

Contractile Tests

Loading (Forced Biting). Loading may be accomplished by having the subject bite down with force onto a soft object such as a cotton roll placed between the posterior teeth (Fig. 8–45). This motion causes compression of the condyle into the mandibular fossa on the opposite side and a distraction of those structures on the same side. This maneuver can have two outcomes:

1. Complaints of increased pain on the side of forced biting indicate tension forces on the capsule and ligament.
2. No complaint of increased pain on the side of forced biting represents reduction of the load on retrodiscal tissue.

Loading (Forced Retrusion). The examiner pushes the anterior tip of the patient's mandible in a posterior and superior direction (Fig. 8–46). The initial force is delivered through the midline, the second to the right, and the third to the left. This test is used to assess retrodiscal tissues, but it may provide false-negative results (no pain) if the strong muscles of mastication inhibit mandibular motion.

Special Tests

The examiner can listen to the TMJ with a stethoscope placed over the joint, as the patient opens and closes the mouth. Normally, a single, solid occlusion sound is heard, but a slipping sound is heard when the teeth are not coming together simultaneously. Crepitus, usually heard during the end stage of opening, may be associated with arthritic changes, as apparent roughening of the condyle and articular eminence is present. Subluxation

Figure 8–46. Forced retrusion.

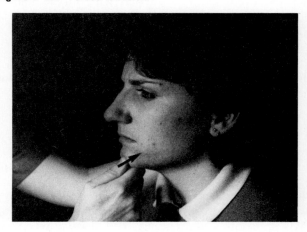

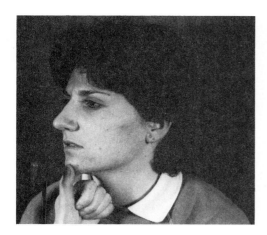

Figure 8–47. Jaw reflex.

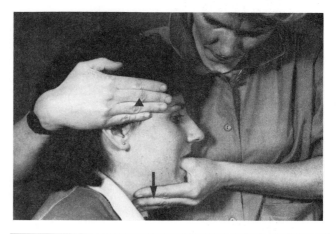

Figure 8–48. Distraction of the TMJ.

of the disc commonly results in a simultaneous clicking sound.

Jaw Reflex

The integrity of the trigeminal nerve is assessed via the jaw jerk. The subject's mouth is relaxed and open in the resting posture. The examiner places a thumb on the mandible, then lightly taps the thumb with the pointed end of the reflex hammer (Fig. 8–47). A normal response is one in which the mouth closes.

Tests of Muscles of Mastication

Successful testing of the muscles of mastication requires that certain principles be observed.

1. The mouth must be open approximately 1 cm during the examination.
2. The head must be supported to prevent movement of the head and rotation of the neck.
3. The force imparted should be applied gradually to ensure a maximum buildup of tension by the subject.
4. Contact with the TMJ should be avoided during the examination, so the subject will not confuse pain associated with contact and pain arising from some dysfunction or pathology.

Testing the Lateral Pterygoid. The lateral pterygoid is important in opening the mouth. This structure is assessed by having the patient slightly open the mouth and then resist the therapist's attempt to forcefully close it. The musculature involved in closing the mouth is assessed by having the subject's mouth slightly open while the examiner attempts to open it further. The examiner places the thumbs on the lower anterior teeth and applies a downward force.

Testing the Medial and Lateral Pterygoid Muscles. Both the lateral and medial pterygoid muscles may be tested by assessing lateral excursion of the mandible. The medial pterygoid also functions to elevate the mandible. The upper head of the lateral pterygoid functions to influence the relationship between the condyle and the disc. The lower head of the lateral pterygoid serves to protrude and deviate the mandible to the opposite side. Protrusion of the mandible may also be accomplished by bilateral contraction of the lateral pterygoid.

Testing the Medial Pterygoid and Musculature Involved in Opening the Jaw. The subject is relaxed, with the mouth slightly open and the jaw slightly protruded. The examiner supports the head while attempting to move the jaw posteriorly as the subject resists. The medial pterygoid also functions to elevate the mandible.

Testing the Digastric and Posterior Fibers of the Temporalis. The subject resists the attempt by the examiner to move the mandible forward by pushing anteriorly on the lingual surface of the lower anterior teeth. The anterior digastric muscle is also involved in the function of mandibular depression, while the temporalis also acts to elevate the mandible.

Joint Play (Accessory Movement)

Distraction (Fig. 8–48)

Restriction. General hypomobility.

Open-Packed Position. Subject is seated with back and shoulders supported and mouth slightly open.

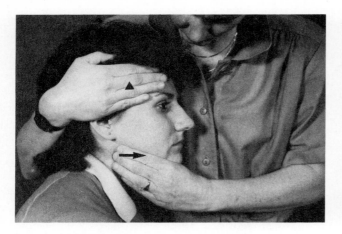

Figure 8–49. Ventral glide of the mandible.

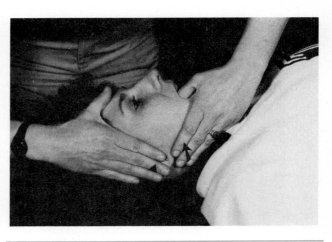

Figure 8–50. Medial-lateral glide of the mandible.

Fixed Segment. Examiner stabilizes subject's head (temporal bone) with one hand, placing the ulnar border of the little finger just superior to the joint space of the TMJ.

Moving Segment. With the other hand, the examiner holds the ramus of the mandible with the radial side of the index finger while placing the thumb inside the mouth onto the lower molars.

Ventral Glide (Fig. 8–49)

Restriction. Inability to open mouth fully.

Open-Packed Position. Subject is seated with back and shoulders supported and mouth slightly open.

Fixed Segment. Examiner holds subject's head (temporal bone) with one hand, placing the ulnar border of the little finger just superior to the joint space of the TMJ.

Moving Segment. Examiner grasps the subject's mandible with the other hand, with the fingers pointed dorsally and gripping the angle of the mandible.

Medial-Lateral Glide (Fig. 8–50)

Restriction. Lateral excursion.

Open-Packed Position. Subject is supine with mouth slightly open.

Fixed Segment. Examiner's one hand holds subject's head (temporal bone), with the distal interphalangeal joints of the fingers just superior to the joint space.

Moving Segment. Examiner's other hand is placed along the mandible with the thenar eminence immediately inferior to the joint space.

Summary of Joint Play of the Temporomandibular Joint

Table 8–1 provides a summary of TMJ play.

Bibliography

Daniels L, Worthingham C: Muscle Testing Techniques of Manual Examination. Philadelphia, WB Saunders, 1986

Friedman MH, Weisberg J: Screening procedures for temporomandibular joint dysfunction. Am Fam Physician 25:157, 1982

Friedman MH, Weisberg J: Application of orthopedic principles in evaluation of the temporomandibular joint. Phys Ther 62:597, 1982

Table 8–1. Summary of TMJ Play

GLIDE	RESTRICTION	FIXED BONE	MOVING BONE
Distraction	General hypomobility	Temporal	Mandible
Ventral	Inability to open mouth fully	Temporal	Mandible
Medial-lateral	Lateral deviation	Temporal	Mandible

Gelb H: Patient Evaluation. In Gelb H (ed): Clinical Management of Head, Neck, and TMJ Pain and Dysfunction. Philadelphia, WB Saunders, 1977

Gould A III, Davies G (eds): Orthopedic and Sports Physical Therapy. St Louis, CV Mosby, 1985

Helland NM: Anatomy and function of the temporomandibular joint. J Orthoped Sports Phys Ther 1:145, 1980

Hollinshead WH, Jenkins DB: Functional Anatomy of the Limbs and Back. Philadelphia, WB Saunders, 1981

Kaltenborn M: Mobilization of the Extremity Joints. Oslo, Bygdoy Alle, 1980

Kendall FP, McCreary EK: Muscle Testing and Function. Baltimore, Williams & Wilkins, 1983

Magee J: Orthopedic Physical Assessment. Philadelphia, WB Saunders, 1987

Maitland GD: The Peripheral Joints: Examination and Recording Guide. Adelaide, Australia, Virgo Press, 1973

Norkin CC, White DJ: Measurement of Joint Motion: A Guide to Goniometry. Philadelphia, FA Davis, 1985

Travell J: Temporomandibular joint pain referred muscles of the head and neck. J Prosthet Dent 10:745, 1960

Williams P, Warwick R (eds): Gray's Anatomy, 36th British ed. Philadelphia, WB Saunders, 1980

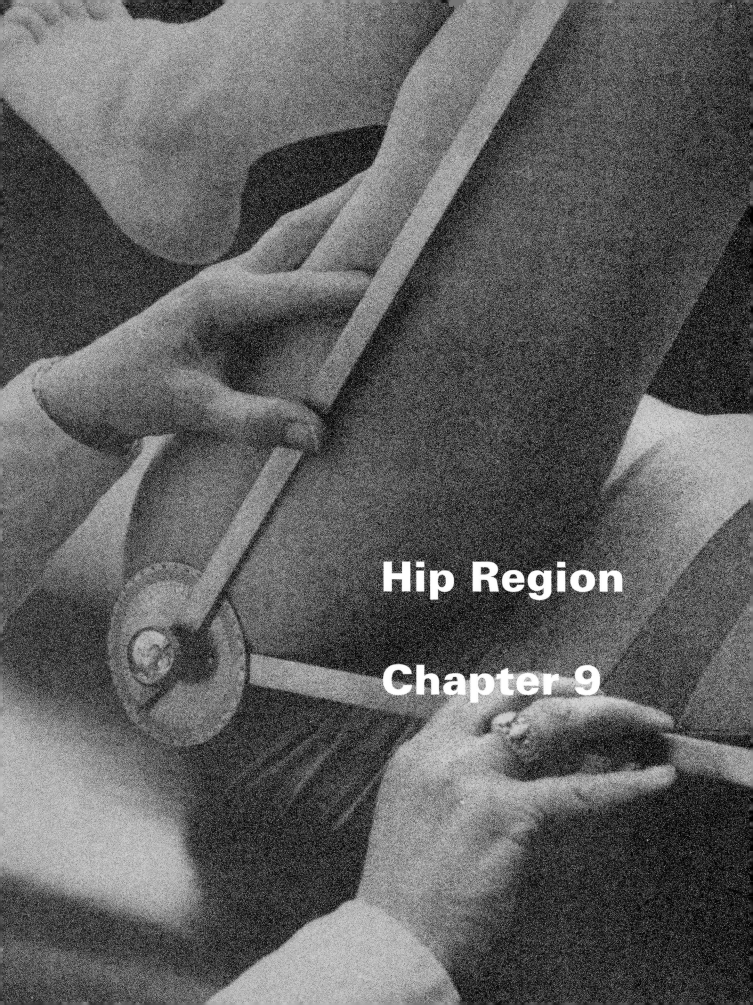

Hip Region

Chapter 9

The hip joint is a synovial ball-and-socket type of joint with the head of the femur articulating with the acetabulum. It has greater congruency than any other joint in the body. The hip joint transmits a great force between the trunk and the floor; in addition, it plays a major role in ambulation. The articular arrangement is designed for stability but does permit limited mobility. The hip joint has three degrees of freedom of motion. The true axis of motion goes through the center of the femoral head. Clinically, the axis is at the level of the greater trochanter.

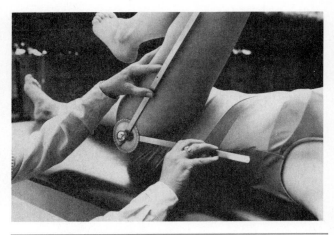

Figure 9–1. End position for measuring hip flexion.

Goniometry

Hip Flexion

Hip flexion occurs in the sagittal plane between the head of the femur and the acetabulum of the os coxa. As the hip moves into flexion, the head of the femur glides in a posterior and inferior direction. Hip flexion motion is accompanied by secondary movements such as posterior pelvic tilt and lumbar vertebral flexion. The subject is stabilized so that the secondary motions do not affect hip joint flexion and are not included in the measurement.

to find trochanter pass. rot. pt's leg.

Motion. 0 to 115 to 125 degrees into a position of hip flexion with knee flexion.

Position
- Preferred: Subject lies supine with the opposite lower limb flat on the table top (Fig. 9–1).
- Alternate: Subject is in sidelying position on the opposite side (Fig. 9–2).

Goniometric Alignment

Axis. Placed on the lateral aspect of the hip approximately a fingerbreadth anterior and superior to the greater trochanter of the femur.

Stationary Arm. Placed parallel to the long axis of the trunk, in line with the greater trochanter of the femur.

Moving Arm. Placed along the lateral midline of the femur toward the lateral epicondyle.

Stabilization. The pelvis is stabilized.

Precautions
- Allow the knee to flex to prevent a stretch on the hamstring muscles.
- Keep the opposite lower limb flat on the table to control posterior pelvic tilt.
- Avoid lumbosacral motion.

Hip Extension and Hyperextension

ASIS stay on table

Extension and hyperextension motion occurs in the sagittal plane as the return from hip flexion. The test position for hip joint hyperextension is lying on the side opposite the hip joint being measured. As the femur extends and hyperextends, the head glides in an anterior and inferior direction in the acetabulum of the os coxa. The extension-hyperextension motion at the hip is usually accompanied by anterior pelvic tilt and increased lumbar lordosis. The subject is stabilized, and the secondary motions are not included in the measurement.

Hyperextension of the hip joint is rare as a true motion. Careful analysis of the motion will show that it is in reality extension of the lumbar vertebrae with forward tilt of the pelvis.

Motion. From 115 to 125 degrees to 0 degrees of hip extension and 0 to 10 to 15 degrees of hip hyperextension. In the prone test position, the subject must keep the anterior superior iliac spines (ASIS) flat on the table to ensure that the motion is occurring at the hip joint and not at the lumbar vertebrae.

Position
- Preferred: Subject lies supine with both lower limbs in the anatomical position.
- Alternate:
  1. Subject is in sidelying position on the opposite side with the non-test hip flexed to 90 degrees to prevent anterior rotation of the pelvis (Fig. 9–3).
  2. Subject lies prone with the hip and knee joints in the anatomical position (Fig. 9–4).

Goniometric Alignment

Axis. Placed laterally on the femur approximately a fingerbreadth anterior and superior to the greater trochanter.

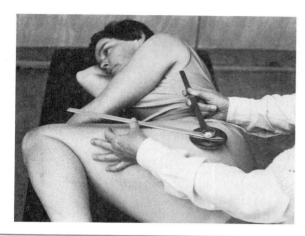

Figure 9–2. End position for measuring hip flexion in the alternate sidelying position.

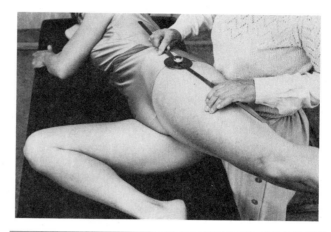

Figure 9–3. End position for measuring hip extension.

Stationary Arm. Placed parallel to the long axis of the trunk in line with the greater trochanter of the femur.

Moving Arm. Placed along the lateral midline of the femur toward the lateral epicondyle.

Stabilization. The pelvis and lumbar vertebrae are stabilized.

Precautions
- Avoid lumbar extension.
- Keep the knee joint extended to prevent stretch on the rectus femoris muscle.
- Avoid anterior pelvic tilt.

Hip Abduction

In the anatomical position, hip abduction motion occurs in the frontal plane; however, in the test position, the motion occurs in the transverse plane. The motion of hip joint abduction occurs between the head of the femur gliding in an inferior direction in the acetabulum of the pelvis. Hip joint abduction is usually accompanied by contralateral pelvic tilt, which is not included in the measurement.

Motion. 0 to 45 degrees of hip abduction.

Position. Subject lies supine with the lower limb to be tested in the anatomical position (Figs. 9–5 and 9–6).

Goniometric Alignment

Axis. Placed on the anterior surface of the hip joint in line with the greater trochanter of the femur.

Stationary Arm. Placed parallel to and below the ASIS at the level of the hip joint.

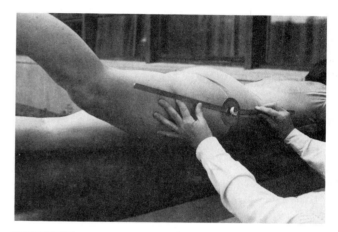

Figure 9–4. End position for measuring hip hyperextension in the alternate prone position.

Moving Arm. Placed on the anterior surface of the thigh parallel to the dorsal midline of the femur, toward the midline of the patella.

Stabilization. The pelvis is stabilized.

Precautions
- Prevent lateral rotation at the hip joint.
- Prevent lateral tilt of the pelvis (hip hiking).

Hip Adduction

In the test position adduction of the hip joint occurs in the transverse plane; in the anatomical position, the motion occurs in the frontal plane. The head of the femur glides in a superior direction in the acetabulum. The adduction motion of the hip is usually accompanied by ipsilateral tilt of the pelvis, which is not included in the measurement.

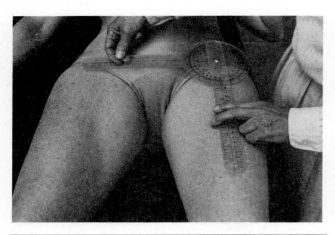

Figure 9–5. Starting position for measuring hip abduction.

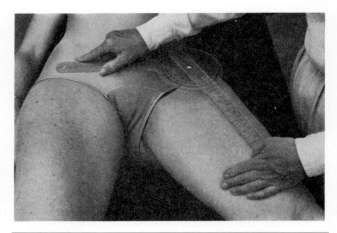

Figure 9–6. End position for measuring hip abduction.

Motion. 0 to 20 to 30 degrees of hip joint adduction.

Position. Subject lies supine with the hip and knee joints in the anatomical position. The opposite lower limb is abducted to allow full range of motion on the test side (Fig. 9–7).

Goniometric Alignment

Axis. Placed inferior to the ASIS in line with the greater trochanter.

Stationary Arm. Placed parallel to and inferior to the ASIS at the level of the hip joint.

Moving Arm. Placed on the anterior surface of the thigh, parallel to the dorsal midline of the femur, toward the midline of the patella.

Stabiliation. The pelvis is stabilized.

Precautions
- Prevent medial rotation of the hip joint.
- Prevent ipsilateral tilt of the pelvis.

Hip Medial Rotation

In the test position hip medial rotation motion occurs in the frontal plane, and in the anatomical position, it occurs in the transverse plane. The motion of medial rotation is produced between the head of the femur and the acetabulum. The head of the femur glides in a posterior direction in the acetabulum during medial rotation of the joint. In the alternate test position, the hip is flexed and not in the anatomical position. Greater range of motion occurs with the hip joint flexed because it is in the open-packed position.

Motion. 0 to 30 to 45 degrees of hip joint medial rotation. The total range of motion varies depending on whether the hip joint is flexed or extended.

Position towel under test knee
- Preferred: Subject lies supine with the hip joint in the anatomical position and the knee flexed to 90 degrees over the edge of the table. The opposite hip and knee are flexed, and the foot lies flat on the table (Figs. 9–8 and 9–9).
- Alternate: more range-hip loose packed
  1. Subject sits with the knee flexed over the edge of the table. The femur is parallel with the table top, and the hip joint is flexed 90 degrees.
  2. Subject lies prone with the hip joint in the anatomical position and the knee joint flexed 90 degrees (Figs. 9–10 and 9–11).
  3. Subject lies supine the knee joints flexed 90 degrees and the stationary arm of the goniometer perpendicular to the floor (Fig. 9–12).

Figure 9–7. End position for measuring hip adduction.

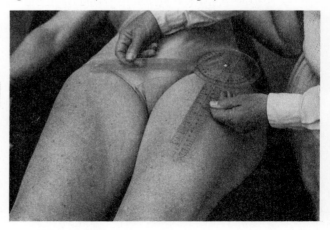

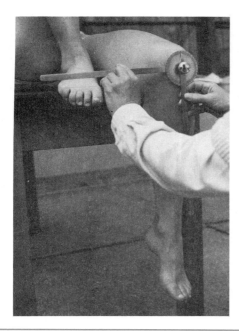

Figure 9–8.   Starting position for measuring hip medial rotation.

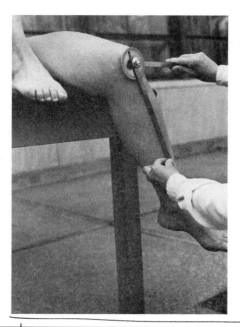

Figure 9–9.   End position for measuring hip medial rotation.

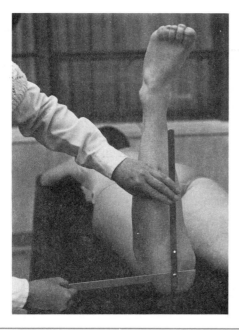

Figure 9–10.   Starting position for measuring hip medial rotation in the alternate prone position.

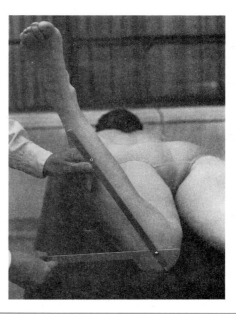

Figure 9–11.   End position for measuring hip medial rotation in the alternate prone position.

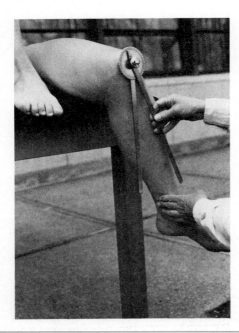

Figure 9–12. End position for measuring hip medial rotation in the alternate supine position, using the effects of gravity on the stationary arm of the goniometer.

Goniometric Alignment

Axis. Placed over the anterior midpatella to project through the shaft of the femur to the femoral head.

Stationary Arm
- Preferred: Placed parallel to the table top.
- Alternate: Placed perpendicular to the floor or parallel to the midline of the tibia.

Moving Arm. Placed along the crest of the tibia to a point midway between the malleoli.

Stabilization. Stabilize the distal end of the thigh.

Precautions
- Avoid rotation and lateral tilting of the pelvis toward the same side.
- Prevent the pelvis from lifting off the table.
- In the sitting position, prevent contralateral trunk flexion.
- Prevent adduction at the hip joint.

Hip Lateral Rotation

In the anatomical position, lateral rotation of the hip occurs in the transverse plane. In the test position, the motion occurs in the frontal plane. As the motion of hip lateral rotation occurs, the head of the femur glides in an anterior direction in the acetabulum. In the preferred test position, the hip joint is in the anatomical position. Less range of motion in lateral rotation occurs because the hip joint is in a closed-packed position.

Motion. 0 to 30 to 45 degrees of hip joint lateral rotation. In the preferred test position, the hip joint is in the anatomical position.

Position
- Preferred: Subject is supine, with the knee flexed to 90 degrees over the edge of the table. The "non-test" hip and knee joint are flexed, and the foot is flat on the table (Fig. 9–13).
- Alternate:
  1. Subject sits with the hip and knee joints flexed to 90 degrees.
  2. Subject lies prone with the test knee joint flexed to 90 degrees (Fig. 9–14).
  3. Subject lies supine with the stationary arm of the goniometer perpendicular to the floor (Fig. 9–15).

Goniometric Alignment

Axis. Placed over the anterior aspect of the midpatella projecting through the shaft of the femur toward the hip joint.

Stationary Arm
- Preferred: Placed parallel to the tabletop.
- Alternate: Placed perpendicular to the floor or parallel to the tibial crest.

Moving Arm. Placed along the crest of the tibia to a point midway between the malleoli.

Figure 9–13. End position for measuring hip lateral rotation.

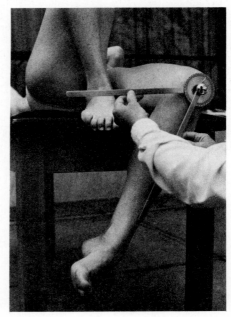

Stabilization. The distal end of the femur and the pelvis are stabilized.

Precautions

- Avoid rotation of the pelvis toward the opposite side.
- Prevent hip joint adduction or flexion.
- Avoid contralateral tilt of the pelvis.
- Prevent ipsilateral trunk flexion or rotation.

Functional Muscle Testing

Hip Flexion

The hip flexor muscles lie anterior to the axis of motion in the sagittal plane. The hip flexor muscle group contracts both concentrically and eccentrically during activities of daily living such as walking, running, and ascending and descending stairs. As a group, the muscles tend to be more type II phasic muscles. In an erect standing posture, the hip flexors contact because the gravity line lies slightly posterior to the hip joint.

Position. Subject stands.

Activity. Subject places the foot of the test limb onto a step of 8 inches and returns the foot to the floor or ascends a flight of stairs (Fig. 9–16).

Muscles. Iliacus, psoas major, sartorius, tensor fasciae latae, pectineus, adductor longus, gracilis.

Types of Contraction

- Concentric: Flexing the hip when placing foot onto the step.
- Eccentric: Extending the hip when returning foot to the floor.

Resistance

- The weight of the limb against gravity offers the resistance.
- Functional: 5 repetitions.
- Functionally Fair: 3 to 4 repetitions.
- Functionally Poor: 1 to 2 repetitions.
- Nonfunctional: 0 repetitions.

Hip Extension

The extensor muscles of the hip lie posterior to the axis in the sagittal plane. The hip extensor muscles are more of a type I static, or postural, muscle. The muscles contract during activities of daily living both concentrically and eccentrically. Common activities involving eccentric contraction are sitting down, descending stairs, and decelerating the lower limb during ambulation. The muscle group contracts concentrically in rising from a seated position, ascending stairs, and during the stance phase of gait. During normal walking, the extension motion is

Figure 9–14. End position for measuring hip lateral rotation in the alternate prone position.

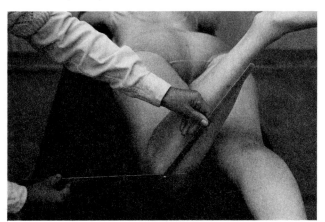

Figure 9–15. End position for measuring hip lateral rotation in the alternate supine position, using the effects of gravity on the stationary arm of the goniometer.

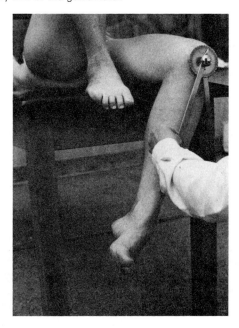

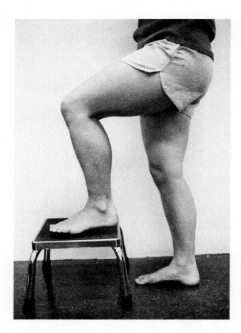

Figure 9–16. Hip flexion.

produced by the hamstrings, and the gluteus maximus is not involved.

Position. Subject stands.

Activity. Subject slowly lowers self onto the seat of a standard chair and returns to standing without the aid of the upper limbs (Fig. 9–17).

Muscles. Gluteus maximus, hamstrings, posterior gluteus medius, superior portion of the adductor magnus, piriformis.

Types of Contraction
· Eccentric: Flexing the hip when sitting down.
· Concentric: Extending the hip when returning to a standing position.

Resistance
· Body weight offers resistance.
· Functional: 5 repetitions.
· Functionally Fair: 3 to 4 repetitions.
· Functionally Poor: 1 to 2 repetitions.
· Nonfunctional: 0 repetitions.

Hip Abduction

The muscles of hip abduction generally lie lateral and superior to the sagittal plane axis. These muscles are important during the stance phase of gait, providing support for the pelvis so that it remains level and does not drop to the non–weight-bearing side. They contract

functionally through a limited range of motion, performing an isometric to eccentric type of contraction. The abductor muscle group contracts concentrically during sidestepping motions.

Position. Subject stands.

Activity. Subject lifts the "non-test" limb, keeping the pelvis as level as possible on the test (weight-bearing) side. A slight drop (5 degrees) is normal. Lateral pelvic tilt might be observed in ambulation on level surfaces (Fig. 9–18).

Muscles. Gluteus medius, gluteus minimus, tensor fasciae latae, superior portion of the gluteus maximus, piriformis.

Types of Contraction
· Eccentric: Pelvis tilts slightly contralaterally as the hip abductors prevent ipsilateral hip adduction.

Resistance
· Body weight offers the resistance, and subject holds position.
· Functional: 1 minute.
· Functionally Fair: 30 to 59 seconds.
· Functionally Poor: 1 to 29 seconds.
· Nonfunctional: 0 seconds.

Hip Adduction

Adductor muscles of the hip generally lie medial to the sagittal axis. They assist in ambulation during hip flexion and extension and produce type I, phasic, concentric contraction. The muscles maintain a reasonable base of support for the body during motion or in a static posture. The adductor muscles are essential for stabilizing

Figure 9–17. Hip extension.

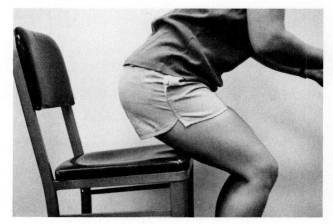

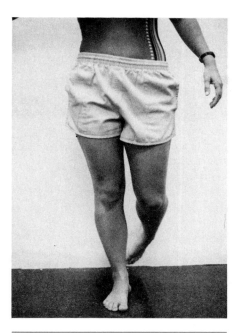

Figure 9–18. Hip abduction on the right.

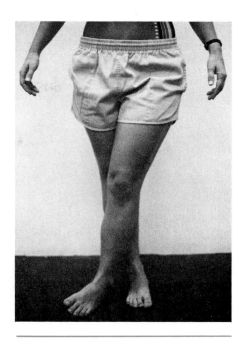

Figure 9–19. Hip adduction on the left.

the pelvis when it is supported on both lower limbs and play an essential part in certain postures and movements in such sports as skiing, horseback riding, and executing a soccer style kick.

Position. Subject stands.

Activity. Subject walks sideways for 20 feet in each direction. The lead lower limb must abduct, and the test lower limb adducts (Fig. 9–19).

Muscles. Adductor longus, adductor magnus, adductor brevis, pectineus, gracilis.

Types of Contraction
· Concentric: Hip adduction in the test limb.

Resistance
· The weight of the test limb offers resistance.
· Functional: 20 feet one way.
· Functionally Fair: 10 to 19 feet.
· Functionally Poor: 1 to 9 feet.
· Nonfunctional: 0 feet.

Hip Medial Rotation

The hip medial rotator muscles are less numerous and powerful than the lateral rotators, and they run anterior to the vertical axis of the hip. The motion of hip medial rotation occurs during the swing phase of gait as a concentric type of contraction. Functionally, medial rotation

occurs on the non–weight-bearing limb when the lateral border of the foot is brought toward the head. In a static bilateral, weight-bearing posture, rotation of the pelvis toward the left will result in hip medial rotation on the left.

Position. Subject stands, with the body weight on the nontest lower limb. The other foot is off the floor. The subject may lightly hold on to the treatment table with the hands for balance but may not support any body weight with the hands. Subject medially rotates the non–weight-bearing hip.

Activity
1. Subject slowly twists the pelvis toward the test side. The trunk follows the pelvis but does not precede pelvic motion (Fig. 9–20).
2. Subject walks forward taking longer than normal strides.

Muscles. Gluteus medius, gluteus minimus, tensor fasciae latae.

Types of Contraction
· Concentric: In the non–weight-bearing position, the lateral border of the test limb is brought toward the head.

Resistance
· The weight of the pelvis, trunk, head, and upper limbs offer resistance.
· Functional: 10 repetitions to each side.

- Funtionally Fair: 5 to 9 repetitions to each side.
- Functionally Poor: 1 to 4 repetitions to each side.
- Nonfunctional: 0 repetitions.

Distance
- The weight of the lower limb in the swing phase of gait offers resistance.
- Functional: 10 steps.
- Functionally Fair: 5 to 9 steps.
- Functionally Poor: 1 to 4 steps.
- Nonfunctional: 0 steps.

Hip Lateral Rotation

The numerous and powerful hip lateral rotators cross posterior to the vertical axis through the hip. The motion of hip lateral rotation tends to accompany hip extension during many functional activities. The lateral rotators of the hip concentrically contract during the stance phase of gait. In a non–weight-bearing position, the lateral rotators of the hip contract concentrically when one wishes to bring the medial border of the foot toward the ipsilateral hip.

Position. Subject stands with the test lower limb bearing the total body weight. The non-test lower limb is off the floor. The subject may use the hands lightly on the treatment table for balance, but not to bear any body weight (Fig. 9–21).

Activity. Subject stands on the non-test lower limb. The other limb is off the floor. Subject laterally rotates the non–weight-bearing hip.

Muscles. Gluteus maximus, piriformis, obturator internus and externus, superior and inferior gemellus, quadratus femoris, posterior portion of the adductor magnus, pectineus.

Types of Contraction
- Concentric: In the non–weight-bearing position, the medial border of the test limb is brought toward the ipsilateral hip.

Resistance
- The body weight offers the resistance.
- Functional: 10 repetitions to each side.
- Functionally Fair: 5 to 9 repetitions to each side.
- Functionally Poor: 1 to 4 repetitions to each side.
- Nonfunctional: 0 repetitions.

Manual Muscle Testing

Psoas Major and Iliacus Muscles

The psoas major and the iliacus muscles have a common insertion and are called the iliopsoas muscle. The combined muscle produces the motion of hip flexion in the sagittal plane through a test range of 30 degrees from a

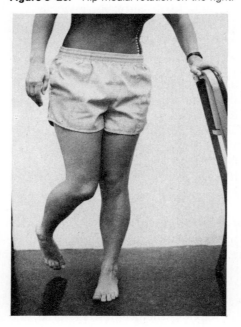

Figure 9–20. Hip medial rotation on the right.

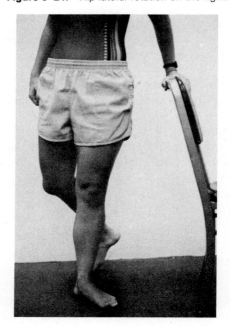

Figure 9–21. Hip lateral rotation on the right.

Attachments of Psoas Major, Iliacus, and Rectus Femoris Muscles

Muscles	Proximal	Distal	Innervation
Psoas major	Transverse processes, bodies, and intervertebral discs of T12 and all lumbar vertebrae	Lesser trochanter of femur	Spinal nerves L1 and L2 (L3)
Iliacus	Iliac fossa and crest, ala of the sacrum	Lesser trochanter of femur	Spinal nerves L2 (L3)
Rectus femoris	Anterior inferior iliac spine (AIIS)	Tibial tuberosity through patellar ligament	Femoral L3 and L4 (L2)

starting position of 90 degrees of flexion. During the movement the pelvis remains fixed in a posterior pelvic tilt.

Palpation

Psoas Major.   With the subject seated and bent forward to relax the abdominal muscles, place fingers deep into the abdomen below the ribs and above the iliac crest, gently pushing toward the posterior abdominal wall (Fig. 9–22).

Iliacus.   It is difficult to palpate the iliac muscle, which lies on the iliac fossa.

Position
- AG: Subject sits with the knees flexed and the pelvis in posterior tilt. Hands should be holding on to the edge of the table (Fig. 9–23).
- GM: Subject is in sidelying position with the upper limb supported on a powder board; the hip is in neutral rotation and the knee is flexed 90 degrees (Fig. 9–24).

Movement.   Flexion of hip in the sagittal plane.

Resistance.   Applied to the proximal knee on the anterior surface of the thigh.

Figure 9–22.   Palpation of the psoas major muscle.

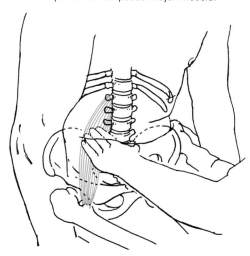

Figure 9–23.   Testing the iliopsoas muscle in the AG position.

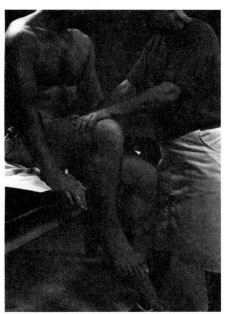

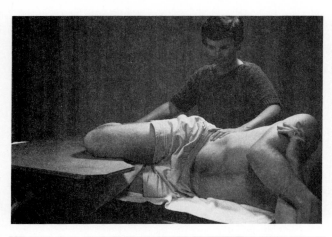

Figure 9–24.   Testing the iliopsoas muscle in the GM position.

Stabilization.   The opposite side of the pelvis is stabilized.

Substitutions

- The hip abducts and laterally rotates as the sartorius flexes.
- The hip abducts and medially rotates as the tensor fasciae latae flexes.
- Rectus femoris is an accessory muscle to hip flexion.

Sartorius Muscle

The sartorius muscle performs hip flexion accompanied by abduction and lateral rotation. It is a two-joint muscle that crosses the knee joint and assists in flexing it.

Palpation.   Palpate below and slightly medial to the anterior superior iliac spine (Fig. 9–25).

Position
- AG: Subject sits with the pelvis in posterior pelvic tilt and both knees flexed to 90 degrees off the edge of the table (Fig. 9–26).
- GM: Subject lies supine with the heel of the test limb on the opposite ankle; the "non-test" limb is in the anatomical position (Fig. 9–27).

Movement.   Subject brings the plantar surface of the heel to the opposite knee. In the GM position, the subject slides the heel along the leg to the knee, keeping the lateral surface of the test limb on the table.

Resistance.   Applied to the medial malleolus to resist hip lateral rotation, and on the lateral surface of the thigh proximal to the knee to resist flexion and abduction.

Stabilization.   When giving resistance as stated above, one hand provides counterpressure for the other.

Substitution
- Iliopsoas and rectus femoris produce straight hip flexion without abduction or lateral rotation.
- Tensor fasciae latae produces hip flexion and abduction with medial rather than lateral rotation.

Figure 9–25.   Palpation of the sartorius muscle.

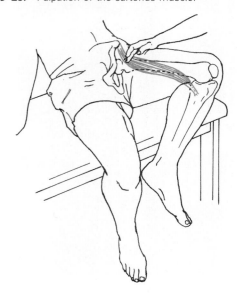

Figure 9–26.   Testing the sartorius muscle in the AG position.

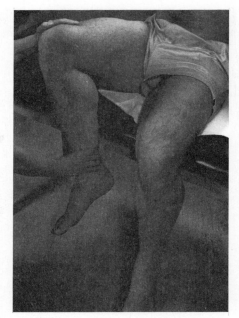

Attachments of Sartorius Muscle

Muscle	Proximal	Distal	Innervation
Sartorius	ASIS	Proximal medial aspect of tibia	Femoral L2 and L3

Attachments of Gluteus Maximus Muscle

Muscle	Proximal	Distal	Innervation
Gluteus maximus	Gluteal line of the ilium, posterior sacrum, coccyx, and sacrotuberous ligament	Iliotibial tract and the gluteal tuberosity of the femur	Inferior gluteal S1 and S2 (L5)

Gluteus Maximus Muscle

The gluteus maximus muscle produces the motion of hip extension from a starting position of hip flexion through a test range of 125 to 140 degrees. The extension action of the gluteus maximus is increased if the hip is laterally rotated and may be tested as a lateral rotator of the hip. With the knee in extension, as the angle of hip flexion decreases, the hamstrings contribute more to the motion. If the knee is flexed the gluteus maximus contributes more to the action of extension until the hip is flexed less than 45 degrees. Others test the gluteus maximus muscle in the prone position, moving into 15 degrees of hip hyperextension.

Palpation. Palpate between the sacrum and the greater trochanter, with the hip in lateral rotation (Fig. 9–28).

Position
- AG: Subject stands with trunk flexed over a table and knee flexed (Fig. 9–29).
- GM: Subject is in sidelying position with test limb supported and hip flexed 90 degrees and flexes knee for gluteus maximus action (Fig. 9–30).

Figure 9–27. Testing the sartorius muscle in the GM position.

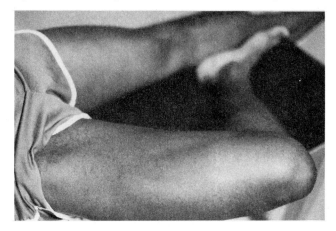

Figure 9–28. Palpating the gluteus maximus muscle.

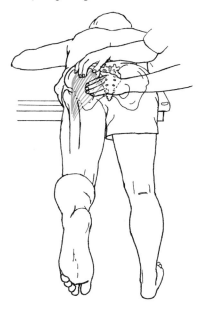

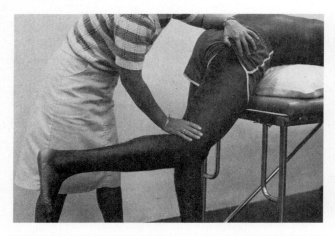

Figure 9–29. Testing the gluteus maximus muscle in the AG position.

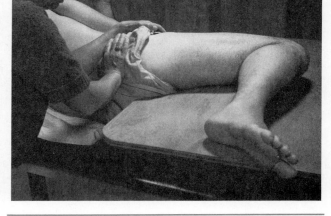

Figure 9–30. Testing the gluteus maximus muscle in the GM position.

Movement. Extension of the hip from a flexed position.

Resistance. Applied proximal to the knee joint on the posterior thigh.

Stabilization. The pelvis is stabilized and hyperextension of the lumbar spine is prevented.

Substitutions
- Hamstrings extend the hip without any action from the gluteus maximus.
- Stabilize the lumbar vertebrae to prevent an increase in lordosis.

Gluteus Medius and Minimus Muscles

Both the gluteus medius and minimus muscles produce the movement of hip abduction. The test position is with the hip extended and in neutral rotation. The motion produced is through a test range of 45 degrees. The pelvis should remain motionless. Both the gluteus medius and gluteus minimus muscles may be tested as medial rotators of the hip through a test range of 45 degrees.

Palpation

Gluteus Medius. Only the anterior and middle portions are palpable, either laterally below the crest of the ilium or immediately proximal to the greater trochanter (Fig. 9–31).

Figure 9–31. Palpating the gluteus medius muscle.

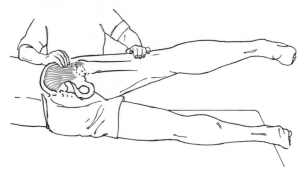

Figure 9–32. Testing the gluteus medius and minimus muscles in the AG position.

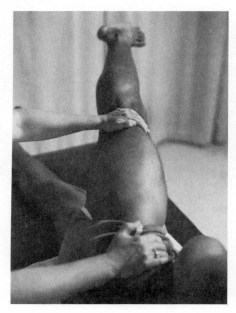

Attachments of Gluteus Medius and Minimus Muscles

Muscle	Proximal	Distal	Innervation
Gluteus medius	Lateral surface of ilium between crest and line	Lateral surface of greater trochanter of femur	Superior gluteal L5 (S1)
Gluteus minimus	External surface of ilium and inferior gluteal line	Anterior surface of greater trochanter of femur	Superior gluteal L5 (S1)

Gluteus Minimus. It lies deep to the gluteus maximus and the gluteus medius, and therefore is not palpable.

Position
- AG: Subject is in sidelying position with the lower hip and knee flexed to 90 degrees. The test limb rests on the table behind the lower limb; the hip is neutral and the knee is extended (Fig. 9–32).
- GM: Subject is supine, with the opposite lower limb in neutral, and the test lower limb supported on a powder board (Fig. 9–33).

Movement. Abduction of the hip without flexion or lateral rotation.

Resistance. Applied proximal to the knee joint on the lateral side of the thigh.

Stabilization. The pelvis is stabilized.

Substitutions
- The quadratus lumborum and the lateral abdominal tilt the pelvis laterally giving the appearance of abduction.
- If the patient rolls slightly to the supine position, the tensor fasciae latae is in a more favorable position to abduct the hip as it will be in a flexed position.
- Gluteus maximus (superior portion) is an accessory to hip abduction.

Alternate Testing of the Gluteus Medius and Minimus Muscles

Alternate testing of the gluteus medius and minimus as medial rotators of the hip is possible.

Position
- AG: Subject lies supine or is sitting, with the knees flexed over the edge of the table (Fig. 9–34).

Figure 9–33. Testing the gluteus medius and minimus muscles in the GM position.

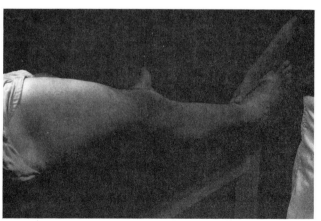

Figure 9–34. Testing the gluteus medius and minimus muscles during hip medial rotation in the alternate AG position.

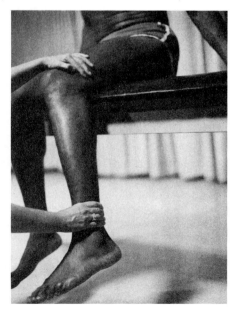

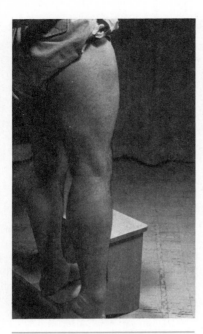

Figure 9–35. Testing the gluteus medius and minimus muscles during hip medial rotation in the alternate GM position.

- GM: Subject lies supine with the test knee extended and the hip laterally rotated. If the subject is able to stand, then the position is non–weight-bearing on the test limb, the knee is extended, and the hip laterally rotated (Fig. 9–35).

Movement.   Medial rotation of the hip joint. In the GM position, the knee must move beyond the midline. In the AG position, the leg moves in a lateral direction.

Resistance.   Applied proximal to the lateral malleolus into lateral rotation. If knee pathology is present, resistance should be applied proximal to the knee to prevent torque forces from below.

Stabilization.   The knee joint is stabilized on the medial side.

Substitutions
- Patient may elevate the buttock on the test side.
- Subject may evert the foot, extend the knee, or abduct the hip, giving the appearance of medial rotation.
- In the GM standing position, the subject may laterally rotate on the supporting limb.

Tensor Fasciae Latae Muscle

The tensor fasciae latae muscle produces the motion of hip flexion accompanied by abduction and medial rotation. It may also assist in knee extension.

Palpation.   Palpate below and slightly lateral to the ASIS (Fig. 9–36).

Position
- AG: Subject is in the sidelying position with the non-test limb in the anatomical position. The test limb is in 45 degrees of hip flexion, the knee is extended with the limb resting on the table in front of the "non-test" limb (Fig. 9–37).
- GM: Subject is semisitting with the hips flexed 45 degrees, in neutral rotation, and the arms supporting the trunk. The test leg is on a powder board (Fig. 9–38).

Movement.   Abduction of the hip joint while maintaining 45 degrees of hip flexion.

Resistance.   Applied to the distal thigh on the lateral side.

Stabilization.   The pelvis is stabilized.

Substitutions
- Prevent substitution by stabilizing the pelvis.
- The hip flexors produce only flexion at the hip joint with no abduction.

Figure 9–36.   Palpating the tensor fasciae latae muscle.

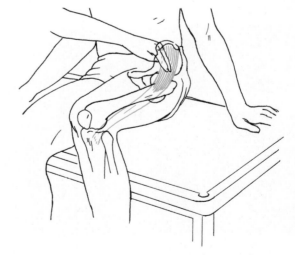

Attachments of Tensor Fasciae Latae Muscle

Muscle	Proximal	Distal	Innervation
Tensor fasciae latae	Lateral surface of anterior superior iliac spine, anterior outer crest of ilium	Iliotibial tract to proximal, lateral aspect of tibia	Superior gluteal L4 and L5

Adductor Longus, Magnus, and Brevis, and Gracilis and Pectineus Muscles

The adductor muscles as a group produce adduction of the hip with the hip extended through a test range of 20 to 25 degrees. The adductor longus and brevis and the pectineus may act as synergists in flexion of the hip joint. The adductor magnus muscle (vertical portion) acts as a synergist to hip joint extension. The subject may use the hands on the table to stabilize the trunk.

Palpation
- Palpate the adductor longus on the medial side of the thigh immediately below the pubic arch (Fig. 9–39).
- Palpate the adductor magnus along the medial aspect of the thigh in the middle to lower half (Fig. 9–40).
- The adductor brevis is too deep for accurate assessment.

- Palpate the round tendon of the gracilis on the medial aspect of the knee (Fig. 9–41).
- The pectineus is difficult to palpate and uncomfortable for the patient.

Position
- AG: Subject is in the sidelying position with the non-test limb supported in 25 degrees of abduction. The lower limb is the test limb (Fig. 9–42).
- GM: Subject lies supine with the opposite limb in 25 degrees of abduction. The test lower limb is in a position of slight abduction, supported on a friction-free surface (Fig. 9–43).

Movement.   Adduct the hip to 25 degrees.

Resistance.   Applied proximal to the knee joint into abduction.

Stabilization.   The pelvis is stabilized.

Figure 9–37. Testing the tensor fasciae latae muscle in the AG position.

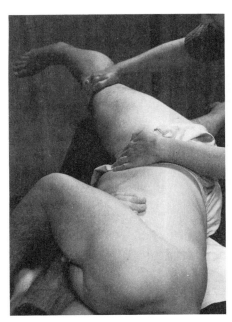

Figure 9–38. Testing the tensor fasciae latae muscle in the GM position.

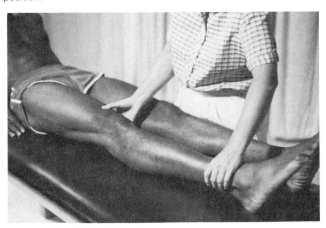

Attachments of the Adductor Longus, Magnus, and Brevis, and Gracilis and Pectineus Muscles

Muscle	Proximal	Distal	Innervation
Adductor longus	Anterior surface of pubis at crest	Middle third of medial lip of linea aspera of femur	Obturator L3 (L2 and L4)
Adductor magnus	Inferior ramus of pubis and ischium and ischial tuberosity	Gluteal tuberosity, linea aspera, medial supracondylar line, and adductor tubercle of femur	Obturator L3 (L2) Tibial portion of sciatic L3 and L4 (L2)
Adductor brevis	Inferior pubic ramus	Distal pectineal line and superior portion of medial lip of linea aspera of femur	Obturator L3 (L2 and L4)
Gracilis	Inferior pubic ramus and symphysis	Distal to medial condyle of tibia	Obturator L2 (L3)
Pectineus	Superior pubic ramus	Pectineal line of femur	Femoral L2 (L3) Obturator (L2 and L3)

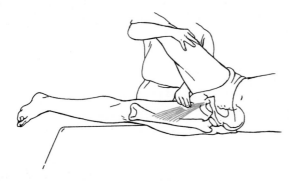

Figure 9–39.   Palpating the hip adductor longus muscle.

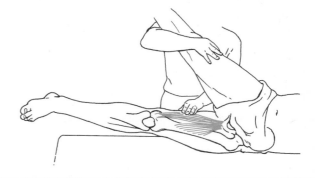

Figure 9–40.   Palpating the adductor magnus muscle.

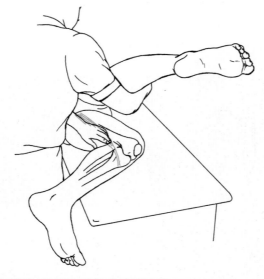

Figure 9–41.   Palpating the gracilis muscle.

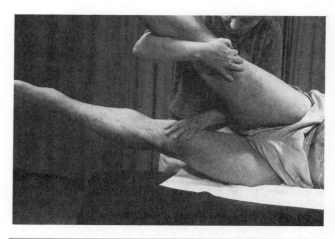

Figure 9–42.   Testing the adductor muscle group in the AG position.

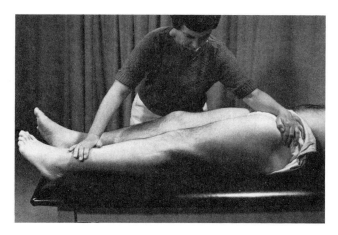

Figure 9–43. Testing the adductor muscle group in the GM position.

Substitutions

- The hamstrings can substitute. Hip adduction is accompanied by lateral rotation of the hip.
- The quadratus lumborum can substitute by elevating the pelvis on the test side.
- Flexing the trunk to the opposite side may give the appearance of hip adduction.
- Medial and lateral rotators allow no rotation during the motion of hip.

Obturator Internus and Externus, Superior and Inferior Gemellus, Quadratus Femoris, and Piriformis Muscles

The short gluteal, or lateral rotator muscles produce the motion of lateral rotation of the hip through a test range of 45 degrees.

Palpation. Most of the lateral rotators are too deep to the gluteus maximus to be palpated accurately. The tendon of the piriformis muscle may be palpated as it approaches the greater trochanter posteriorly.

Position
- AG: Subject lies supine with the knee flexed over the edge of the table and the opposite hip and knee flexed with the foot supported on the table (Fig. 9–44).
- GM: Subject lies supine with the test limb's knee extended and the hip medially rotated (Fig. 9–45). The subject is standing non–weight-bearing on the test limb with the knee extended and the hip medially rotated (Fig. 9–46).

Movement. Lateral rotation of the hip. In the GM position, the knee must move beyond the midline. In the AG position the foot and leg move in a medial direction.

Resistance. Applied to the distal leg proximal to the medial malleolus or proximal to the knee joint if pathology exists.

Stabilization. The knee joint is stabilized on the lateral side.

Substitutions
- Subject may elevate the buttock on the opposite side.
- Subject may invert the foot, flex the knee, or adduct the hip, giving the appearance of lateral hip rotation.
- In the standing GM position, subject may laterally rotate on the supporting lower limb.

Figure 9–44. Testing the hip lateral rotator muscles in the AG position.

Figure 9–45. Testing the hip lateral rotator muscles in the GM position.

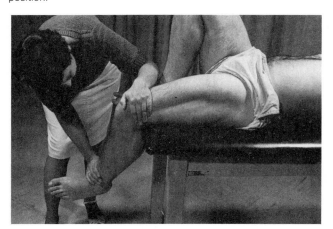

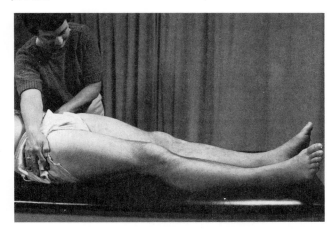

Attachments of Obturator Internus and Externus, Superior and Inferior Gemellus, Quadratus Femoris, and Piriformis Muscles

Muscles	Proximal	Distal	Innervation
Obturator internus	Internal surface of obturator foramen, pelvic surface of ischium, and internal surface of obturator membrane	Medial surface of greater trochanter of femur	Sacral plexus S1 (L5)
Obturator externus	Rami of pubis and ischium and external surface of obturator membrane	Trochanteric fossa of femur	Obturator L4 (L3)
Superior gemellus	Spine of ischium	With obturator internus muscle to greater trochanter of femur	Sacral plexus S1 (L5)
Inferior gemellus	Ischial tuberosity	With obturator internus muscle to greater trochanter of femur	Sacral plexus S1 (L5)
Quadratus femoris	Lateral ischial tuberosity	Intertrochanteric crest	Sacral plexus L5 and S1
Piriformis	Anterior surface of sacrum, border of greater sciatic foramen, and anterior of sacrotuberous ligament	Superior surface of greater trochanter of femur	Sacral plexus S1 (S2)

Clinical Tests

Palpation

Examination of the hip region requires the examiner to observe and palpate certain structural landmarks to determine the source of pathology. The structures that should be located and identified include:

1. Anterior superior iliac spine.
2. Anterior inferior iliac spine.
3. Iliac crest.
4. Umbilicus.
5. Posterior superior iliac spine.
6. Ischial tuberosity.
7. Gluteal fold.
8. Greater trochanter.
9. Pubic symphysis.

Figure 9–46. Testing the hip lateral rotator muscles in the GM position.

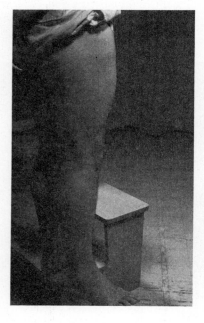

Passive and Active Movements and Contractile Testing

The motions of the hip to be assessed actively and passively and by contractile testing include:

1. Flexion.
2. Extension.
3. Abduction.
4. Adduction.
5. External rotation.
6. Internal rotation.

Special Tests

Thomas Test

Indication. Thomas test assesses hip flexion contractures in subjects who may have developed compensatory lumbar lordosis masking the flexion contracture.

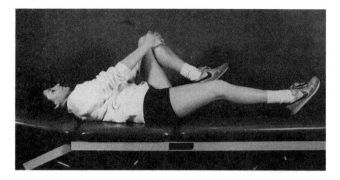

Figure 9–47. Thomas test.

Method. The subject lies supine and flexes both knees toward the chest. While holding one hip in the flexed posture, the subject releases the contralateral limb and extends it toward the table (Fig. 9–47). In a variation, the subject lies supine and flexes the contralateral hip and knee to flatten the lumbar lordosis. The examiner observes whether the extended hip remains so or is drawn up into flexion.

Results. Inability of the extended or extending limb to rest flat on the table is an indication of hip flexor tightness. To be more specific, if the hip and knee of the extended limb remain in a position of flexion, the tightness could be in either the iliopsoas or the rectus femoris muscle.

In order to delineate the source of tightness, the knee is passively extended. If the limb drops further into hip extension as it moves closer to the table, the tightness is in the rectus femoris. If passive extension of the knee does not affect the degree of hip flexion, the tightness is not in the rectus femoris but rather in the iliopsoas muscle.

If the hip joint is in a position of abduction and internal rotation while remaining in a flexed posture,

tightness of the tensor fasciae latae muscle may be indicated.

Other means of assessing a tight rectus femoris muscle include having the subject lie supine with the knees flexed over the edge of the table at approximately 90 degrees. The subject then flexes one knee to the chest and holds it. If the contralateral knee moves into extension, rectus femoris tightness is probably present. If the examiner attempts to passively flex the knee to the position of 90 degrees and encounters no resistance or palpable tightness, then the probable cause of restriction is tightness in the joint structures.

Ely's test for rectus femoris muscle tightness involves having the subject lie prone while the examiner passively flexes the knee (Fig. 9–48). If, during the passive knee flexion, the subject simultaneously flexes the ipsilateral hip, tightness of the rectus femoris is evident.

Ober's Test

Indication. Ober's test is designed to detect tightness in the tensor fascia lata muscle and iliotibial band.

Method. The subject is in a sidelying position with the limb to be tested on top. The hip and knee of the lower limb should be flexed in order to stabilize the subject on the table. The uppermost limb is passively positioned in abduction and some extension, so that the iliotibial band crosses over the greater trochanter (Fig. 9–49). The knee may be either flexed or extended, although greater stretch of the tensor and iliotibial band is elicited in extension. It is important that the examiner stabilize the pelvis in the sidelying position to avoid substitution. The examiner then slowly lowers the uppermost limb, observing to what degree the limb adducts toward the table.

Results. The flexibility of the tensor and iliotibial band is to be considered within normal limits if the

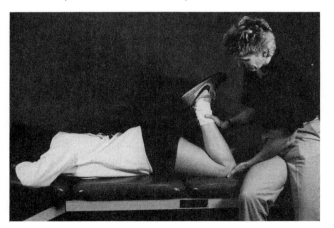

Figure 9–48. Ely's test. Flexion of the ipsilateral hip during simultaneous passive knee flexion is a positive result.

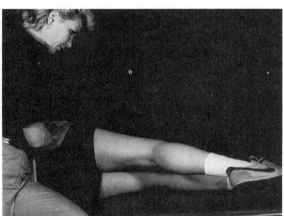

Figure 9–49. Ober's test.

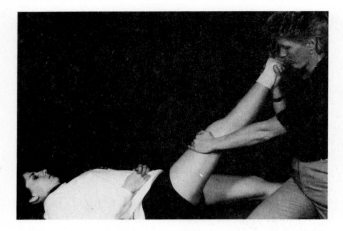

Figure 9–50. Conventional straight leg raise.

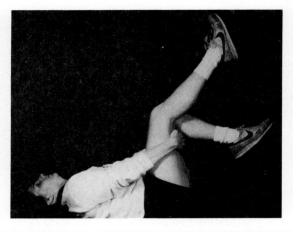

Figure 9–51. The 90-90 straight leg raise.

uppermost limb adducts and returns to the table. Tightness of this structure is indicated if the limb remains in an abducted posture.

Conventional Straight Leg Raise

Indication. The conventional straight leg raise (SLR) is measured to determine the status of the sciatic nerve as well as the flexibility of the hamstring muscles.

Method. The subject is supine. The examiner passively raises the limb into hip flexion, making sure to keep the knee extended (Fig. 9–50).

Results. In assessing hamstring flexibility, the angle of hip flexion necessary to be considered within normal limits is 80 to 90 degrees. Less is an indication of hamstring muscle tightness.

90–90 Straight Leg Raise

Indication. The 90–90 SLR assesses hamstring flexibility.

Method. The subject is positioned as in the conventional SLR test. The subject flexes the hip to 90 degrees and grasps behind the knees to maintain the hip position. The subject's knee is passively extended through its range of motion (Fig. 9–51).

Results. Knee extension from 20 degrees of flexion to full extension is considered to be within normal limits for hamstring flexibility. Hamstring tightness is indicated if the knee remains flexed beyond 20 degrees.

Trendelenburg Sign

Indication. Trendelenburg sign indicates weakness of the gluteus medius muscle during unilateral weight bearing.

Method. The examiner either stands or kneels behind the subject in an optimal positon to view the relationship of posterior pelvic structures. The subject stands with weight evenly distributed on the lower limbs. Assuming that there are no postural abnormalities, bony and soft tissue landmarks should be symmetrical throughout the pelvis and lower limbs. The patient is directed to stand on one limb. A gluteus medius muscle that is functionally strong is able to stabilize the pelvis on the weight-bearing side by maintaining the level of the pelvis on the unsupported side. This balance mechanically is accomplished by the distal attachment of the gluteus medius pulling and holding the pelvis level (Fig. 9–52A and B).

Results. Trendelenburg sign is negative when the pelvis remains level during unilateral weight bearing. A positive sign is indicated when, during unilateral weight bearing, the pelvis drops toward the unsupported limb (9–52*C, D*). The result of the test is positive, therefore, for the gluteus medius muscle of the weight-bearing limb, indicating that the muscle is either nonfunctional or weak. A Trendelenburg gait, which is evident during unsupported ambulatory activities, is also a positive result.

Leg-Length Discrepancies

Detecting a True Discrepancy

Indication. Measurement of leg length assesses whether an actual difference in leg length exists, secondary to bony inequality of the pelvis, femur, or tibia.

Method. The subject lies supine. Care must be taken to ensure that the pelvis is level, that the subject is lying relatively straight, and that the lower limbs are approximately 15 to 20 cm apart and parallel to one another. If an abduction or adduction contracture is present in one hip, the opposite hip should be assessed in a similar

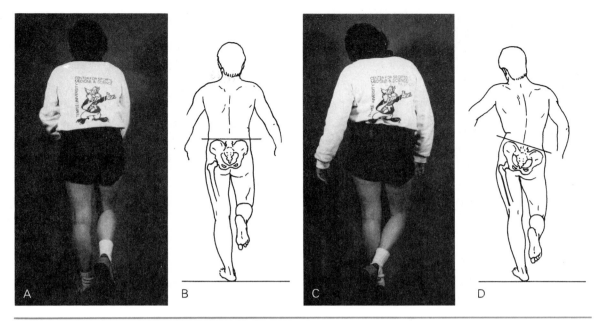

Figure 9–52. *(A, B)* Trendelenburg sign. Normally, during unilateral weight bearing, the pelvis remains level. *(C, D)* A positive result is present when the pelvis drops toward the unsupported limb during unilateral weight bearing.

position to ensure accuracy of measurement. Care must also be taken to be consistent in the specific point of the landmarks chosen to measure for discrepancy. Carelessness in replicating points during testing and comparison will yield inaccurate information.

The initial measurement is taken from the ASIS to the medial malleolus (Fig. 9–53). If excessive hypertrophy or atrophy of one thigh is present, the examiner may choose to use the lateral malleolus for measurement rather than the medial malleolus, in hopes of minimizing error due to circumferential soft tissue differences. If a leg-length discrepancy is found, specific measurements may be taken and compared from various landmarks.

1. ASIS to greater trochanter in assessment of varus or valgus of the hip.
2. Greater trochanter to the lateral joint line of the femur, indicating length of the femoral shaft.
3. Medial joint line of the knee to medial malleolus, indicating tibial shaft length.

Results. Different measurements on the left and right demonstrate leg-length inequality due to skeletal differences. The specific measurements described above allow the examiner to identify the skeletal component responsible for the discrepancy.

The examiner also can visually assess whether a difference in limb length is present at the femur or the tibia, by flexing the subject's hips and knees, making sure that the feet are lined up evenly and symmetrically with one another. A longer femur will cause the ipsilateral knee to project more distally than the other knee when viewed

from the side. A longer tibia will cause the knee to lie more proximal than the opposite one.

Identifying an Apparent Discrepancy

Indication. Apparent leg-length discrepancy is assessed to determine whether it is due to some type of pelvic obliquity or a postural abnormality. This test is used only after it has been determined that an actual difference in limb length does not exist.

Method. The subject is positioned in the manner described for true leg-length discrepancy. A measurement is taken from the umbilicus to the medial malleolus, indicating the actual distance from a soft tissue to a bony landmark.

Figure 9–53. True leg-length measurement. Measure from the ASIS to the medial malleolus.

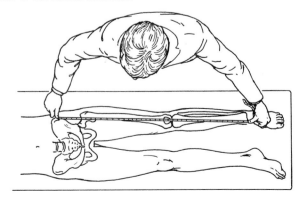

Results. Inequality of the measurements between the left and right sides indicates an apparent leg-length discrepancy secondary to pelvic obliquity or postural abnormality.

Patrick's Test (FABER Test)

Indication. Patrick's test is designed to alert the examiner to the possibility of hip pathology or involvement of the sacroiliac joint. Clinically, this test does not yield useful information regarding specific pathology.

Method. The subject is supine, and the examiner positions the limb to be tested in *flexion*, *ab*duction, and *external rotation* (FABER), so that the foot of the test limb rests on the subject's opposite knee (Fig. 9–54). The examiner then slowly and passively presses the limb being tested toward the table while applying counter-pressure to the opposite ilium.

Results. A negative result is indicated if the tested limb drops to the table or comes to lie parallel to the plane of the opposite limb without pain. A positive result is confirmed if there is pain in the back or hip or the tested limb remains in a plane above the opposite limb.

Sign of the Buttock

Indication. The sign of the buttock test is beneficial in determining whether a patient's pain has its origin in the buttock, as opposed to the hip, the sciatic nerve, or the hamstring muscles.

Method. The examiner performs an SLR test on the subject. If the SLR is limited, the examiner flexes the hip and knee simultaneously.

Results. If the subject's hip flexion is limited with the knee both extended and flexed, then pathology is present

Figure 9–54. Patrick's test.

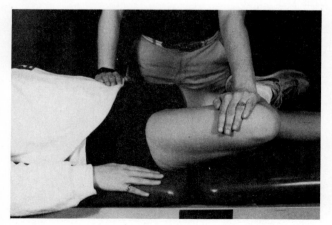

in the buttock and not in the hip, sciatic nerve, or hamstring muscles. Performing SLR causes all of the structures mentioned above to stretch; however, when the knee is allowed to flex as the hip is flexing, stress is taken off of the hip, sciatic nerve, and hamstrings.

Noble's Compression Test

Indication. Noble's compression test is performed to determine whether iliotibial band syndrome is present in the knee. As the knee moves through the range of flexion and extension, the iliotibial band moves posterior to the femoral epicondyle during flexion, and anterior to the epicondyle during extension. This movement may cause friction between the epicondyle and the band, resulting in reactive inflammation.

Method. The subject lies supine with the knee flexed 90 degrees. The examiner applies pressure to the lateral femoral condyle and maintains that pressure while the subject slowly extends the knee.

Results. If at approximately 30 degrees from full extension, the subject complains of pain over the lateral femoral condyle, the test result is positive.

Tests to Assess Congenital Hip Dislocation

Barlow's Test

Indication. Barlow's test is designed to assess the presence of congenital hip dislocation.

Method. The infant lies supine; the examiner stands at the foot of the table facing the subject's lower limbs. The hips are flexed to 90 degrees while the knees are held in full flexion. The examiner's middle fingers are placed over the greater trochanters of each thigh. The examiner's thumbs are placed along the medial side of the thigh and knee, opposite the lesser trochanter. Each hip is assessed separately while the opposite one is stabilized. The hip being examined is abducted while the examiner applies forward pressure from behind the greater trochanter. The examiner then applies backward and outward pressure by pressing the thumb against the inner thigh.

Results. As forward pressure is being exerted on the infant's thigh, a click or clunk felt by the examiner indicates hip dislocation.

As backward pressure is applied, it causes the femoral head to slip out of the acetabulum. Once this pressure is removed, the hip reduces. This situation suggests that this hip is "dislocatable" but not actually dislocated.

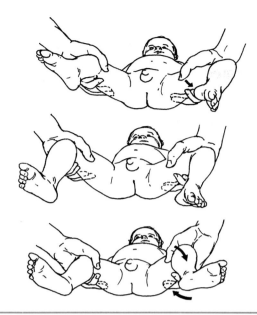

Figure 9–55. Ortolani's sign.

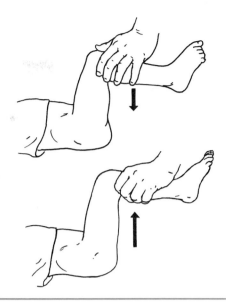

Figure 9–56. Telescoping sign.

Ortolani's Sign

Indication. Ortolani's sign is used to assess congenital hip dislocation.

Method. The infant lies supine while the examiner grips the legs with the thumbs along the medial side of the knee and thigh and the fingers along the lateral thigh to the buttock. The hips are positioned in flexion (Fig. 9–55). As minimal traction is applied, the hips are abducted, while pressure is applied to the greater trochanters laterally.

Results. The examiner may encounter resistance to the abduction and external rotation at approximately 30 to 40 degrees. At this point, a click or clunk may be felt by the examiner, indicating reduction of the hip. Once the hip has reduced, further hip abduction will be possible toward a normal range of 70 to 90 degrees.

Telescoping Sign

Indication. The telescoping sign is used to determine the presence of a dislocated hip.

Method. The subject lies supine while the examiner flexes the hips and knees to 90 degrees (Fig. 9–56). The examiner applies posterior pressure on the knee so that the thigh is forced toward the table. The examiner grasps the upper tibia and applies an anterior force, pulling the thigh upward or away from the table.

Results. In a normal thigh, the forces applied should not result in significant movement of the hip. In a dis-

located hip, however, excessive pistoning or telescoping motion will be seen as these forces are applied.

Galeazzi's Sign

Indication. Galeazzi's sign is used to assess unilateral hip dislocation in infants aged 3 to 18 months only.

Method. The infant lies supine with the hips flexed 90 degrees and the feet resting on the table.

Results. One knee sitting higher than the other when viewed from below indicates unilateral hip dislocation.

Joint Play (Accessory Movement)

Distraction and Caudal Glide (Fig. 9–57)

Restriction. General hypomobility; abduction.

Open-Packed Position. 30 degrees of flexion, 30 degrees of abduction, and slight external rotation.

Positioning. Subject lies supine with a stabilizing strap applied to the pelvis. If the subject has no history of knee pathology, the therapist stands at the bottom of the table facing the subject. A belt is wrapped around the pelvis of the therapist and placed in the web spaces of the therapist's hands. This allows the therapist to apply the distraction force with the body instead of the upper limbs. The therapist's hands are placed around the subject's leg at the ankle.

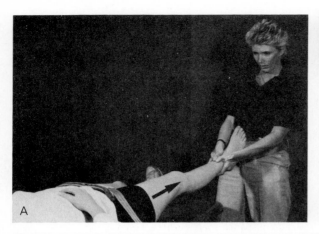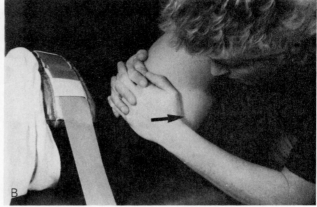

Figure 9–57. (*A*) Distraction and caudal glide of the hip joint. (*B*) Distraction/caudal glide in cases of knee pathology.

Movement. The therapist applies a distracton force by leaning backward, thereby creating a pull through the belt to the therapist's hands.

Posterior Glide (Fig. 9–58)

Restriction. Internal rotation; flexion.

Positioning. The subject lies supine with the ischial tuberosity of the treated limb at the edge of the table and the limb not being treated resting on the floor or footstool. A wedge is placed beneath the ischial tuberosity to provide additional support to the pelvis. The therapist stands between the subject's legs facing the hip being treated. The hip is maintained in the open-packed position by a strap suspended from the therapist's shoulder. The therapist's one hand is placed on the posterolateral aspect of the distal thigh to assist in support and

maintenance of position. The other hand is placed anteriorly on the proximal thigh.

Movement. The therapist applies a posteriorly directed force to the subject's anterior proximal thigh.

Anterior Glide (Fig. 9–59)

Restriction. External rotation; extension.

Positioning. The subject lies prone with the anterior pelvis at the edge of the table and the limb not being treated resting on the floor or footstool. A wedge is placed beneath the distal pelvis to provide additional support to the pelvis. The therapist stands between the subject's limbs facing the hip being treated. The hip is maintained in the open-packed position by a strap suspended from the therapist's shoulder. The therapist's one

Figure 9–58. Posterior glide of the femur.

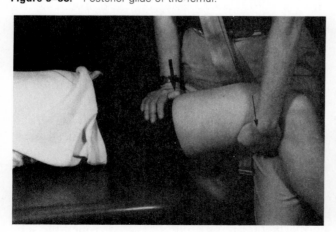

Figure 9–59. Anterior glide of the femur.

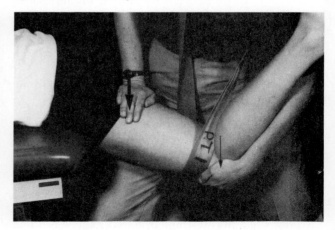

Table 9–1. Summary of Hip Joint Play

GLIDE	RESTRICTION	FIXED BONE	MOVING BONE
Distraction	General hypomobility	Acetabulum	Femur
Caudal	Abduction and flexion	Acetabulum	Femur
Dorsal	Internal rotation and flexion	Acetabulum	Femur
Ventral	External rotation	Acetabulum	Femur
Lateral	Adduction	Acetabulum	Femur

hand is placed on the anterolateral aspect of the distal thigh or lower leg to assist in support and maintenance of position. The therapist's other hand is placed posteriorly on the proximal thigh.

Movement. The therapist applies an anteriorly directed force to the subject's posterior proximal thigh.

Summary of Hip Joint Play

Table 9–1 provides a summary of joint play of the hip.

Bibliography

Backhouse KM, Hutchings RT: Color Atlas of Surface Anatomy. Baltimore, Williams & Wilkins, 1986

Corrigan B, Maitland GD: Practical Orthopedic Medicine. Boston, Butterworth & Co, 1983

Daniels L, Worthingham C: Muscle Testing Techniques of Manual Examination. Philadelphia, WB Saunders, 1986

Gould A III, and Davies G (eds): Orthopedic and Sports Physical Therapy. St Louis, CV Mosby, 1985

Hollinshead WH, Jenkins DB: Functional Anatomy of the Limbs and Back. Philadelphia, WB Saunders, 1981

Hoppenfeld S: Physical Examination of the Spine and Extremities. New York, Appleton-Century-Crofts, 1976

Kaltenborn M: Mobilization of the Extremity Joints. Oslo, Bygdoy Alle, 1980

Kendall FP, McCreary EK: Muscle Testing and Function. Baltimore, Williams & Wilkins, 1983

Kessler R, Hertling D: Management of Common Musculoskeletal Disorders. Philadelphia, Harper & Row, 1983

Kisner C, Colby LA: Therapeutic Foundations: Foundations and Techniques. Philadelphia, FA Davis, 1985

Magee J: Orthopedic Physical Assessment. Philadelphia, WB Saunders, 1987

Maitland GD: The Peripheral Joints: Examination and Recording Guide. Adelaide, Australia, Virgo Press, 1973

Norkin CC, White DJ: Measurement of Joint Motion: A Guide to Goniometry. Philadelphia, FA Davis, 1985

Saunders H: Evaluation, Treatment, and Prevention of Musculoskeletal Disorders. Minneapolis, H Duane Saunders, 1985

Williams P, Warwick R (eds): Gray's Anatomy, 36th British ed. Philadelphia, WB Saunders, 1980

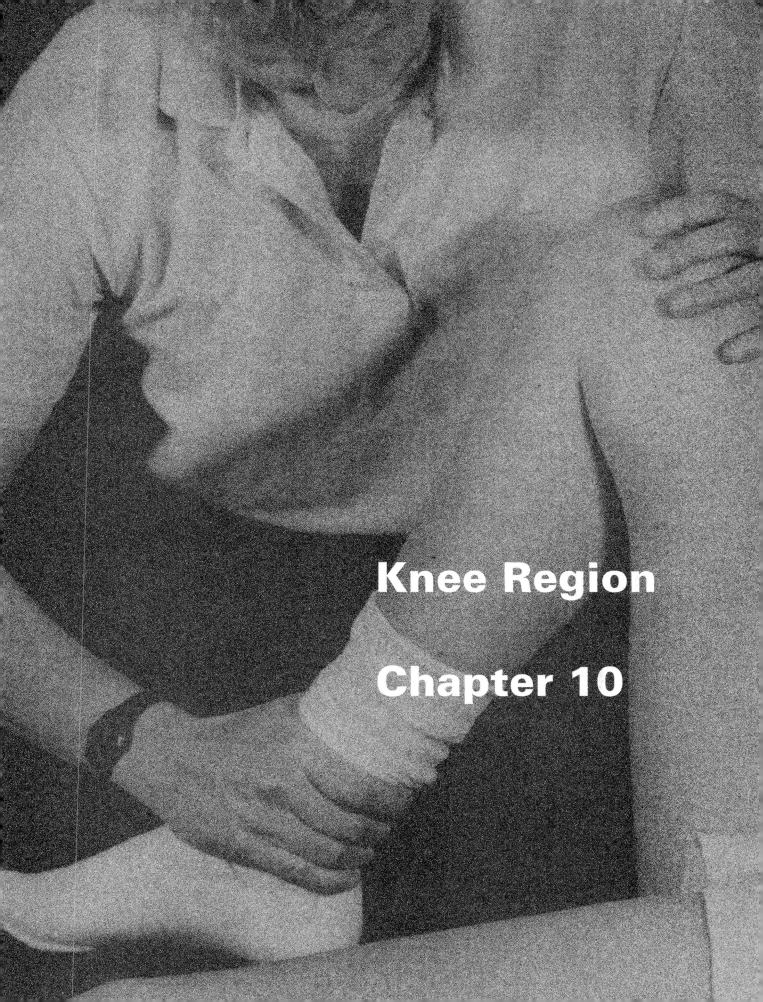

Knee Region

Chapter 10

The knee joint, like the elbow, allows shortening and lengthening of the limb. It is a large, complex, and unstable condyloid synovial joint formed by three bones, the distal femur, the proximal tibia, and the patella. There are two degrees of freedom of movement. Motions of flexion and extension occur in the sagittal plane, and axial rotation occurs in the transverse plane. The axis of motion in the coronal plane is located immediately above the joint surfaces through the femoral condyles.

The knee functions in a closed chain, in conjunction with the hip and ankle joints, for supporting the body weight during such activities as squatting, walking, and sitting. In an open kinematic chain, the knee provides mobility for the lower limb. Mobility is provided by bony structures, and stability is provided primarily by soft tissue structures, such as ligaments and muscles. The knee joint is most stable in the full extended position and least stable in flexion, when the soft tissue structures are slack and the articular surfaces are least congruent.

Goniometry

Knee Flexion

Knee joint motion occurs in the sagittal plane between the condyles of the femur and the tibia. As the tibial condyles flex on the femoral condyles, the tibia glides in a posterior direction. As knee flexion begins, the tibia rotates medially on the femur. If the tibia is fixed, as in ambulation, the femur rotates laterally to provide knee flexion.

Figure 10–1. End position for knee flexion measurement.

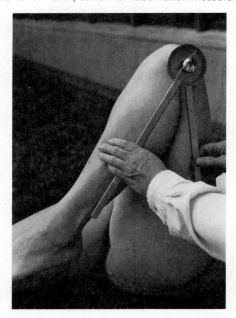

Motion. 0 to 120 to 130 degrees of flexion.

Position
- Preferred: Subject lies supine with the hip flexed 90 degrees (Fig. 10–1).
- Alternate: Subject is in sidelying position on the "non-test" side. The hip and knee flex simultaneously.

Goniometric Alignment

Axis. Placed over the lateral epicondyle of the femur.

Stationary Arm. Placed parallel to the lateral midline of the femur on a line from the lateral epicondyle to the greater trochanter.

Moving Arm. Placed parallel to the lateral midline of the fibula toward the lateral malleolus.

Stabilization. The thigh is stabilized.

Precautions
- Prevent hip joint rotation and extension, and further flexion.
- Note degree of hip flexion if not 90 degrees.
- Keep the hip joint flexed to prevent stretching of the rectus femoris muscle.

Knee Extension

The motion of knee joint extension, the return from knee joint flexion, occurs in the sagittal plane. As the knee extends, the tibial condyles glide on the femoral condyles anteriorly. At the end of the range of motion the tibia rotates laterally on the femoral condyles. If the tibia is fixed, the femur rotates medially on the tibial condyles.

Motion. 130 to 120 degrees to 0 degrees of extension.

Position *& towel roll under ankle*
- Preferred: Subject lies supine with the hip joint in extension (Fig. 10–2).
- Alternate:
  1. Subject is in sidelying position on the non-test side, with the hip joint in the anatomical position.
  2. Subject is prone, with the hip joint in the anatomical position (Fig. 10–3).

Goniometric Alignment

Axis. Placed over the lateral epicondyle of the femur.

Stationary Arm. Placed parallel to the lateral midline of the femur on a line from the lateral epicondyle to the greater trochanter.

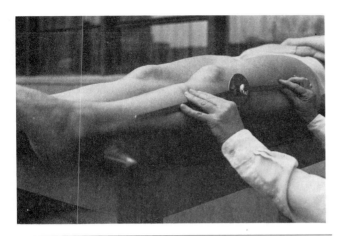

Figure 10–2. End position for knee extension measurement.

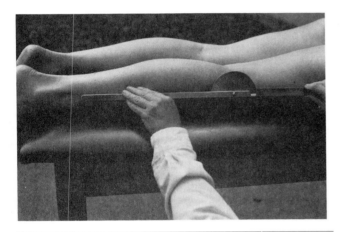

Figure 10–3. End position for knee extension measurement in the alternate prone position.

Moving Arm. Placed parallel to the lateral midline of the fibula toward the lateral malleolus.

Stabilization. The weight of the lower limb provides sufficient stabilization.

Precaution. Prevent hip joint rotation and flexion.

Functional Muscle Testing

Knee Flexion

The action of the hamstring muscles at the knee depends on the position of the hip. When they are stretched by hip flexion, their efficiency as knee flexors increases. The action of the knee flexor muscles is to decelerate the lower limb during the swing phase of gait. During this action, the knee flexors use an eccentric type of contraction. Functionally, the knee flexor muscles may contract concentrically when the subject is on hands and knees,

by pulling the buttocks back onto the heels. The flexor muscles are also rotators of the knee joint.

Position. Subject stands.

Activity. Subject walks backward or runs forward 20 feet.

Muscles. Hamstrings (biceps femoris, semitendinosus, and semimembranosus, popliteus, sartorius, and gracilis).

Types of Contraction
- Concentric: The knee flexes when the subject initiates the backward swing phase.
- Eccentric: The knee extends when the subject lowers the foot to the floor. In forward running, the muscles decelerate the lower limb.

Resistance
- The weight of the leg and foot offer the resistance.
- Functional: 20 feet.
- Functionally Fair: 10 to 19 feet.
- Functionally Poor: 1 to 9 feet.
- Nonfunctional: 0 feet.

Knee Extension

The quadriceps femoris muscles cross anterior to the axis of the knee joint and are powerful extensors. The knee extensor muscles perform eccentric as well as concentric contraction for many activities of daily living. They are considered postural, or type I, muscles. They perform eccentrically many of the same functions as the hip extensor muscles, such as sitting down in a chair and descending stairs or ramps. Concentrically, they function in ascending stairs, and rising from a sitting position and during both the stance and swing phases of gait.

Position. Subject stands.

Activity
- Subject squats 20 to 30 degrees and returns to standing. Both right and left knees are tested simultaneously.
- Subject, with knees flexed, jumps, lifting the body off the floor.

Muscles. Quadriceps (rectus femoris, vastus lateralis, medialis, and intermedius)

Types of Contraction
- Eccentric: The knees flex when squatting.
- Concentric: The knees extend when standing up and during a low jump.

Resistance
- Body weight offers the resistance.
- Functional: 5 repetitions.
- Functionally Fair: 3 to 4 repetitions.
- Functionally Poor: 1 to 2 repetitions.
- Nonfunctional: 0 repetitions.

Manual Muscle Testing

Quadriceps Femoris Muscles: Rectus Femoris, Vastus Intermedius, Medialis, and Lateralis

The quadriceps femoris muscles produce the motion of knee joint extension from a starting position of 90 degrees of flexion. In the break test method of evaluating knee joint extension, the knee is unlocked to approximately 10 degrees short of full extension.

Palpation
- Palpate the rectus femoris in the V-shaped area between the sartorius and tensor fasciae latae muscles (Fig. 10–4). The vastus intermedius lies deep to the rectus femoris and is difficult to palpate with accuracy. Lift the rectus femoris muscle and palpate beneath it from the medial or lateral side.

Figure 10–4. Palpating the rectus femoris muscle.

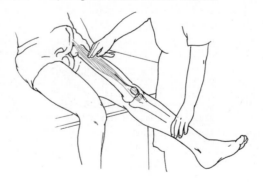

Figure 10–5. Palpating the vastus medialis muscle.

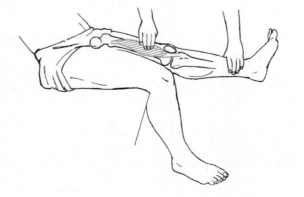

- Palpate the vastus medialis along the medial thigh. The bulky portion is proximal to the patella (Fig. 10–5).
- Palpate the vastus lateralis along the lateral thigh (Fig. 10–6).

Position
- AG: Subject is semi-sitting with the hip flexed 45 degrees and the knee flexed 90 degrees over the edge of the table with support under the knee (Fig. 10–7).
- GM: Subject is in sidelying position with the test leg supported on friction-free surface. The hip is flexed 45 degrees and the knee 90 degrees (Fig. 10–8).

Movement. Extend the knee joint to 0 degrees, or complete extension.

Resistance. Applied to the anterior surface, proximal to the ankle joint.

Stabilization. The thigh is stabilized.

Substitutions
- In the GM position, the subject may extend the hip, causing passive extension of the knee joint.
- The subject may quickly flex the knee, then relax.
- The articularis genu is an accessory muscle for knee extension and acts to pull the joint capsule superiorly during the motion, to prevent the capsule from becoming trapped in the joint.

Hamstring Muscles (Biceps Femoris, Semimembranosus, Semitendinosus)

The hamstring muscles produce the motion of knee flexion from a starting position of 10 degrees of knee flexion, which unlocks the knee joint. The test range is approximately 90 degrees, and the hip may or may not be flexed

Figure 10–6. Palpating the vastus lateralis muscle.

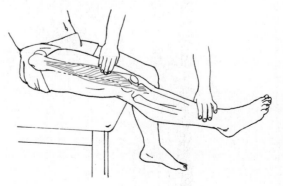

Attachments of Quadriceps Femoris Muscles

Muscle	Proximal	Distal	Innervation
Rectus femoris	Anterior inferior iliac spine (AIIS); superior rim of acetabulum	Tibial tuberosity through patellar ligament	Femoral L3 and L4 (L2)
Vastus intermedius	Anterior and lateral proximal two thirds of femoral shaft, distal half of linea aspera	Tibial tuberosity through patellar ligament	Femoral L3 and L4 (L2)
Vastus medialis	Distal intertrochanteric line, medial lip of linea aspera, proximal supracondylar line, and tendon of adductor longus and magnus muscles	Tibial tuberosity through patellar ligament	Femoral L3 and L4 (L2)
Vastus lateralis	Proximal aspect of intertrochanteric line, inferior greater trochanter, and proximal half of lateral lip of linea aspera of femur	Tibial tuberosity through patellar ligament	Femoral L3 and L4 (L2)

on a pillow or over the edge of the table. Hip flexion is necessary if the rectus femoris muscle shows tightness. If one of the hamstring muscles is weak, the tibia will rotate toward the strong side.

Palpation
- Palpate the biceps femoris along the lateral posterior thigh; the tendon lies immediately proximal to the back of the knee (Fig. 10–9).
- Palpate the semimembranosus immediately proximal to the knee posteriorly on either side of the semitendinosus tendon (Fig. 10–10). This muscle is best palpated during the initial 45 degrees of knee flexion.

- Palpate the semitendinosus tendon immediately proximal to the knee joint posteriorly on the medial side (Fig. 10–11).

Position
- AG: Subject lies prone with the hip flexed and in neutral rotation and the knee flexed 10 degrees (Fig. 10–12).

Alternate:
- GM: Subject is in sidelying position with the test leg on a friction-free surface. The hip is slightly flexed, and the knee is flexed 10 degrees (Fig. 10–13).

Figure 10–7. Testing the quadriceps femoris muscles in the AG position.

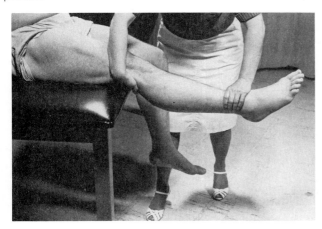

Figure 10–8. Testing the quadriceps femoris muscles in the GM position.

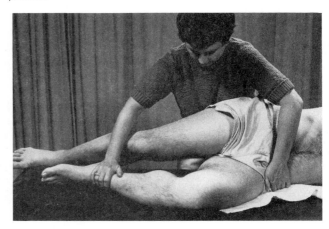

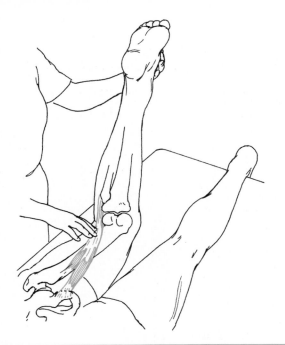

Figure 10–9. Palpating the biceps femoris muscle.

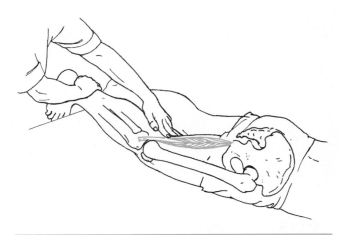

Figure 10–10. Palpating the semimembranosus muscle.

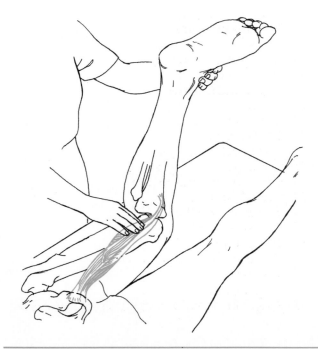

Figure 10–11. Palpating the semitendinosus muscle.

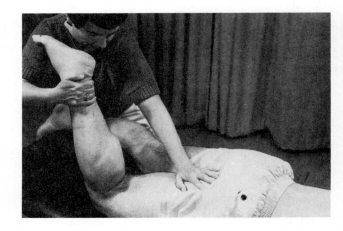

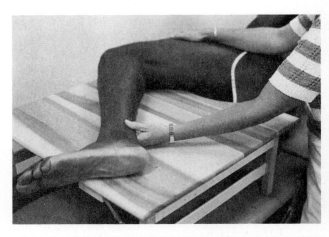

Figure 10–13. Testing the hamstring muscles in the GM position.

Attachments of Hamstring Muscles

Muscle	Proximal	Distal	Innervation
Biceps femoris, long head	Ischial tuberosity and sacrotuberous ligament	Head of fibula and lateral tibial condyle	Tibial portion of sciatic nerve S1 (L5 and S2)
Biceps femoris, short head	Lateral lip of linea aspera, proximal supracondylar line of the femur		Peroneal portion of sciatic nerve S1 (L5 and S2)
Semimembranosus	Ischial tuberosity	Posteromedial aspect of medial tibial condyle	Tibial portion of sciatic nerve L5 and S1 (S2)
Semitendinosus	Ischial tuberosity	Proximal medial tibial shaft	Tibial portion of sciatic nerve L5 and S1 (S2)

Movement. Flex the knee joint to 90 degrees.

Resistance. Applied posteriorly, proximal to the ankle joint with the tibia in lateral rotation for the biceps femoris and in medial rotation for the semimembranosus and the semitendinosus muscles.

Stabilization. The thigh is stabilized. If weakness exists, the subject will increase flexion of the hip.

Substitutions

- The gastrocnemius is an accessory knee flexor. To mimimize its action, do not allow the ankle to plantar-flex.
- The gracilis is an accessory knee flexor; therefore do not allow the hip to adduct.
- The sartorius is an accessory knee flexor; therefore prevent the hip from flexing and abducting.
- The plantaris is an accessory muscle to knee flexion; therefore do not allow the ankle to plantar-flex.
- In the GM position, the subject may flex the hip, causing passive flexion of the knee.

Clinical Tests

Palpation

Examintion of the knee joint requires that the therapist be familiar with the location of various structures and landmarks. Among the structures to be observed or palpated are:

1. Medial tibial plateau.
2. Tibial tuberosity.
3. Medial femoral condyle.
4. Adductor tubercle.
5. Lateral tibial plateau.
6. Lateral femoral condyle.
7. Head of the fibula.
8. Patella.
9. Quadriceps tendon.
10. Prepatellar bursae.
11. Suprapatellar bursae.
12. Infrapatellar bursae.
13. Pes anserine bursae.
14. Medial meniscus.
15. Medial collateral ligament.
16. Semitendinosus tendon.
17. Semimembranosus tendon.
18. Lateral meniscus.
19. Lateral collateral ligament.
20. Biceps femoris tendon.
21. Iliotibial band.
22. Common peroneal nerve.
23. Popliteal fossa.
24. Popliteal artery.
25. Origin of the heads of the gastrocnemius muscle.

Active and Passive Movements and Contractile Testing

The active and passive movements that need to be assessed during examination of the knee and contractile testing include:

1. Flexion.
2. Extension.
3. External tibial rotation.
4. Internal tibial rotation.

Special Tests

Patellofemoral Tests

Q Angle

Indication.   The **Q** angle test should be performed in all evaluations of knee pathology, especially in cases of patellofemoral pathomechanics and dysfunction. The **Q** angle is also extremely important in the biomechanical examination of the lower limb for determining postural malalignment syndromes.

Method.   The **Q** angle is a static measurement of the angle that the patellar tendon makes with the rectus femoris. It provides an indication of the lateral vector force applied to the patella.

The subject lies supine with the lower limb relaxed and in the anatomical position. Positioning is important as it has been demonstrated that various positions of the hip and foot may alter the **Q** angle. The examiner places the axis of the goniometer over the midpoint of the patella with the proximal arm positioned over the thigh, citing the anterior superior iliac spine (ASIS) (Fig. 10–14). The distal arm lies over the tibial tubercle. The **Q** angle may be measured with the subject in the long sitting position if the subject cannot lie supine.

Results.   Normally, the **Q** angle in males should range from 10 to 15 degrees and in females from 10 to 19 degrees. Typically, women's **Q** angles fall toward the higher end of the range, while those of men fall toward the lower end. Angles found to be lower than the norms may be related to chondromalacia patellae and patella alta, while angles greater than the norms are associated with patellofemoral dysfunction, increased femoral anteversion, genu valgum, or increased external tibial torsion. If assessed in the sitting position, the **Q** angle should measure 0 degrees.

Patellofemoral Grinding Test (Clarke's Sign)

Indication.   The patellofemoral grinding test should be performed in suspected cases of patellofemoral dysfunction and is designed to determine the integrity of the posterior patella and the trochlear groove of the femur.

Method.   The subject lies supine with the knee extended and the lower limb in a relaxed posture. The examiner places the web space of the hand around the superior pole of the patella (Fig. 10–15). The patient is then asked to do a "quad set" (isometric quadriceps contraction) while the examiner resists the tendency of the patella to glide superiorly. It is important that the

---

Figure 10–14.   (*A*) Measurement of Q angle. (*B*) Q angle is the difference in measurement between the anatomical and mechanical axes of the knee.

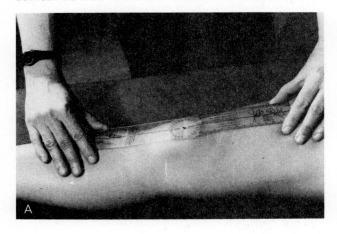

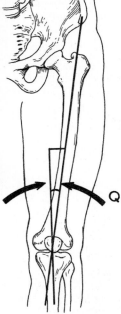

A

B

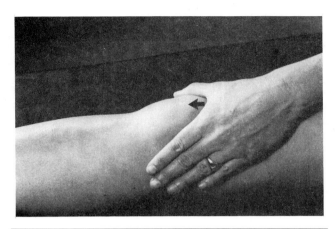

Figure 10–15.   Patellofemoral grinding test.

examiner not exert a straight posterior force on the patella, which would press the patella against the femur, causing pain.

Results.   A negative result is one in which the subject is able to sustain the contraction without pain while the examiner is applying force. A positive result is manifested in retropatellar pain and the subject's inability to maintain the contraction. Because normal subjects experience pain if the examiner's force is too great, this test should be repeated a few times and compared to responses elicited in the uninvolved knee.

Waldron's Test

Indication.   Waldron's test helps diagnose chondromalacia patellae.

Method.   The subject begins this test in the standing position. While the examiner palpates the patella, the subject is instructed to do several deep knee bends or squats in a slow, controlled manner.

Results.   The examiner should be palpating the patella, noting where in the range pain is felt and crepitus is detected. In order for this test to be positive for chondromalacia, the pain and crepitus must occur simultaneously. Patellar tracking should also be observed during this procedure.

Patellar Apprehension Test

Indication.   The patellar apprehension test is used to assess patellofemoral subluxation or dislocation.

Method.   The subject lies supine with the knee in a slightly flexed posture of approximately 30 degrees. With the knee relaxed, the examiner places the thumbs along the medial patellar border and applies a laterally directed force (Fig. 10–16*A*).

Results.   If the subject feels as though the knee is beginning to dislocate, the quadriceps will suddenly contract to pull the patella back in line, and the subject will look apprehensive (Fig. 10–16*B*). These findings constitute a positive result.

McConnell's Test

Indication.   McConnell's test may be performed where patellofemoral pain is suspected.

Method.   The subject is asked to perform an activity that creates patellofemoral compressive forces, thereby reproducing pain. This activity may be a quadriceps contraction while the knee is in a flexed position, ascending and descending stairs, or squatting. Once the pain is reproduced, the examiner gently glides the patella medially while the subject performs the activity.

Figure 10–16.   (*A*) Patellar apprehension test. (*B*) Positive test is indicated by a look of apprehension on the subject's face.

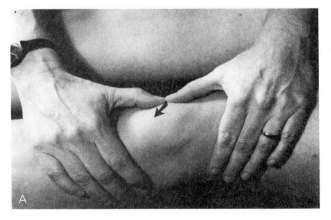
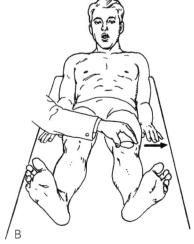

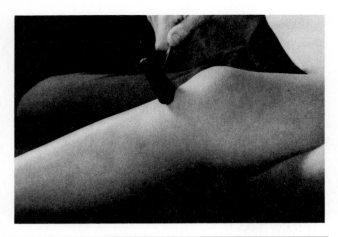

Figure 10–17. Patellar tendon reflex.

Results. A positive test result for patellofemoral pain is diminished pain response when the patella has been glided medially. One must be aware that a positive result yields no information regarding the specific source or etiology of the pain; it tells only that patellofemoral pathology is present.

Patellar Tendon Reflex

Indication. The patellar tendon reflex is assessed in order to determine the integrity of the neurologic function of the L4 level.

Method. The subject may be either supine or seated for this test. In either case, the knee should be in a position of flexion and the quadriceps muscle relaxed. The examiner taps the patellar tendon with the broad side of the reflex hammer and observes the response (Fig. 10–17).

Results. The normal response should be one of a jerking into knee extension. As in other reflex tests, one should compare the reaction of the uninvolved side. A diminished or heightened response indicates similar findings, as noted in previous reflex tests.

Wilson's Test

Indication. Wilson's test is performed in suspected cases of osteochondritis dissecans.

Method. The subject sits, with the knee to be examined flexed over the edge of the table. The subject is asked to rotate the tibia inward and to maintain that rotation while actively extending the knee. The subject is instructed to stop extending the knee at approximately 30 degrees from full extension, where the pain noticeably increases. The subject is then asked to rotate the tibia outward, and the examiner observes for fluctuation of pain.

Results. If, during the outward tibial rotation, the subject's pain disappears, the test for osteochondritis dissecans is positive. The pain experienced during this test must be located in the medial femoral condyle. Pain felt in any other area of the knee during the course of this examination is not representative of osteochondritis dissecans.

Tests for Effusion of the Knee

Patellar Ballotment Test (Patellar Tap Test)

Indication. The patellar ballotment test may be used with persons whose presenting symptom is gross effusion of the knee.

Method. The subject is supine with the knee in extension or as close to extension as the subject can comfortably tolerate. The examiner gently pushes the patella in a posterior direction and then releases it (Fig. 10–18).

Results. When the examiner releases the patella of a patient with significant effusion, it will spring back or rebound anteriorly. This rebound effect is due to the dispersion of the fluid from between the patella and the femur when the examiner pushes posteriorly, followed by a rapid flush of fluid back beneath when the patella is released.

Fluctuation Test

Indication. The fluctuation test is indicated for persons with subtle, minimal effusion.

Method. The subject is positioned as for the patellar ballottment test. The examiner milks the fluid caudally from the suprapatellar pouch, simultaneously pushing it from the medial side of the knee to the lateral side (Fig.

Figure 10–18. Patellar ballotment test.

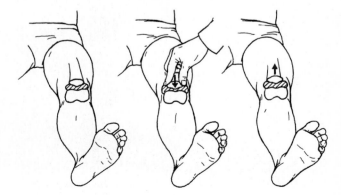

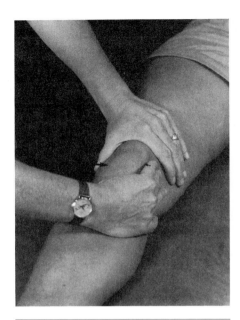

Figure 10–19. Fluctuation test.

10–19). One or two fingers are placed without pressure along the lateral aspect of the knee to be examined.

Results. As the fluid is milked first inferiorly and then laterally, the examiner feels a slight bulging or an increase in pressure laterally, secondary to flushing of the fluid to the lateral side.

Tests for Plica

Hughston's Plica Test

Indication. Plica testing is performed when symptoms suggest involvement of the synovial plica. Plica testing should also be done to differentiate between plica pathology and questionable meniscal lesions.

Method. The subject lies supine. The examiner's one hand flexes the knee and medially rotates the leg, and the heel of the other hand is placed along the lateral aspect of the patella (Fig. 10–20). The examiner then pushes the patella medially while simultaneously palpating the medial femoral condyle with the fingers. The knee is then passively flexed and extended while the examiner palpates the plica.

Results. Palpable "popping" of the plica under the examiner's fingers while the testing maneuver is being performed indicates pathology.

Mediopatellar Plica Test

Indication. The indication is suspected inflammation of the synovial plica.

Method. The subject lies supine. The examiner passively flexes the knee to approximately 30 degrees and attempts to move the patella in a medial direction, noting any pain response (Fig. 10–21).

Results. Pain indicates that the edge of the mediopatellar plica is becoming pinched between the medial femoral condyle and the patella.

"Stutter" Test

Indication. The "stutter" test is indicated when plica involvement is suspected and the subject shows no evidence of joint effusion.

Method. The subject is seated with both knees flexed over the edge of the table to 90 degrees. The examiner instructs the subject to extend one knee slowly as the examiner palpates the patella during the movement.

Results. Pathology is present if the patella jumps, or "stutters," at some point in the range between 60 and

Figure 10–20. Hughston's plica test.

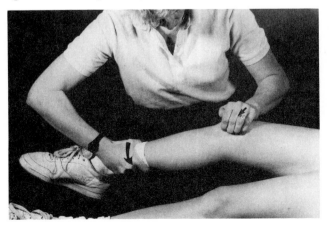

Figure 10–21. Mediopatellar plica test.

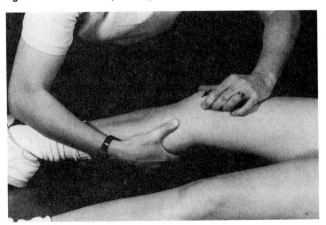

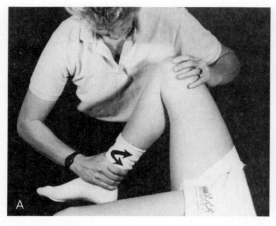
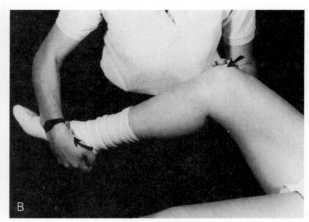
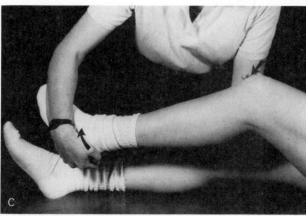

Figure 10–22. (*A*) McMurray's test. (*B*) Lateral tibial rotation combined with a valgus force to the knee during knee extension assesses the medial meniscus. (*C*) Medial tibial rotation combined with a varus force to the knee during knee extension assesses the lateral meniscus.

45 degrees from full extension, interrupting what would normally be smooth, fluid motion.

Meniscal Tests

All procedures described in the following six tests are indicated when a subject's history or mechanism of injury leads the examiner to suspect damage to the medial or lateral meniscus. These tests, although clinically diagnostic of meniscal tears, many times are not definitive. Therefore arthrography or arthroscopic examination is necessary for definitive diagnosis.

McMurray's Test

Method. The subject relaxes supine, and the examiner places the knee being examined into as much flexion as the subject's range of motion will allow (Fig. 10–22*A*). In examining the right knee, the examiner grasps the patient's right heel with the right hand while the left hand controls the joint. The left hand is positioned so that the thumb and index finger firmly grip either side of the joint posterior to the lateral and medial ligaments.

The heel is then rotated, causing relative internal and external tibial rotation.

This test has many variations, including the addition of an abduction-adduction force and gradual extension of the knee, which may be combined or imposed separately. Lateral tibial rotation with an abduction or valgus force is associated with testing the medial meniscus, while internal rotation with an adduction or varus force stresses the lateral meniscus (Fig. 10–22*B* and *C*).

Results. The examiner may palpate and listen over the meniscus for evidence of clicking or snapping, often accompanied by pain, which indicates pathology. It is important for the examiner to realize that structures other than menisci may produce the clicking or snapping, so the test result may be false positive.

Apley's Grinding Test

Method. The subject lies prone with the knee joint flexed to 90 degrees (Fig. 10–23). The examiner stabilizes the posterior distal thigh with one hand while the other hand grasps the plantar surface of the calcaneus.

The examiner transmits a compressive force through the calcaneus and the leg to the knee while simultaneously rotating the leg laterally and medially.

Results. Pain reproduced with compression and lateral tibial rotation may indicate a positive finding for a lateral meniscal tear, while pain associated with compression and medial rotation may indicate medial meniscal pathology. Pain evident on tibial distraction and rotation has been associated with ligament injury.

O'Donoghue's Test

Method. The examiner flexes the supine subject's knee to 90 degrees and then rotates the leg inward and outward a few times. The examiner then fully flexes the subject's knee and again rotates it in both directions.

Results. Increased pain on rotation with the knee fully flexed as compared with 90-degree flexion indicates a meniscal tear or capsule irritation.

Screw Home Mechanism (Helfet's Test)

Indication. The screw home mechanism provides information on the normal biomechanical lateral rotation of the tibia on the femur during extension in an open kinematic chain. Absence of this normal rotation may be associated with a torn meniscus or patellofemoral dysfunction.

Method. The subject sits with the knees flexed approximately 90 degrees over the edge of the table. A skin pencil is used to mark the midpoint of the patella and the tibial tuberosity. In this sitting position, the two markings should align vertically. The subject then slowly

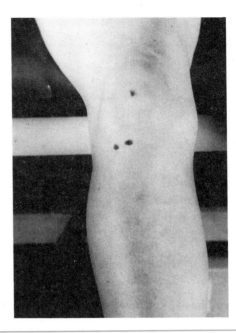

Figure 10–24. Screw home mechanism: In the position of knee extension, the second mark on the tibial tubercle should lie lateral to the initial mark made with the knee in flexion.

extends the knee, and at full extension, the landmarks are palpated and marked again (Fig. 10–24). The relationship between the first set of markings and the second set is examined.

Results. During normal biomechanical extension of the knee, the leg moves from a relatively neutral position to one of external rotation. Therefore, the second mark on the tibial tuberosity should lie lateral to the first mark on the tibia. If this is not the finding, normal lateral tibial rotation during extension is decreased or absent. This abnormal biomechanical situation may be related to the torn meniscus or to patellofemoral pathology.

Bounce Home Test

Indication. The bounce home test is used to determine whether a structure (the meniscus) may be preventing complete extension of the joint.

Method. The subject is supine as the examiner cups the heel of the foot with the hand. The examiner then maximally flexes the subject's knee and from that position allows passive motion into extension.

Results. Normally, the knees move smoothly into full extension. In a knee with a meniscal tear, extension is either not complete or has a springy end feel, which is classically associated with meniscal tears.

Figure 10–23. Apley's grinding test: Compression force through the leg combined with medial tibial rotation assesses the medial meniscus; lateral tibial rotation during compression tests the lateral meniscus.

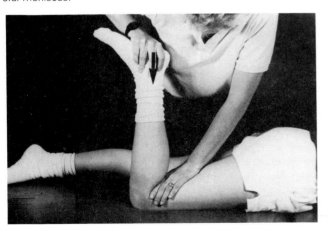

Test for Retracting Meniscus

Indication.   This test is indicated in suspected cases of a retracting meniscus.

Method.   The subject lies supine as the examiner flexes the knee 90 degrees. The examiner palpates the area of the tibial plateau corresponding to the anatomical location of the medial meniscus. The subject's leg is then rotated laterally and medially while the examiner carefully palpates for the meniscus.

Results.   In a normal biomechanical situation, the medial meniscus should be impalpable during lateral tibial rotation and should reappear during medial rotation. A torn medial meniscus will not be felt to disappear during lateral rotation.

Ligamentous Testing

Ligamentous testing of the knee is an integral part of the total joint assessment. For ease in organization, the examination of the ligamentous structures may be divided into the following classifications: straight-plane medial, lateral, anterior, and posterior instability; and anteromedial, anterolateral, posterolateral, and posteromedial rotatory instability.

Tests for Straight-Plane Instability

Apley's Distraction Test

Indication.   Apley's test is indicated in suspected cases of medial or lateral collateral ligament injury.

Method.   The subject lies prone with the knee flexed 90 degrees. The examiner stabilizes the femur by placing the leg on the distal posterior surface of the thigh. The examiner grasps the distal portion of the leg with both hands, using the malleoli as prominences to which leverage may be applied. The leg is distracted and simultaneously moved into lateral and medial tibial rotation (Fig. 10–25).

Results.   Pain on the medial aspect of the knee joint during distraction and lateral tibial rotation may indicate a lesion of the medial collateral ligament. Lateral knee pain experienced during distraction and internal tibial rotation may represent a lateral collateral ligament injury.

Valgus (Abduction) Stress Test

Indication.   The valgus and abduction stress test is used to assess the integrity of the structures responsible for medial stability of the joint.

Method.   The subject lies supine with the limb in a relaxed position. This test should be performed in both full extension and in an unlocked position of about 20 to 30 degrees of flexion to allow testing of both the primary and secondary restraints. In the position of flexion, the posterior capsule is relaxed, thereby allowing for isolated testing of the medial collateral ligament.

The examiner places one hand along the lateral side of the knee joint and the other medially on the subject's leg (Fig. 10–26). Using the lateral hand as a fulcrum, the examiner applies a valgus force to the knee by pulling the leg from the midline of the body.

Results.   Medial gapping and/or pain during the procedure is evidence of dysfunction. A positive result with the knee in the unlocked flexed position could mean dysfunction of the medial collateral ligament, the middle third of the medial capsule, the posterior cruciate ligament, or the posterior oblique ligament.

Gapping or pain noted when testing the knee in full extension represents more extensive joint damage in

Figure 10–25.   Apley's distraction test.

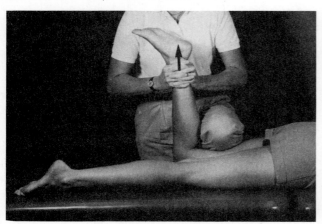

Figure 10–26.   Valgus stress test of the knee.

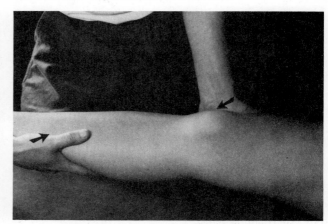

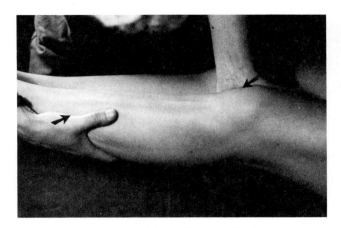

Figure 10–27. Varus stress test of the knee.

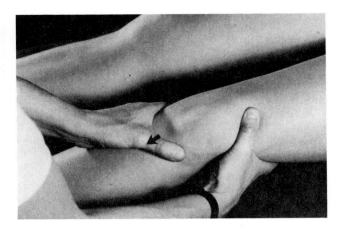

Figure 10–28. Lachman's test.

terms of stability. Structures that may be damaged in association with this instability may include superficial and deep fibers of the medial collateral ligament, the posteromedial capsule, the posterior oblique ligament, the anterior and posterior cruciate ligaments, the semimembranosus muscle, and the medial quadriceps expansion.

Varus (Adduction) Stress Test

Indication. The varus stress test is indicated in persons who may have sustained damage to the lateral stabilizing structures of the knee.

Method. The subject is relaxed and supine. The examiner places one hand along the medial aspect of the joint and the other on the lateral side of the leg (Fig. 10–27). With the hand on the knee acting as a fulcrum, the examiner imparts a varus force on the joint by pulling the leg into adduction.

This test is performed with the knee in extension as well as in an unlocked position of 20 to 30 degrees. As in the valgus stress test, laxity in the completely extended position represents a more serious injury.

Results. Gapping or pain while the test is performed in the unlocked position indicates possible injury to the lateral collateral ligament, the middle third of the lateral capsule, the posterolateral capsule, the arcuate complex (lateral collateral ligament, short lateral ligament, arcuate ligament, tendinous aponeurotic expansion of the popliteus muscle), the iliotibial band, and the biceps femoris tendon.

Lachman's Test

Indication. Lachman's test is the most reliable clinical assessment of anterior cruciate insufficiency, especially of the posterolateral band.

Method. The subject lies supine with the limb in slight external rotation and the knee in approximately 15 degrees of flexion (Fig. 10–28). This position allows the posterior meniscal horns to clear the femoral condyles, thereby obviating a false-negative finding for anterior cruciate ligament tear. The examiner stabilizes the distal thigh with one hand while creating an anterior "drawer" force on the proximal tibia with the other.

Results. The lack of firm end feel while drawing the tibia forward or more draw on the test leg than on the normal limb represents a positive test for anterior cruciate ligament insufficiency. The following structures may be involved: the anterior cruciate ligament, the arcuate complex, or the posterior oblique ligament.

Dynamic Extension Test

Indication. The dynamic extension test may also be used to evaluate a knee with anterior cruciate ligament insufficiency. It is a variation of Lachman's test, performed dynamically with a quadriceps contraction.

Method. The subject lies supine, with the knee extended and the examiner's closed fist under the distal thigh (Fig. 10–29A). The subject raises the leg from the table as the examiner observes the tibial movement (Fig. 10–29B); the subject then lowers the leg back onto the examiner's fist, and again tibial motion is noted.

Results. If the anterior cruciate ligament is deficient, as the subject extends the knee the tibia moves anteriorly onto the femur. When the leg is then lowered and relaxed on the closed fist, the tibia falls backward onto the femur into its resting position. This test may prove beneficial on the acutely injured knee where more intricate assessment methods are difficult, if not impossible, to carry out.

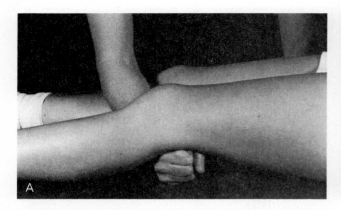
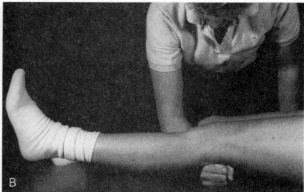

Figure 10–29. Dynamic extension test: (A) The closed fist of the examiner is positioned under the distal femur of the subject, whose knee is extended. (B) Closed fist of examiner under distal femur while subject extends knee.

Anterior Drawer Test

Indication. Suspicion of anterior cruciate ligament laxity or rupture is an indication for the anterior drawer examination. It is important to realize that this test may yield a false-negative result.

Method. The subject lies supine with the knee flexed to 90 degrees. The examiner stabilizes the foot on the table in neutral rotation by sitting on it (Fig. 10–30). The examiner grasps the proximal tibia, ensuring relaxation of the hamstrings, and attempts to pull the tibia anteriorly on the femur. Simultaneous palpation of the anterior joint line with the thumbs allows the examiner to feel the forward translation of the tibia accurately.

Results. Approximately 6 mm anterior translation of the tibia on the femur is normal. A positive straight drawer test is one in which there is excessive, equal forward displacement of both tibial condyles on the femoral condyles. The examiner must be sure that the posterior cruciate ligament is not lax or torn, as such a condition may result in a false-positive anterior drawer test (see Drop Back Sign, below).

Excessive anterior displacement of the tibia may represent involvement of any of the following structures: the anterior cruciate ligament (notably the anteromedial band), the posterolateral or posteromedial capsule, the deep fibers of the medial collateral ligament, the posterior oblique ligament, the iliotibial band, and the arcuate complex.

Anterior Drawer in External Rotation

Method. The subject is positioned as in the anterior drawer test, but the foot and leg are stabilized in external rotation. This externally rotated position causes tightening of the medial structures. The examiner imposes an anterior "drawing" force on the tibia.

Results. If any laxity of the medial compartment structures exists—most notably in the medial collateral ligament—the medial tibial condyle displaces farther forward than the lateral condyle of the tibia (Fig. 10–31).

Figure 10–30. Anterior drawer test.

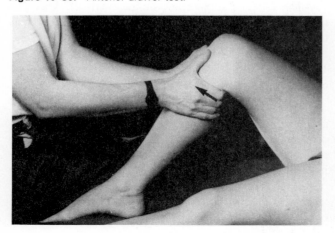

Figure 10–31. Anterior drawer in external rotation.

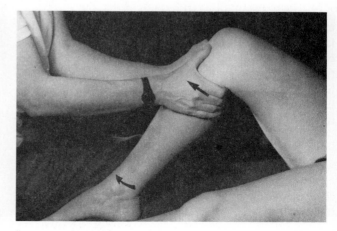

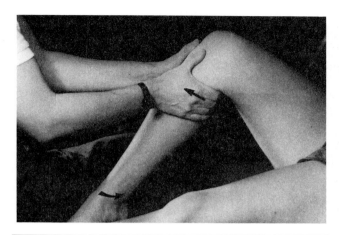

Figure 10–32. Anterior drawer in internal rotation.

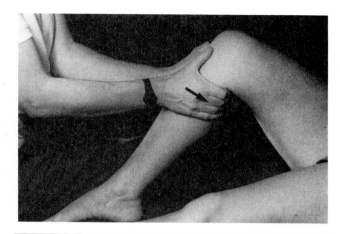

Figure 10–33. Posterior drawer sign.

This movement is associated with external tibial rotation, all of which is found to be present with anteromedial rotatory instability.

Anterior Drawer in Internal Rotation

Method. The subject is positioned as for the straight anterior drawer, except that the foot and tibia are placed in internal rotation. This position tightens the lateral collateral ligament and other lateral compartment structures.

Results. If, during this drawer test, the lateral tibial condyle displaces anteriorly and medially with respect to the medial tibial condyle and the femoral condyles, anterior cruciate and lateral compartment laxity are evident (Fig. 10–32). The combined anterior motion and internal tibial rotation is typical of anterolateral rotatory instability.

Posterior Drawer Test

Indication. The posterior drawer examination technique should be performed in cases of suspected posterior cruciate ligament tear.

Method. The subject lies supine, with the knee being examined flexed to 90 degrees and the foot resting on the examining table (Fig. 10–33). The examiner sits on the foot to stabilize it, grasps the proximal tibia, and pushes the tibia posteriorly on the femur.

Results. Excessive posterior translation of the tibia backward on the femur represents a positive result. Any of the following structures may be damaged and associated with a positive finding: the posterior cruciate or posterior oblique ligament, the arcuate complex, or the anterior cruciate ligament.

Drop Back Sign (Posterior "Sag" Sign)

Indication. The drop back sign should be assessed in all cases of suspected anterior or posterior cruciate ligament laxity or rupture.

Method. The subject is placed in the drawer test position of 90 degrees of knee flexion with the foot resting on the table. In this position, the relationship of the tibia to the femur is examined.

Results. If the posterior cruciate ligament is intact, a normal biomechanical relationship will exist between the tibia and femur. With ligament laxity or a tear, gravity in this testing posture will cause the tibia to "drop back" and come to lie farther posterior than normal with respect to the femur (Fig. 10–34).

In the patient with a "drop back" sign, accuracy of the assessment of the anterior cruciate ligament becomes important. The examiner must first restore the normal femoral and tibial alignment before performing the anterior drawer test. If the normal relationship is not established prior to assessment of the anterior cruciate ligament, it will result in a false-positive result for the anterior drawer.

Figure 10–34. Drop back sign.

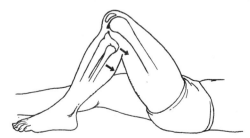

Anteromedial Rotatory Instability Test

Slocum's Test

Indication. Slocum's test may be performed to diagnose anteromedial rotatory instability.

Method. The subject is positioned supine, with the knee flexed about 85 degrees and the foot resting on the table with the leg in 15 degrees of lateral rotation. The external tibial rotation causes increased tension in the intact posteromedial structures and thereby diminishes anterior tibial displacement, even with a lax anterior cruciate ligament. The examiner grips the proximal tibia and attempts to draw it forward.

An alternate testing position is sitting with the knees flexed over the table edge. Again the leg is rotated laterally 15 degrees and an anterior drawing force is applied to the proximal tibia.

Results. Anterior motion of the tibia, primarily on the medial side, indicates anteromedial rotatory instability.

Structures that may be implicated with this type of instability include the medial collateral ligament (especially the superficial fibers), the posteromedial capsule, the posterior oblique ligament, and the anterior cruciate ligament.

Anterolateral Rotatory Instability Tests

Slocum's Test

Indication. Slocum's test is indicated when assessing anterolateral rotatory instability of the knee.

Method. The subject may be either supine or seated, with the knee flexed 80 to 90 degrees. The leg, with the foot resting on the table, is placed in 30 degrees of medial rotation, and the examiner imposes an anterior force on the proximal tibia.

Results. When the lateral aspect of the tibia displaces farther anteriorly than the uninvolved side of the knee, anterolateral rotatory instability is indicated.

The following structures may be involved with this type of instability: the anterior or posterior cruciate ligament, the lateral collateral ligament, the posterolateral capsule, the arcuate complex, and the iliotibial band.

Losee's Test

Indication. Losee's test is indicated in suspected anterolateral rotatory instability.

Method. The subject lies supine. The examiner laterally rotates the leg by grasping the foot and ankle (Fig. 10–35). This tibial rotation reduces the subluxation of

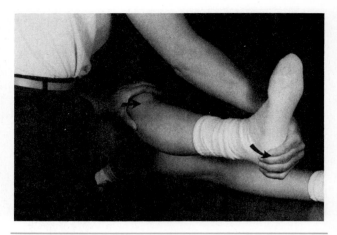

Figure 10–35. Losee's test: The examiner applies a valgus force to the knee while extending the joint and applies anterior force to the head of the fibula.

the knee. Stabilizing the leg against the trunk, the examiner flexes the subject's knee to 30 degrees, to relax the hamstring muscle. The examiner places the other hand anterolaterally on the knee so that the fingers lie over the patella, and the thumb wraps around the fibular head. The examiner applies a valgus force to the knee using the examiner's trunk as a fulcrum while extending the subject's knee and applying an anterior force to the fibular head. The purpose of the valgus stress is to make any anterior subluxation more pronounced by compressing the structures of the lateral side. Simultaneously, the ankle and foot are allowed to move into medial rotation, which ensures the anterior subluxation of the lateral tibial condyle.

Results. As the examiner goes through the testing maneuver, a "clunk" of the knee just prior to full extension indicates anterior tibial subluxation typical of anterolateral rotatory instability. Structures implicated in this instability may include the anterior cruciate and lateral collateral ligaments, the posterolateral capsule, the arcuate complex, and the iliotibial band.

Lateral Pivot Shift

Indication. The pivot shift is the test of choice in the assessment of anterolateral rotatory instability of the knee.

Method. The subject is relaxed and supine with the hip flexed 20 degrees and held in slight internal rotation. The examiner flexes the knee approximately 5 degrees by placing the heel of one hand behind the fibula, over the lateral gastrocnemius muscle. The examiner's other hand holds the leg in slight internal rotation by grasping the ankle. A valgus stress is then applied to the knee while maintaining the medial tibial rotation (Fig. 10–36A). If

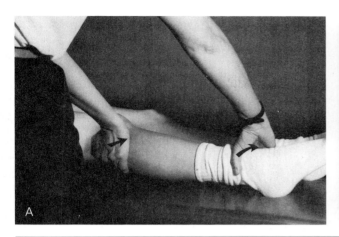 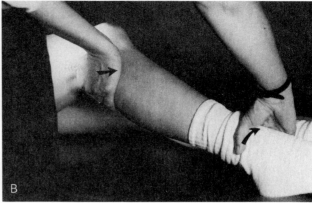

Figure 10–36. (*A*) Lateral pivot shift: While maintaining the tibia in slight medial rotation, the examiner flexes the knee about 5 degrees and applies valgus force. (*B* The knee is then moved into flexion, where reduction of the tibia occurs at 30 to 40 degrees.

the leg is then passively moved into flexion, the tibia will reduce posteriorly at about 30 or 40 degrees (Fig. 10–36*B*).

Results. Tibial reduction at 30 to 40 degrees represents anterolateral rotatory instability. The reduction is a result of the iliotibial bands becoming a flexor as it moves posterior to the axis of the knee. Because of its distal attachment, the flexion moment causes the tibia to be pulled posteriorly with contraction of the tensor muscle and iliotibial band.

The same structures that are implicated as being damaged in Losee's test are associated with the pivot shift.

Hughston's Jerk Test

Indication. Anterolateral rotatory instability is an indication for this test.

Method. The subject and examiner are positioned as described for the pivot shift, except that the subject's hip is flexed 45 degrees (Fig. 10–37). At 90 degrees of knee flexion, the leg is then extended while maintaining the valgus stress and internal tibial rotation.

Results. In a positive test, the lateral tibial condyle shifts anteriorly with a sudden movement at approximately 25 degrees of knee flexion. If the knee is extended more, the tibia reduces spontaneously. Structures named above in Losee's test are associated with a positive finding here.

Slocum's ALRI Test

Indication. Slocum's ALRI test provides another means of assessment of *anterolateral rotary instability* (ALRI).

Method. The subject is positioned between supine and sidelying, with the uppermost limb being involved (Fig. 10–38). The bottom limb is flexed to provide stabilization during the test. The foot of the test limb rests on the table in a position of medial rotation, with the knee in 10 degrees of flexion. The valgus force is created by the knee hanging freely as a result of the leg position. When anterior tibial subluxation is present, the lateral tibial condyle may be palpated as being displaced forward on the femur.

The examiner stands behind the subject and positions a thumb and index finger behind the fibular head and the lateral tibial plateau, respectively. The thumb of the other hand is placed behind the lateral femoral condyle. As even pressure is applied to the condyle and the fibular head, the knee is gently moved into flexion.

Figure 10–37. Hughston's jerk test: With the hip flexed 45 degrees and slightly medially rotated and the knee flexed 90 degrees, valgus stress is applied as the knee is extended.

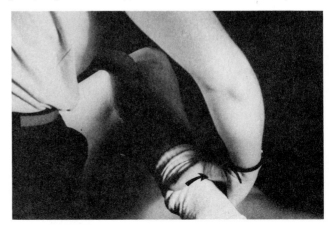

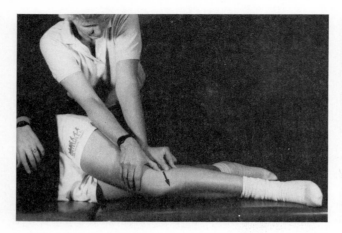

Figure 10–38. Slocum's ALRI test: With even anteriorly directed pressure applied to the lateral femoral condyle and fibular head, the knee is moved into flexion. A clunk felt as the knee passes through the range of 25 to 45 degrees indicates lateral tibial condyle reduction.

Results. A positive test result is demonstrated when the lateral tibial condyle reduces as the knee flexes through the range between 25 and 45 degrees. As reduction occurs, a clunk can be felt by the examiner.

The Slocum ALRI test may prove useful in the patient who is unable to relax the hamstrings or in the overweight person who may be difficult to handle in other testing positions. Damaged structures associated with other tests of anterolateral rotatory instability are tested by this examination.

Flexion-Rotation Drawer Test

Indication. The flexion-rotation drawer test is a variation of the pivot shift for the assessment of anterolateral rotatory instability. It is a combination of Lachman's test and the lateral pivot shift.

Method. While keeping the tibia in neutral rotation, the examiner flexes the subject's knee to 15 degrees by supporting the calf and grasping the ankle (Fig. 10–39A). In this position, the examiner observes any abnormal tibial motion. The knee is then gently flexed an additional 15 degrees, and again, the tibial motion is noted (Fig. 10–39B).

Results. In the knee with anterolateral rotatory instability, the initial position of 15 degrees of flexion causes the lateral portion of the femur to move posteriorly and rotate laterally. After the knee is flexed another 15 degrees, the tibia drops from its position of relative anterior subluxation to neutral. The structures associated with anterolateral rotatory instability are also involved here.

Posterolateral Rotatory Instability Tests

Jakob's Test (Reverse Pivot Shift)

Indication. Jakob's test is indicated in suspected cases of posterolateral rotatory instability.

Method. The subject lies supine with the knee muscles relaxed. The examiner stands at the end of the table facing the subject's leg, lifts it with one hand, and stabilizes it against the pelvis. The other hand, placed proximally on the fibula, supports the lateral side of the leg. The knee is flexed 70 to 80 degrees, and the tibia is externally rotated at the ankle, producing posterolateral subluxation of the lateral tibial condyle (Fig. 10–40A). The knee is then allowed to move passively into extension, aided by gravity and the weight of the leg. As the knee moves into extension, the examiner leans into the foot, creating a valgus force transmitted through the leg to the knee (Fig. 10–40B).

Results. In posterolateral rotatory instability, the lateral tibial condyle reduces by shifting anteriorly to the

Figure 10–39. Flexion rotation drawer test: Testing involves knee flexion to 15 degrees with neutral tibial rotation (A), followed by additional knee flexion another 15 degrees with observation of tibial motion (B).

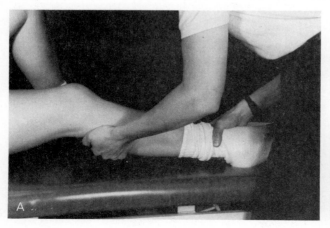

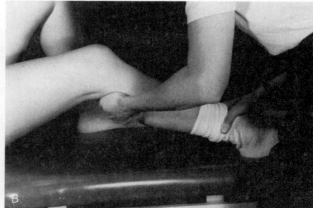

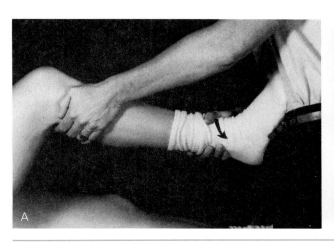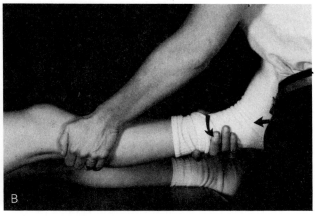

Figure 10–40. Jakob's test: The knee is flexed 70 to 80 degrees with external tibial rotation. (*A*) As the knee is passively moved into extension, the examiner leans into the foot, putting valgus force on the knee (*B*).

neutral position at about 20 degrees from full extension. As the knee is again flexed, the lateral tibial condyle moves into posterior subluxation and lateral rotation.

The following structures may be damaged, thereby contributing to posterolateral rotary instability: the posterior or anterior cruciate or the lateral collateral ligament, the posterolateral capsule, the arcuate complex, or the biceps femoris tendon.

External Rotational Recurvatum Test

Indication. The external rotational recurvatum test assesses posterolateral rotatory instability.

Method 1. The subject lies supine. The examiner places one hand around the subject's foot or heel while the other hand holds the posterolateral portion of the knee (Fig. 10–41*A* and *B*). Beginning in flexion of 30 to 40 degrees, the knee is slowly extended while the examiner palpates for a response.

Results. Hyperextension and lateral rotation of the lateral tibial condyle not palpable on the uninvolved side indicate posterolateral rotatory instability.

Method 2. The subject lies supine with both lower limbs extended. The examiner lifts both limbs from the table by grasping the great toe (Fig. 10–41*C*).

Results. Subjects with posterolateral rotatory instability demonstrate relative hyperextension of the knee and external tibial rotation in the test limb compared with the uninvolved side. As a result of the external tibial rotation, the tibial tuberosity lies more laterally on the affected side. There is also noticeable bowing of the medial side of the involved limb.

Hughston's Posterolateral Drawer Sign

Indication. Suspicion of anterolateral rotatory instability is an indication for this test.

Method. The subject is supine with the hip flexed 45 degrees and the knee flexed 80 to 90 degrees. The examiner rotates the tibia laterally at the ankle and then sits on the foot in order to stabilize it. The examiner pushes the tibia posteriorly as in the drawer test.

Results. If, during the posterior drawer test, the lateral tibial condyle of the test leg rotates excessively or moves posteriorly as compared with the uninvolved knee, the result is positive. This test can only be positive in the presence of anterior cruciate ligament rupture. Other structures that when damaged produce this form of instability include those described with Jakob's test.

Posteromedial Rotatory Instability Tests

Hughston's Posteromedial Drawer Sign

Indication. Hughston's posteromedial drawer sign is used in the assessment of posteromedial rotatory instability.

Method. The subject is positioned as for Hughston's posterolateral drawer sign, except that the tibia is internally rotated. The examiner performs a posterior drawer to the proximal tibia.

Results. Excessive posterior movement or rotation of the medial tibial condyle on the test leg as compared to the uninvolved knee indicates posteromedial rotatory instability. The structures listed below may be involved with this form of rotatory instability: posterior and an-

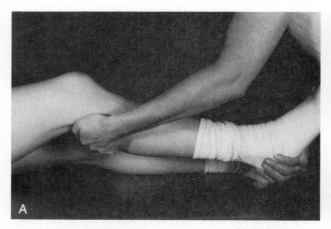

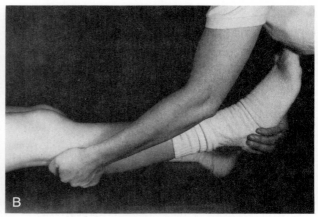

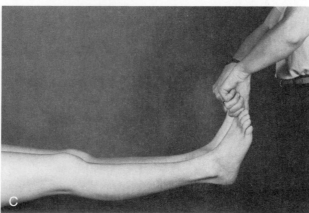

Figure 10–41. (*A*) External rotational recurvatum test: One method is with the knee flexed 30 to 40 degrees and supported by the examiner. (*B*) The knee is slowly extended as the examiner palpates for a response of hyperextension and lateral tibial rotation. (*C*) In an alternate method the examiner grasps the great toes and lifts the extended limbs off the table.

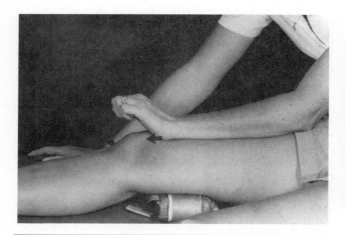

Figure 10–42. Inferior glide of the patella.

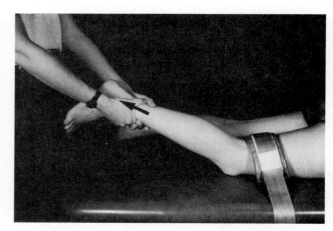

Figure 10–43. Distraction of the tibiofemoral joint.

terior cruciate, medial collateral, and posterior oblique ligaments, posteromedial capsule, and semimembranosus muscle.

If the posterior cruciate is intact, the tibia will demonstrate only posterolateral rotation. If the posterior cruciate is torn, the tibia will not only rotate posterolaterally, but will sublux posteriorly.

Joint Play (Accessory Movement)

Patellofemoral Joint

Inferior Glide (Fig. 10–42)

Restriction.   Knee flexion.

Open-Packed Position.   Slight knee flexion.

Positioning.   The subject lies supine with the knee slightly flexed over a small roll beneath the joint. The examiner places the heel of the mobilizing hand on the superior border of the patella, with the palm and fingers resting over the patellar area. The other hand is placed on top of the mobilizing hand to assist in the movement.

Movement.   The examiner moves the patella in an inferior direction.

Tibiofemoral Joint

Distraction (Fig. 10–43)

Restriction.   General hypomobiity.

Open-Packed Position.   25 degrees of knee flexion.

Positioning.   The subject lies prone with the distal thigh stabilized by a strap. The examiner stands at the foot of the table facing the subject. The examiner grasps the distal leg of the subject above the malleoli.

Movement.   The examiner applies a distraction force to the subject's knee as the examiner leans backward, pulling on the subject's leg.

Ventral Glide (Fig. 10–44)

Restriction.   Knee extension.

Positioning.   The subject lies prone so that the distal thigh rests at the edge of the treatment table. A wedge is placed beneath the distal thigh to help support the distal thigh. The examiner stands beside the knee being treated with one hand on the posterior proximal leg as close to the joint line as possible. The other hand holds the distal leg to provide support and to maintain the resting position.

Movement.   The examiner applies a ventral force to the proximal posterior leg.

Dorsal Glide (Fig. 10–45)

Restriction.   Knee flexion.

Positioning.   The subject lies supine so that the distal thigh rests at the edge of the treatment table. A wedge is placed beneath the distal thigh to support the distal femur. The examiner stands beside the knee being treated. One hand is placed on the anterior proximal leg as close to the joint line as possible. The other hand holds the distal leg to provide support and to maintain the resting position.

Movement.   The examiner applies a dorsal force to the proximal posterior leg.

Superior Tibiofibular Joint

Ventral Glide (Fig. 10–46)

Restriction.   Foot pronation.

Open-Packed Position.   Anatomical position.

Figure 10–44.   Ventral glide of the tibia.

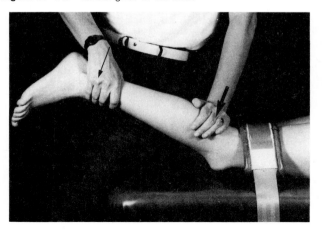

Figure 10–45.   Dorsal glide of the tibia.

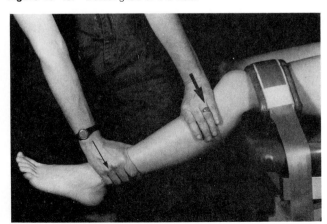

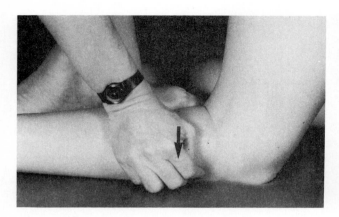

Figure 10–46. Ventral glide of the fibula.

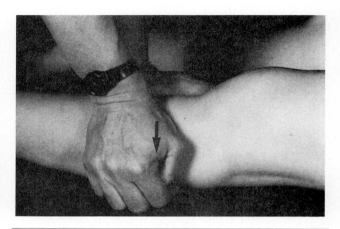

Figure 10–47. Dorsal glide of the fibula.

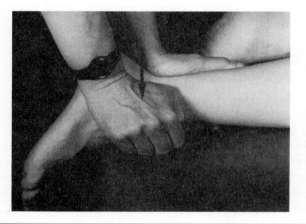

Figure 10–48. Ventral glide of the fibula.

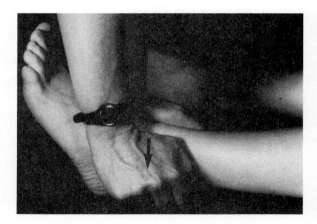

Figure 10–49. Dorsal glide of the fibula.

Positioning. The subject is placed in a weight-bearing position of knee flexion to 90 degrees. The examiner places the thenar eminence of one hand on the posterior proximal fibula of the subject. The other hand may be positioned on top of the mobilizing hand to assist in the movement.

Movement. The examiner applies a ventrally directed force to the posterior surface of the proximal fibula.

Dorsal Glide (Fig. 10–47)

Restriction. Foot supination.

Positioning. The subject lies supine with the knee joint resting in extension. The examiner places the thenar eminence of the mobilizing hand on the anterior surface of the proximal fibula. The other hand may be used to assist in the movement by placing it on top of the mobilizing hand.

Movement. The examiner applies a dorsally directed force to the anterior surface of the proximal fibula.

Inferior Tibiofibular Joint

Ventral Glide (Fig. 10–48)

Restriction. Foot pronation.

Open-Packed Position. Anatomical position.

Positioning. The subject lies prone. A wedge may be placed beneath the distal tibia to aid in stabilization. The examiner places the thenar eminence of one hand posteriorly on the subject's lateral malleolus to apply the mobilizing force. The other hand may be positioned on top of the mobilizing hand to assist in the movement.

Movement. The examiner applies a ventrally directed force to the posterior surface of the distal fibula.

Dorsal Glide (Fig. 10–49)

Restriction. Foot supination.

Positioning. The subject lies supine. The examiner places the thenar eminence of the mobilizing hand on

Table 10–1.   Summary of Joint Play of the Knee

GLIDE	RESTRICTION	FIXED BONE	MOVING BONE
Patellofemoral Joint			
Inferior	Flexion	Femur	Patella
Superior	Extension	Femur	Patella
Medial	General hypomobility	Femur	Patella
Tibiofemoral Joint			
Distraction	General hypomobility	Femur	Tibia
Ventral	Extension	Femur	Tibia
Dorsal	Flexion	Femur	Tibia
Superior/Inferior Tibiofibular Joints			
Dorsal	Supination of foot	Tibia	Fibula
Ventral	Pronation of foot	Tibia	Fibula

the anterior surface of the lateral malleolus to apply the mobilizing force. The other hand may be used to assist in the movement by placing it on top of the mobilizing hand.

Movement.   The examiner applies a dorsally directed force to the anterior surface of the distal fibula.

Summary of Joint Play of the Knee

Table 10–1 provides a summary of joint play of the patellofemoral, tibiofemoral, superior tibiofibular, and inferior tibiofibular joints.

Bibliography

Backhouse KM, Hutchings RT: Color Atlas of Surface Anatomy. Baltimore, Williams & Wilkins, 1986

Corrigan B, Maitland GD: Practical Orthopedic Medicine. Boston, Butterworth & Co, 1983

Daniels L, Worthingham C: Muscle Testing Techniques of Manual Examination. Philadelphia, WB Saunders, 1986

Gould JA III, Davies GG (eds): Orthopedic and Sports Physical Therapy. St Louis, CV Mosby, 1985

Hollinshead WH, Jenkins DB: Functional Anatomy of the Limbs and Back. Philadelphia, WB Saunders, 1981

Hoppenfeld S: Physical Examination of the Spine and Extremities. New York, Appleton-Century-Crofts, 1976

Jackson DW, Drez D Jr: The Anterior Cruciate Deficient Knee: New Concepts in Ligament Repair. St Louis, CV Mosby, 1987

Kaltenborn M: Mobilization of the Extremity Joints. Oslo, Bygdoy Alle, 1980

Kendall FP, McCreary EK: Muscle Testing and Function. Baltimore, Williams & Wilkins, 1983

Kessler R, Hertling D: Management of Common Musculoskeletal Disorders. Philadelphia, Harper & Row, 1983

Kisner C, Colby LA: Therapeutic Foundations: Foundations and Techniques. Philadelphia, FA Davis, 1985

Losee RE: Diagnosis of chronic injury to the anterior cruciate ligament. Orthop Clin North Am 16:1, 1985

Magee DJ: Orthopedic Physical Assessment. Philadelphia, WB Saunders, 1987

Maitland GD: The Peripheral Joints: Examination and Recording Guide. Adelaide, Australia, Virgo Press, 1973

Norkin CC, White DJ: Measurement of Joint Motion: A Guide to Goniometry. Philadelphia, FA Davis, 1985

Saunders DH: Evaluation, Treatment, and Prevention of Musculoskeletal Disorders. Minneapolis, H Duane Saunders, 1985

Schneider RC, Kennedy JC, Plant ML: Sports Injuries: Mechanisms, Prevention, and Treatment. Baltimore, Williams & Wilkins, 1985

Turek SL: Orthopedics: Principles and Their Application, vol 2. Philadelphia, JB Lippincott, 1984

Williams P, Warwick R (eds): Gray's Anatomy, 36th British ed. Philadelphia, WB Saunders, 1980

Ankle and
Foot Region

Chapter 11

Danny DiSabatino, P.T., contributed to this chapter.

The ankle and foot are flexible enough to adapt to uneven terrain but sufficiently stable to bear the body weight. Ankle injuries occur frequently. The ankle and foot have to make continuous adjustments to the ground during ambulation to compensate for the motion of deviation at the knee and hip joints in order to keep the center of gravity over the relatively small base of support.

The talocrural joint is composed of the distal ends of the tibia and fibula, and the trochlea of the talus. A hinge joint, it permits one degree of freedom of motion. The medial and lateral surfaces of the joint are guarded by the medial malleolus of the tibia and the lateral malleolus of the fibula. The axis of motion lies transversely and passes through the talus, connecting the two malleoli. The plane of the axis is oblique in that the lateral malleolus extends more distally and is posterior to the medial malleolus. The posterior alignment of the lateral malleolus is due to the torsion of the tibia. Movements at the talocrural joint are described as dorsiflexion and plantar flexion. During the motion at the talocrural joint, the fibula moves on the tibia both superiorly and inferiorly.

The superior surface of the calcaneus and the inferior surface of the talus form the subtalar joint. The talus also articulates with the tarsal navicular anteriorly. The motions of supination and pronation occur around an oblique axis, allowing the foot to conform to the surface of the terrain. The axis for supination and pronation motion is described by a line that begins on the lateral posterior aspect of the heel and proceeds anterior, superior, and medial.

The bones that form the articulation for the midtarsal joint are the talus and calcaneus proximally and the navicular and cuboid distally. This joint permits coordinated movement of the forefoot with the hindfoot.

The structure of the transtarsal joint has been analyzed frequently, but the joint axis has not been agreed upon. Manter and Hicks have suggested longitudinal and oblique axes around a relatively fixed naviculocuboid unit. The longitudinal axis is nearly horizontal, permitting the motion of pronation and supination. The oblique axis is relatively transverse, also permitting supination and pronation with dorsiflexion and plantar flexion and accompanying abduction and adduction. The two axes provide the total range of motion for supination and pronation.

Triplanar movement occurs at the talocrural, the subtalar, and the midtarsal joints. In an open kinematic chain the movement of supination includes the components of plantar flexion, adduction, and inversion, while pronation includes the components of dorsiflexion, abduction, and eversion. Clinicians often measure goniometric triplanar motion as subtalar inversion and eversion.

The metatarsophalangeal joints of the foot are condyloid synovial joints with two degrees of freedom of motion allowing flexion and extension and abduction and adduction. The motion of flexion is limited, and extension and hyperextension motion is 90 degrees or more in combination with plantar flexion of the first ray. This motion is important for the weight-bearing functions of the foot. Great toe hyperextension is important for toe-off during ambulation.

The interphalangeal joints of the toes are hinge synovial joints with one degree of freedom of motion permitting flexion and extension.

Goniometry

Tibial Torsion

The distal end of the tibia is angled approximately 25 degrees lateral to the proximal end. This angulation in the transverse plane produces toe-out in postural stance and during ambulation. Tibial torsion may be measured with a goniometer. The angle of the malleoli to the talus is measured.

Figure 11–1. Starting position for tibial torsion measurement.

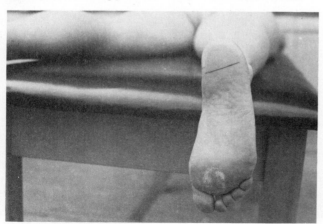

Figure 11–2. End position for tibial torsion measurement.

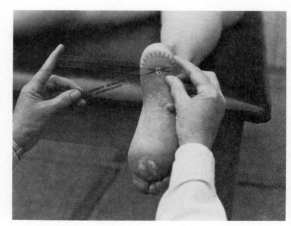

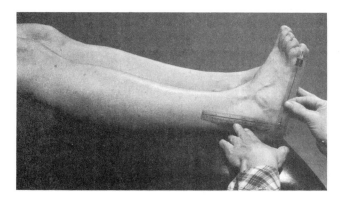

Figure 11–3. Starting position for measuring ankle dorsiflexion.

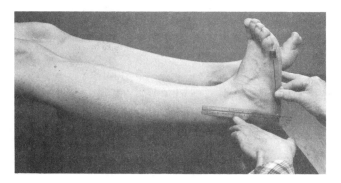

Figure 11–4. End position for measuring ankle dorsiflexion.

Motion.   20 to 30 degrees of torsion.

Position.   Subject lies prone or supine, with the foot over the edge of the treatment table. A line is drawn on the heel horizontal to the table's edge. A second line may be drawn on the heel in line with the malleolus (Figs. 11–1 and 11–2).

Goniometric Alignment

Axis.   Placed at the intersection of the two lines.

Stationary Arm.   Placed parallel to the table top in line with the horizontal line drawn on the heel.

Moving Arm.   Placed along the oblique line, in line with the two malleoli.

Stabilization.   The leg is stabilized, with the femoral condyles in the frontal plane.

Precautions
- Prevent hip rotation.
- Prevent forefoot motion.
- Align the talus squarely with the tibia.

Ankle Joint Dorsiflexion

The motion of ankle joint dorsiflexion occurs in the sagittal plane between the distal ends of the tibia and fibula and the articular surface of the talus. The talus moves on the tibia into ankle dorsiflexion and the motion is accompanied by an accessory gliding motion in a posterior direction. There is an accompanying motion between the superior and inferior tibiofibular joints. The fibula moves superiorly, abducts, and rotates medially with the tibia during ankle dorsiflexion.

Motion.   0 to 20 degrees of ankle dorsiflexion.

10° to be final

Position
- Preferred: Subject lies supine with the knee joint flexed 20 to 30 degrees and supported by a pillow

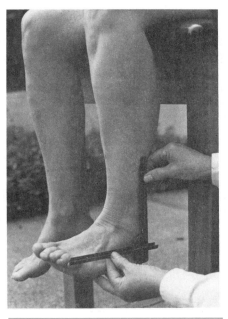

Figure 11–5. End position for measuring ankle dorsiflexion in the alternate sitting position.

to put gastroc. on stretch

or towel roll. The ankle joint is in the anatomical position (Figs. 11–3 and 11–4).
- Alternate: Subject is sitting or in any position that allows the knee to be slightly flexed, and the ankle is in the anatomical position (Fig. 11–5).

Goniometric Alignment

Axis.   Placed over the lateral malleolus *distal to* of the fibula.

Stationary Arm.   Placed parallel to the lateral midline of the fibula projecting toward the fibular head.

Moving Arm.   Placed parallel to the lateral midline of the calcaneus. *5th met. head*

Stabilization.   The leg is stabilized.

Precautions
- Prevent hip and knee joint motion.
- Avoid inversion and eversion.
- Keep the knee flexed to prevent stretching of the gastrocnemius muscle.
- Align the moving arm of the goniometer with the lateral calcaneus, not with the forefoot.

Ankle Joint Plantar Flexion

The motion occurs in the sagittal plane between the distal tibia and fibula and the superior surface of the talus. As the motion of plantar flexion occurs, the talus glides anteriorly on the tibia. During ambulation, the tibia glides posteriorly on the talus. Motion at the tibiotalar joint is accompanied by motion at the superior and inferior tibiofibular joints. The fibula adducts and glides inferiorly on the tibia during plantar flexion.

Motion. 0 to 45 degrees of plantar flexion at the talotibial (talocrural) joint.

Position
- Preferred: Subject lies supine with the hip and knee joints extended and the ankle in the anatomical position (Fig. 11–6).
- Alternate: Subject sits with the knee flexed and the foot in the anatomical position (Fig. 11–7).

Goniometric Alignment

Axis. Placed over the lateral malleolus of the fibula.

Stationary Arm. Placed parallel to the lateral midline of the leg projecting to the head of the fibula.

Moving Arm. Placed parallel to the bottom of the ~~calcaneus.~~ 5th met.

Stabilization. The leg is stabilized.

Precautions
- Avoid forefoot flexion.
- Prevent hip joint rotation.
- Prevent inversion and eversion of the foot.

Midtarsal-Subtalar Inversion (Pronation)

Midtarsal-subtalar motion occurs between talus and calcaneus, talus and navicular, and calcaneus and cuboid. The motion occurs in the transverse, sagittal, and frontal planes.

Motion. 0 to 30 degrees of inversion.

Position
- Preferred: Subject lies supine with the hip in the anatomical position and the ankle relaxed. The knee may be either flexed or extended (Fig. 11–8).
- Alternate: Subject sits with the knee flexed 90 degrees (Figs. 11–9 and 11–10).

Goniometric Alignment

Axis
- Preferred: Placed over the dorsal surface of the foot, midway between the malleoli.

Figure 11–6. End position for measuring ankle plantar flexion.

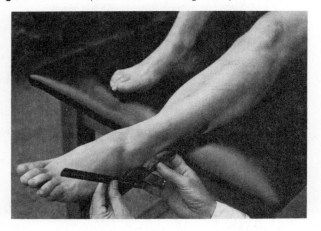

Figure 11–7. End position for measuring ankle plantar flexion in the alternate sitting position.

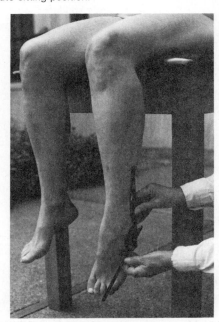

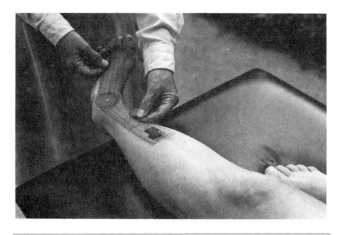

Figure 11–8. End position for triplanar inversion measurement.

- Alternate: Placed on the lateral side of the foot, at the level of the fifth metatarsophalangeal joint.

Stationary Arm
- Preferred: Placed along the anterior surface over the crest of the tibia in line with the tibial tuberosity.
- Alternate: Placed parallel to the longitudinal axis of the tibia laterally.

Moving Arm
- Preferred: Placed along the dorsal surface of the second metatarsal shaft.
- Alternate: Placed parallel to the plantar surface of the heel.

Stabilization.   The leg is stabilized.

Precautions
- Prevent medial rotation and extension of the knee joint.
- Prevent hip joint lateral rotation and abduction.
- Allow ankle joint plantar flexion.

Midtarsal (Transtarsal)-Subtalar Eversion (Supination)

In the test position, the motion is assessed in the frontal plane between talus and calcaneus, talus and navicular, and calcaneus and cuboid.

Motion.   0 to 25 degrees of foot eversion.

Position
- Preferred: Subject lies supine with the hip in neutral position and the ankle joint relaxed. The knee may be either flexed or extended (Fig. 11–11).
- Alternate: Subject sits, with the knee flexed 90 degrees, and the ankle in the anatomical position (Figs. 11–12 and 11–13).

Goniometric Alignment

Axis
- Preferred: Placed over the dorsal aspect of the foot midway between the malleoli.
- Alternate: Placed medial to the head of the first metatarsal bone.

Figure 11–9. End position for measuring eriplanar inversion in the alternate sitting position.

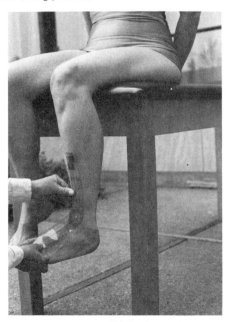

Figure 11–10. Alternate end position for measuring triplanar inversion in the sitting position.

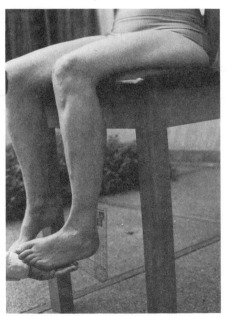

Stationary Arm
- Preferred: Placed on the crest of the tibia.
- Alternate: Placed parallel to the longitudinal axis of the tibia on the medial side.

Moving Arm
- Preferred: Placed on the dorsum of the foot in line with the dorsal shaft of the second metatarsal.
- Alternate: Placed parallel to the plantar surface of the sole of the foot.

Stabilization. The leg is stabilized.

Figure 11–11. End position for measuring triplanar eversion.

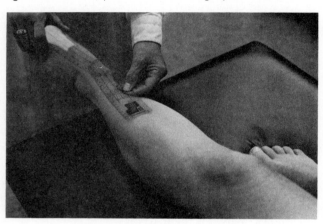

Precautions
- Prevent lateral rotation of the knee.
- Prevent hip joint medial rotation and abduction.
- Allow for dorsiflexion at the ankle.

The Toes

The position for measurement of toe motion may be any comfortable position for the subject in which the ankle is in the anatomical position. It is best if the subject is able to see the procedure. Usually the mobility of the toes is measured not specifically, but grossly. Observations should identify deformities such as hallux valgus and hammer toes. Extension and hyperextension motion of all toes is important for ambulation.

Flexion of the First Metatarsophalangeal Joint

Great toe flexion occurs in the sagittal plane between the head of the first metatarsal and the base of the proximal phalanx. As the motion of flexion occurs, the base of the proximal phalanx glides in a plantar direction.

Motion. 0 to 45 degrees of flexion.

Goniometric Alignment

Axis. Placed over the dorsal aspect of the metatarsophalangeal joint (Fig. 11–14).

Figure 11–12. End position for measuring triplanar eversion in the alternate sitting position.

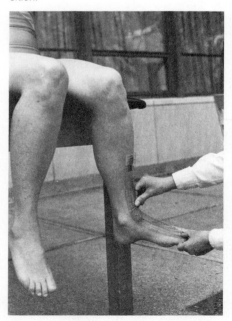

Figure 11–13. Alternate end position for measuring triplanar eversion in the sitting position.

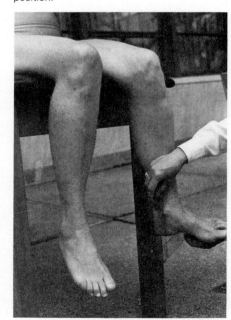

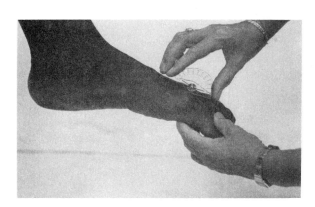

Figure 11–14. End position for metatarsophalangeal joint flexion measurement of the first digit.

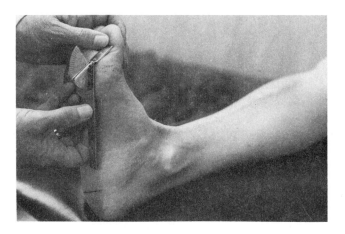

Figure 11–15. End position for metatarsophalangeal joint extension and hyperextension measurements.

Stationary Arm. Placed over the dorsal aspect of the shaft of the first metatarsal bone.

Moving Arm. Placed along the dorsal surface of the shaft of the proximal phalanx.

Stabilization. The metatarsal bones are stabilized.

Precautions
• Prevent ankle joint plantar flexion.
• Prevent midtarsal motions.
• Allow the lateral toes to flex as well.

Extension and Hyperextension of the First Metatarsophalangeal Joint

Extension of the great toe is the return from flexion, whereas hyperextension moves beyond the anatomical position. As the base of the proximal phalanx extends on the first metatarsal bone, the motion is accompanied by a dorsal glide.

Motion. 45 to 0 degrees of extension and 0 to 90 degrees of hyperextension at the first metatarsophalangeal joint.

Goniometric Alignment

Axis. Placed over the plantar aspect of the first metatarsophalangeal joint (Fig. 11–15).

Stationary Arm. Placed over the plantar midline shaft of the first metatarsal bone.

Moving Arm. Placed along the plantar shaft of the proximal phalanx.

Stabilization. The metatarsal bones are stabilized.

Precautions
• Prevent ankle joint dorsiflexion.

• Prevent forefoot inversion or eversion.
• Allow the lateral four digits to extend.
• Permit interphalangeal joint flexion.

Flexion of the Lateral Four Metatarsophalangeal Joints

Metatarsophalangeal flexion of the lateral four digits occurs in the sagittal plane between the metatarsals and the proximal phalanges. As the proximal phalanx moves into flexion, it glides in a plantar direction. Each joint is measured individually.

Motion. 0 to 40 degrees of metatarsophalangeal joint flexion.

Goniometric Alignment

Axis. Placed over the dorsal aspect of the metatarsophalangeal joints (Fig. 11–16).

Stationary Arm. Placed along the dorsal midline longitudinal shaft of each metatarsal bone.

Moving Arm. Placed along the dorsal midline longitudinal shaft of each proximal phalanx.

Stabilization. The metatarsal bones are stabilized.

Precautions
• Prevent ankle joint and forefoot motions.
• Allow toes not being tested to flex.

Extension and Hyperextension of the Lateral Four Metatarsophalangeal Joints

Metatarsophalangeal joint extension occurs between the proximal phalanges and the metatarsal bones. As the motion occurs, the bases of the proximal phalanges glide in a dorsal direction.

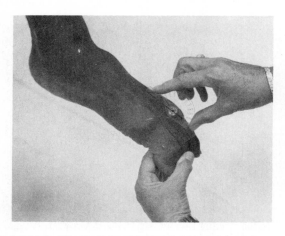

Figure 11–16. End position for measuring metatarsophalangeal joint flexion of the second digit.

Motion. 40 to 0 degrees of extension and 0 to 45 degrees of hyperextension.

Goniometric Alignment

Axis. Placed over the plantar aspect of the metatarsophalangeal joint (Fig. 11–17).

Stationary Arm. Placed along the plantar midline shaft of the metatarsals.

Moving Arm. Placed along the plantar midline aspect of the shaft of the proximal phalanx of each digit.

Stabilization. The metatarsals are stabilized.

Precautions
• Prevent ankle joint and forefoot motion.
• Permit interphalangeal joint flexion.
• Allow the other digits to extend or hyperextend.

Figure 11–17. End position for measuring metatarsophalangeal joint extension for the second digit.

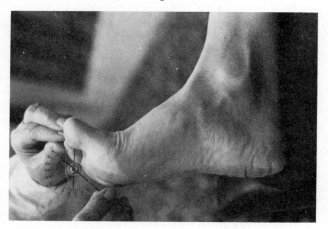

Flexion of the First Interphalangeal Joint and the Lateral Four Proximal Interphalangeal Joints

As the distal phalanx flexes on the proximal phalanx of the first digit, the base of the distal phalanx glides in a plantar direction. The middle phalanges of the lateral four digits glide in a plantar direction during proximal interphalangeal joint flexion.

Motion. 0 to 90 degrees for the great toe; 0 to 35 degrees for the lateral four toes.

Goniometric Alignment

Axis. Placed over the dorsal aspect of the interphalangeal joints (Fig. 11–18).

Stationary Arm. Placed on the dorsal midline shaft of the proximal phalanges for each digit.

Moving Arm. Placed on the dorsal midline shaft of the distal phalanx of the great toe and the dorsal midline shaft of the middle phalanges of the lateral four toes.

Stabilization. The proximal phalanges and the metatarsals are stabilized.

Precautions
• Prevent ankle and forefoot motion.
• Avoid metatarsophalangeal joint motion.
• Allow the distal interphalangeal joint to flex.

Extension and Hyperextension of the First Interphalangeal Joint and Extension of the Lateral Four Proximal Interphalangeal Joints

Extension of the interphalangeal joints is the return from flexion. Hyperextension is a motion in the sagittal plane beyond the anatomical position. The distal phalanx of the first digit glides in a dorsal direction during extension and hyperextension. The middle phalanges of the lateral four digits also glide in a dorsal direction during extension and hyperextension.

Motion. 90 to 0 degrees for the great toe and 35 to 0 degrees for the lateral four toes. Hyperextension is minimal at the interphalangeal joints.

Goniometric Alignment

Axis. Placed over the plantar aspect of the interphalangeal joints (Fig. 11–19).

Stationary Arm. Placed over the plantar midline shaft of the proximal phalanges.

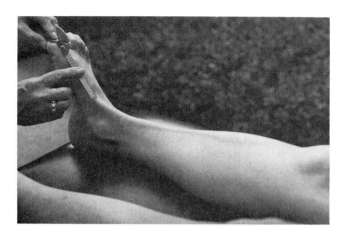

Figure 11–18. End position for measuring interphalangeal joint flexion for the first digit.

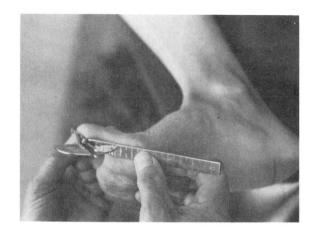

Figure 11–19. End position for measuring interphalangeal joint extension for the first digit.

Moving Arm. Placed over the plantar midline shaft of the distal phalanx of the great toe and over the middle phalanges of the other toes.

Stabilization. The proximal phalanges are stabilized.

Precautions
- Prevent ankle joint and forefoot motions.
- Avoid metatarsophalangeal joint motion.
- Allow the distal interphalangeal joints to extend.

Flexion of the Lateral Four Distal Interphalangeal Joints

Flexion occurs between the middle and distal phalanges of the lateral four digits. The accessory motion that occurs during flexion is plantar gliding of the distal phalanges on the middle phalanges.

Motion. 0 to 60 degrees of distal interphalangeal joint flexion.

Goniometric Alignment

Axis. Placed over the dorsal aspect of the distal interphalangeal joints.

Stationary Arm. Placed along the dorsal midline shaft of the middle phalanges.

Moving Arm. Placed along the dorsal midline shaft of the distal phalanges (Fig. 11–20).

Stabilization. The metatarsals and the proximal and middle phalanges.

Precautions
- Prevent ankle joint and forefoot motions.
- Avoid metatarsophalangeal and proximal interphalangeal joint motion of the digit being measured.

Extension and Hyperextension of the Lateral Four Distal Interphalangeal Joints

The motion of extension and hyperextension of the distal interphalangeal joint is the return from the flexion motion and beyond the anatomical position for hyperextension. As the extension motion occurs, the bases of the distal phalanges glide in a dorsal direction.

Motion. 60 to 0 degrees of extension; hyperextension is minimal.

Figure 11–20. End position for measuring distal interphalangeal flexion of the second digit.

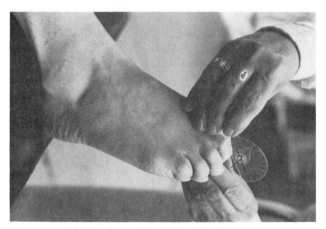

Goniometric Alignment

Axis. Placed over the dorsal aspect of the distal interphalangeal joint.

Stationary Arm. Placed along the dorsal midline shaft of the middle phalanges.

Moving Arm. Placed along the dorsal midline shaft of the distal phalanges.

Stabilization. The proximal and middle phalanges are stabilized.

Precautions
- Prevent ankle and forefoot motions.
- Prevent metatarsophalangeal and proximal interphalangeal joint motions.
- Allow the digits that are not being tested to extend.

Functional Muscle Testing

Ankle

Ankle Dorsiflexion

All the ankle joint muscles that lie anterior to the transverse axis through the joint are dorsiflexors. The ankle dorsiflexor muscles are active during both swing and stance phases of gait. They contract concentrically to clear the toes during swing and eccentrically to lower the foot to the floor at foot contact. During the stance phase of gait, the dorsiflexor muscles move the leg over the fixed foot. When the foot is lifted to be placed on a stool or a stair the dorsiflexors contract.

Position. Subject stands.

Activity. Subject lifts toes and forefoot off the floor and slowly lowers them.

Muscles. Tibialis anterior, extensor digitorum longus, and extensor hallucis longus.

Types of Contraction
- Concentric: The ankle flexes dorsally as the toes and forefoot are raised from the floor.
- Eccentric: Subject lowers the toes and forefoot to the floor from the raised position.

Resistance
- The weight of the forefoot is the resistance.
- Functional: 10 repetitions.
- Functionally Fair: 5 to 9 repetitions.
- Functionally Poor: 1 to 4 repetitions.
- Nonfunctional: 0 repetitions.

Ankle Plantar Flexion

The plantar flexors of the ankle lie posterior to the transverse axis and function in the sagittal plane. The action of ankle plantar flexion is one of the most powerful in the body. The plantar flexors provide the propulsive force during ambulation at push-off. The muscles performing the action of plantar flexion continuously contract during static balance and are considered type I postural, or fatigue-resistant muscles.

Position. Subject stands balanced on one foot and rises up on toes with the hands resting lightly on the treatment table for balance only (Fig. 11–21).

Activity. Subject lifts body weight on the toes, runs a short distance (10 to 15 feet), or jumps five times.

Muscles. Gastrocnemius, soleus, plantaris.

Types of Contraction
- Concentric: Rising on toes, running, and jumping.
- Eccentric: Lowering heels to the floor.

Resistance
- The body weight offers the resistance.
- Functional: 10 repetitions.
- Functionally Fair: 5 to 9 repetitions.
- Functionally Poor: 1 to 4 repetitions.
- Nonfunctional: 0 repetitions.

Figure 11–21. Ankle plantar flexion.

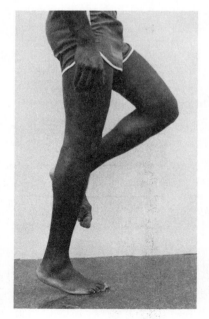

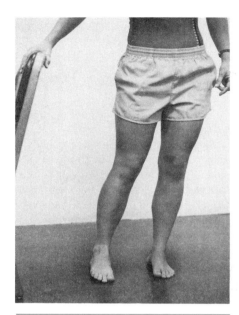

Figure 11–22.   Ankle eversion on the right.

Ankle Eversion

The muscle tendons for eversion lie posterior to the transverse axis through the malleoli. The motion of ankle eversion is primarily for keeping the foot flat on the ground during weight bearing. The lateral muscle group adds stability to the lateral aspect of the ankle and subtalar joints.

Position.   Subject stands, bearing weight on the tested lower limb, with the hands holding lightly on to the treatment table for balance (Fig. 11–22).

Activity.   Subject shifts the body weight toward the opposite side, lifting the lateral edge of the foot off the ground.

Muscles.   Peroneus longus, peroneus brevis, peroneus tertius.

Types of Contraction
- Concentric: Lifting the lateral border of the test foot.
- Eccentric: Controlled return to the starting position.

Resistance
- The body weight offers resistance.
- Functional: 5 repetitions.
- Functionally Fair: 3 to 4 repetitions.
- Functionally Poor: 1 to 2 repetitions.
- Nonfunctional: 0 repetitions.

Ankle Inversion

Ankle inversion keeps the foot flat on the ground during ambulation. The muscles act to provide stability to the medial aspect of the ankle and subtalar joints.

Position.   Subject stands, bearing weight on the tested lower limb. The hands may hold lightly on to the treatment table for balance (Fig. 11–23).

Activity.   Subject shifts the body weight toward the test side, lifting the medial side of the foot off the ground.

Muscles.   Tibialis posterior, tibialis anterior, extensor hallucis longus.

Types of Contraction
- Concentric: Lifting the medial border of the test foot.
- Eccentric: Controlled return to the starting position.

Resistance
- The body weight offers the resistance.
- Functional: 5 repetitions.
- Functionally Fair: 3 to 4 repetitions.
- Functionally Poor: 1 to 2 repetitions.
- Nonfunctional: 0 repetitions.

Figure 11–23.   Ankle inversion on the right.

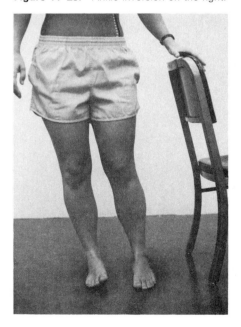

The Toes

Toe Flexion

The toe flexors contract eccentrically during the toe-off phase of gait, after which a concentric contraction follows. The great toe is the primary contributing digit. Otherwise, the toes do not have very significant function because most people wear shoes.

Position. Subject is barefoot and seated.

Activity. Subject uses toes to wrinkle a small towel placed on the floor or to pick up and release a small object (cotton ball, crumpled paper, marble). The subject may be observed walking forward.

Muscles. Flexor hallucis longus, flexor hallucis brevis, flexor digitorum longus, flexor digitorum brevis.

Type of Contraction
· Concentric: Grasping the object.

Resistance
· The object on the floor offers resistance.
· Functional: 10 repetitions.
· Functionally Fair: 5 to 9 repetitions.
· Functionally Poor: 1 to 4 repetitions.
· Nonfunctional: 0 repetitions.

Toe Extension

Toe extension occurs during the swing phase of gait to help the foot clear the floor. Since people usually wear shoes, the functional significance of the toe extensors is limited.

Position. Subject sits, with foot flat on the floor.

Activity. Subject slowly lifts the toes off the floor, keeping the forefoot on the ground.

Muscles. Extensor hallucis longus, extensor hallucis brevis, extensor digitorum longus, extensor digitorum brevis.

Types of Contraction
· Concentric: Lifting toes against gravity.
· Eccentric: Lowering toes to the floor.

Resistance
· The weight of the toes offers the resistance.
· Functional: 10 repetitions.
· Functionally Fair: 5 to 9 repetitions.
· Functionally Poor: 1 to 4 repetitions.
· Nonfunctional: 0 repetitions.

Manual Muscle Testing

Ankle

Gastrocnemius and Plantaris Muscles

The gastrocnemius and plantaris muscles produce 45 degrees of plantar flexion with the knee extended. The motion is tested in the prone position. If no weakness is apparent, a test is performed in the functional position (standing).

Palpation. Palpate the gastrocnemius, with its short, bulky medial and lateral heads immediately distal to the posterior knee joint (Fig. 11–24). (The plantaris is not palpable.)

Position
· AG: (Non–weight-bearing). Subject lies prone with the foot over the edge of the table (Fig. 11–

Figure 11–24. Palpating the gastrocnemius muscle.

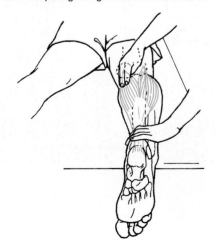

Figure 11–25. Testing the gastrocnemius muscle in the AG position.

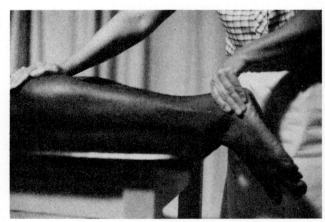

Attachments of Gastrocnemius and Plantaris Muscles

Muscle	Proximal	Distal	Innervation
Gastrocnemius	Medial and lateral condyle of femur	Posterior surface of calcaneus through Achilles tendon	Tibial S2 (S1)
Plantaris	Lateral supracondylar line of femur	Posterior surface of calcaneus through Achilles tendon	Tibial S2 (S1)

25). For the weight-bearing test, the subject stands with the knee extended and the opposite foot off the floor (Fig. 11–26).

- GM: Subject is in sidelying position with the ankle in the anatomical position (Fig. 11–27).

Movement. Plantar flexion of ankle; the heel moves up toward the back of the leg, as in standing on tiptoes.

Resistance. Applied to the plantar surface of the hindfoot. Standing, the body weight provides the resistance.

Stabilization. The leg is stabilized or the standing subject may balance by placing the hands on the table, but may not bear weight on them.

Grades
- Non–weight-bearing:
  P +: Moves through less than half the range.

F −: Moves through more than half the range.
F: Moves through full range.
F +: Cannot take maximal resistance.
G: Takes maximal resistance.

- Standing:
  P +: Less than half the range.
  F −: More than half the range.
  F: 1 repetition.
  F +: 2 to 3 repetitions.
  G: 4 to 6 repetitions.
  G +: 7 to 9 repetitions.
  N: 10 repetitions.

Substitutions
- Do not allow toe flexors to contract.
- Do not allow inversion to occur with the plantar flexion using the tibialis posterior muscle.
- Do not allow eversion with the plantar flexion by using the peroneal muscles.

Figure 11–26. Testing the gastrocnemius muscle in the alternate AG standing position.

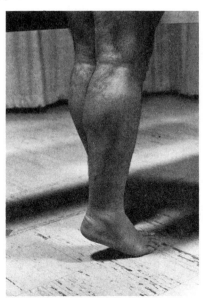

Figure 11–27. Testing the gastrocnemius muscle in the GM position.

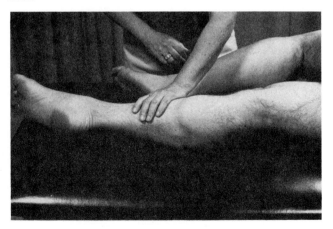

- Soleus is a plantar flexor muscle in any position of the knee joint.
- Subject may quickly dorsiflex, then relax.

Soleus Muscle

The soleus muscle produces plantar flexion of the ankle joint regardless of the position of the knee. To determine the individual functioning of the soleus as a plantar flexor, the knee is flexed to minimize the effect of the gastrocnemius muscle.

Palpation.   The soleus muscle is covered largely by the gastrocnemius muscle, but it is easily palpated distal to the gastrocnemius bulk on either side (Fig. 11–28).

Figure 11–28.   Palpating the soleus muscle.

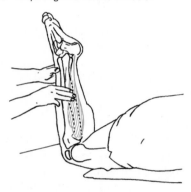

Figure 11–29.   Testing the soleus muscle in the AG position.

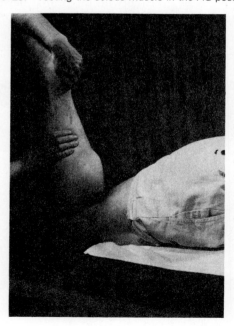

Position
- AG: Subject lies prone with the knees flexed 90 degrees (Fig. 11–29).
- GM: Subject is in sidelying position with the knee flexed 90 degrees (Fig. 11–30).
- Alternate: Subject stands with some degree of knee flexion, while rising up on toes (Fig. 11–31).

Movement.   Plantar flexion of the ankle; the heel moves toward the back of the leg, as in pointing the toes.

Resistance.   Applied to the plantar surface of the hindfoot, unless subject is standing, in which case the body weight provides the resistance.

Stabilization.   Stabilize the leg. A standing subject may balance by placing the hands on the table, but may not bear weight on the hands.

Substitutions
- The gastrocnemius will also plantar flex the foot. To minimize its action, flex the knee.
- Do not allow inversion to occur with the plantar flexion using the tibialis posterior muscle.
- Do not allow eversion with the plantar flexion using the peroneal muscles.
- The patient may quickly dorsiflex, then relax.

Figure 11–30.   Testing the soleus muscle in the GM position.

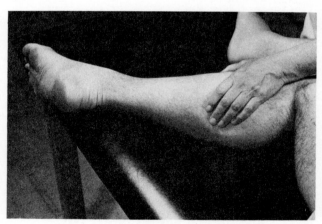

Attachments of Soleus Muscle

Muscle	Proximal	Distal	Innervation
Soleus	Head of fibula, proximal third of shaft, soleal line and midshaft of posterior tibia	Posterior surface of calcaneus through Achilles tendon	Tibial S2 (S1)

Attachments of Tibialis Anterior Muscle

Muscle	Proximal	Distal	Innervation
Tibialis anterior	Distal to lateral tibial condyle, proximal half of lateral tibial shaft, and interosseous membrane	First cuneiform bone, medial and plantar surfaces and base of first metatarsal	Deep peroneal L4 (L5)

Tibialis Anterior Muscle

The tibialis anterior muscle produces the motion of dorsiflexion and inversion through a test range of 15 degrees from the starting (anatomical) position. The knee must remain flexed to allow complete dorsiflexion. If dorsiflexion does not appear to be limited, the test may be conducted with the knee extended.

Palpation. Palpate the tibialis anterior along its course from the lateral side of the tibia. The tendon is also palpated as it crosses the dorsum of the foot from the medial to the lateral side (Fig. 11–32).

Position
- AG: Subject sits with the knee flexed over the edge of the table. The ankle is in the anatomical position (Fig. 11–33).
- GM: Subject is in sidelying position with the test leg uppermost.

Movement. Dorsiflexion and inversion of the ankle.

Figure 11–31. Alternate standing position for testing the soleus muscle against gravity.

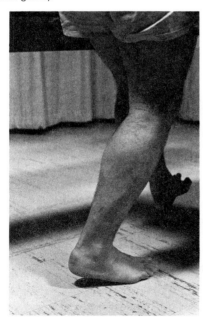

Figure 11–32. Palpating the tibialis anterior muscle.

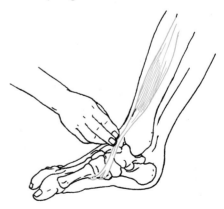

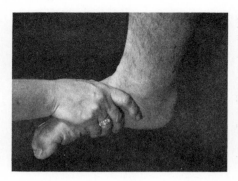

Figure 11–33. Testing the tibialis anterior muscle in the AG position.

Resistance. Applied to the medial dorsal aspect of the forefoot into plantar flexion and eversion.

Stabilization. The leg is stabilized.

Substitutions
- The extensor hallucis longus maintains the big toe in flexion.

Figure 11–34. Palpating the tibialis posterior muscle.

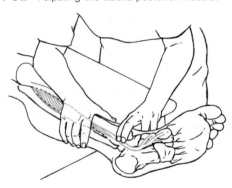

Figure 11–35. Testing the tibialis posterior muscle in the AG position.

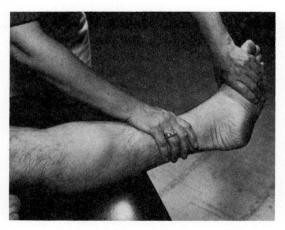

- The extensor digitorum longus dorsiflexes and everts.
- Tibialis posterior will invert without dorsiflexing.
- Together, posterior tibialis and extensor hallucis longus will produce dorsiflexion and inversion.
- The patient may quickly plantar flex, then relax.

Tibialis Posterior Muscle

The tibialis posterior muscle produces the motion of inversion in a plantar-flexed position through a test range of 20 degrees.

Palpation. Palpate the tibialis posterior tendon as it crosses the medial malleolus (Fig. 11–34).

Position
- AG: Subject is in sidelying position with the leg to be tested off the edge of the table (Fig. 11–35).
- GM: Subject lies supine with the foot over the edge of the table. The leg and ankle are in the anatomical position (Fig. 11–36).

Movement. Inversion of the foot while keeping the ankle in slight plantar flexion.

Resistance. Applied to the medial border of the forefoot into eversion and dorsiflexion.

Stabilization. The leg is stabilized.

Substitutions
- The ankle dorsiflexes as it inverts using the tibialis anterior muscle.
- The medial toe flexors contribute to inversion and plantar flexion; keep them relaxed.
- Gastrocnemius and soleus cause plantar flexion.
- Subject may quickly evert, then relax.

Figure 11–36. Testing the tibialis posterior muscle in the GM position.

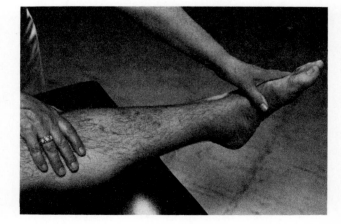

Attachments of Tibialis Posterior Muscle

Muscle	Proximal	Distal	Innervation
Tibialis posterior	Posterior surface of tibia, proximal two thirds posterior of fibula, and interosseous membrane	Tuberosity of navicular bone, tendinous expansion to other tarsals and metatarsals	Tibial L4 and L5

- Extensor hallucis longus is an accessory muscle to inversion, but not plantar flexion.
- Flexor hallucis longus, flexor hallucis brevis, and abductor hallucis muscles invert the forefoot.

Peroneus Longus, Peroneus Brevis, and Peroneus Tertius Muscles

The lateral compartment muscles and the peroneus tertius muscle produce the motion of eversion from a starting position of the ankle in the anatomical position through a test range of 20 degrees.

Palpation
- Palpate the tendon of the peroneus longus, and immediately distal to the lateral malleolus descending to the plantar surface of the foot. Because the two peronei tendons may not appear separated at this point, observe for depression of the great toe (Fig. 11–37).
- The peroneus brevis is covered by the peroneus longus muscle. However, the tendon immediately distal to the lateral malleolus is directed anteriorly toward the fifth metatarsal and is easily identified from the peroneus longus muscle (Fig. 11–38).

- Peroneus tertius may be absent. The tendon is a slip from the extensor digitorum longus muscle. If present, it is palpated laterally on the forefoot toward the fifth metatarsal.

Position
- AG: Subject is in sidelying position. The upper leg is the test leg, with the ankle in the anatomical position (Fig. 11–39).
- GM: Subject lies supine with the foot over the edge of the table and the ankle in the anatomical position (Fig. 11–40).

Movement. Eversion of the foot while maintaining the ankle in a neutral position.

Resistance. Applied to the lateral border of the forefoot.

Stabilization. The leg is stabilized.

Substitutions
- The extensor digitorum longus dorsiflexes the foot while everting.
- The flexor digitorum longus everts the foot, with some plantar flexion.

Figure 11–37. Palpating the peroneus longus muscle.

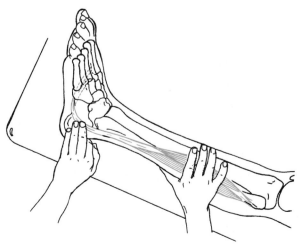

Figure 11–38. Palpating the peroneus brevis muscle.

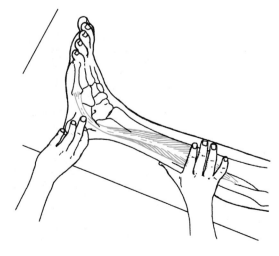

Attachments of Peroneus Longus, Brevis, and Tertius Muscles

Muscles	Proximal	Distal	Innervation
Peroneus longus	Lateral condyle of tibia, head and proximal two thirds of fibula	Base of first metatarsal and first cuneiform, lateral side	Superficial peroneal L5 and S1 (S2)
Peroneus brevis	Distal two thirds of lateral fibular shaft	Tuberosity of fifth metatarsal	Superficial peroneal L5 and S1 (S2)
Peroneus tertius	Lateral slip from extensor digitorum longus	Tuberosity of fifth metatarsal	Deep peroneal L5 and S1

· Subject may quickly invert the foot, then relax.
· The abductor digiti minimi everts the forefoot.

Digits

Because of the shortness of the digits, gravity is not an important factor in the function of the toe muscles. Therefore, all toes are tested with the patient sitting or supine, so that the subject can see the toes and observe the movements. The ankle is in the anatomical position.

Grades for the toes differ from the standard format because gravity is not considered a factor.

O: No contraction.
T or 1: Muscle contraction is palpated but no movement occurs.
P or 2: Subject can partially complete the range of motion.
F or 3: Subject can complete the test range.
G or 4: Subject can complete the test range, but is able to take less resistance on the test side than on the opposite side.

N or 5: Subject can complete the test range and take maximal resistance on the test side as compared with the normal side.

Flexor Hallucis Brevis and Longus Muscles

The flexor hallucis brevis and flexor hallucis longus muscles produce metatarsophalangeal joint flexion through a test range of 30 to 45 degrees and interphalangeal joint flexion through a test range of 90 degrees. The foot must be maintained in midposition.

Palpation
· Palpate the flexor hallucis brevis along the medial arch of the foot, adjacent to the first metatarsal head (Fig. 11–41).
· Palpate the flexor hallucis longus tendon as it crosses the plantar surface of the proximal phalanx of the great toe (Fig. 11–42).

Figure 11–39. Testing the peroneus longus and peroneus brevis muscles in the AG position.

Figure 11–40. Testing the peroneus longus and peroneus brevis muscles in the GM position.

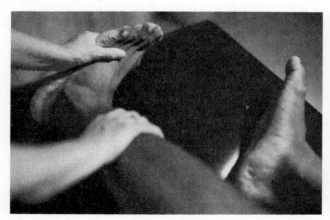

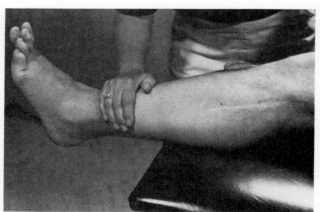

Attachments of Flexor Hallucis Brevis and Longus Muscles

Muscle	Proximal	Distal	Innervation
Flexor hallucis brevis	Plantar surface of cuboid and third cuneiform bones	Base of proximal phalanx of great toe	Medial plantar S3 (S2)
Flexor hallucis longus	Posterior distal two thirds fibula	Base of distal phalanx of great toe	Tibial S2 (S3)

Position.   Subject is sitting or supine (Figs. 11–43 and 11–44).

Movement.   Flexion of the metatarsophalangeal and interphalangeal joints.

Resistance.   Applied beneath the proximal and distal phalanx of the great toe.

Stabilization.   The foot is kept in the anatomical position and the first metatarsal is stabilized.

Substitutions
- The flexor hallucis longus flexes the interphalangeal and metatarsophalangeal joints.
- The subject may quickly extend the toe, then relax.

Flexor Digitorum Brevis and Longus Muscles

The flexor digitorum longus and brevis muscles produce interphalangeal joint flexion through a test range of 75 to 80 degrees. The motion is tested with the foot in the anatomical position. If the gastrocnemius muscle is

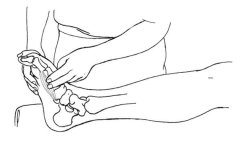

Figure 11–41.   Palpating the flexor hallucis brevis muscle.

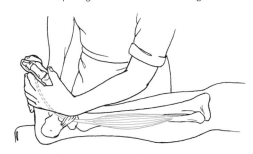

Figure 11–42.   Palpating the flexor hallucis longus muscle.

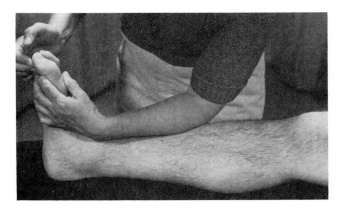

Figure 11–43.   Testing the flexor hallucis longus muscle.

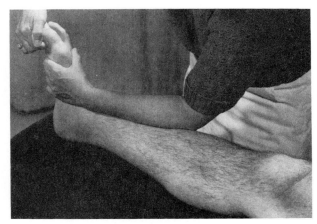

Figure 11–44.   Testing the flexor hallucis brevis muscle.

Attachments of Flexor Digitorum Brevis and Longus Muscles

Muscle	Proximal	Distal	Innervation
Flexor digitorum brevis	Tuberosity of calcaneus	One tendon slip into base of middle phalanx of each of the lateral four toes	Medial and lateral plantar S3 (S2)
Flexor digitorum longus	Middle three fifths of posterior tibia	Base of distal phalanx of lateral four toes	Tibial S2 (S3)

shortened preventing the ankle from assuming the anatomical position, the knee is flexed. The toes may be tested simultaneously.

Palpation
- The flexor digitorum brevis muscle is difficult to palpate. However, the tendon is palpable on the plantar surface of the proximal phalanx of each of the lateral four toes.
- Palpate the flexor digitorum longus tendons on the plantar surface of each middle phalanx of the lateral four toes (Fig. 11–45).

Position.   Subject is sitting or supine (Fig. 11–46).

Movement.   Flexion of the interphalangeal joints of the lateral four toes.

Resistance.   Applied beneath the distal and proximal phalanges. The toes may be tested simultaneously.

Stabilization.   The foot is held in the midposition and the metatarsals are stabilized.

Substitutions
- Alone, the flexor digitorum longus flexes all the joints of the toes.

Extensor Hallucis Longus and Brevis Muscles

The extensor hallucis longus and the extensor hallucis brevis muscles produce the motion of extension of the interphalangeal and metatarsophalangeal joints through a test range of 75 degrees of hyperextension at the metatarsophalangeal joint and from a flexed position to 0

Figure 11–45.   Palpating the flexor digitorum longus muscle.

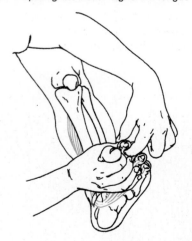

Figure 11–46.   Testing the flexor digitorum longus muscle.

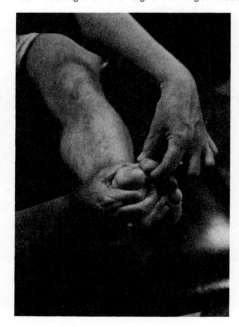

Attachments of Extensor Hallucis Longus and Brevis Muscles

Muscle	Proximal	Distal	Innervation
Extensor hallucis longus	Middle half of anterior shaft of fibula	Base of distal phalanx of great toe	Deep peroneal L5 and S1
Extensor hallucis brevis	Distal superior and lateral surfaces of calcaneus	Dorsal surface of proximal phalanx	Deep peroneal S1 and S2

degrees extension at the interphalangeal joint. The foot is maintained in midposition.

Palpation

- Palpate the extensor hallucis longus tendon on the dorsum of the foot, lateral to the tibialis anterior tendon and as it crosses the dorsum of the first metatarsal (Fig. 11–47).
- The extensor hallucis brevis muscle lies deep to the extensor digitorum longus tendons and is difficult to palpate. The tendon is a medial slip from the extensor digitorum brevis. Palpate the muscle belly on the dorsal lateral surface of the foot.

Position.   Subject is sitting or supine (Fig. 11–48).

Movement.   Extension of the metatarsophalangeal and interphalangeal joints of the first digit.

Resistance.   Applied to the dorsum of both phalanges of the first digit.

Stabilization.   The foot and the first metatarsal are stabilized.

Substitutions

- Plantar flexion of the ankle may stretch the extensor tendons and produce extension of the toes by tendon action.
- The subject may quickly flex the toe, then relax.

Extensor Digitorum Longus and Brevis Muscles

The extensor digitorum longus and the extensor digitorum brevis muscles produce the motion of extension at the metatarsophalangeal and interphalangeal joints of the lateral four digits from a flexed position. The test range for the metatarsophalangeal joints is to 45 degrees of hyperextension and that of the interphalangeal joints, to 0 degrees of extension. The foot is in the anatomical position.

Palpation

- Palpate the four tendons of the extensor digitorum longus as they cross the dorsolateral surface of the foot to each of the lateral four digits (Fig. 11–49).
- The extensor digitorum brevis tendons are difficult to palpate as they lie deep to the extensor digito-

Figure 11–47.   Palpating the extensor hallucis longus muscle.

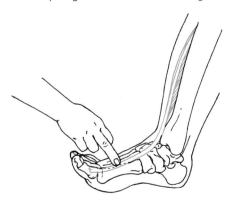

Figure 11–48.   Testing the extensor hallucis longus muscle.

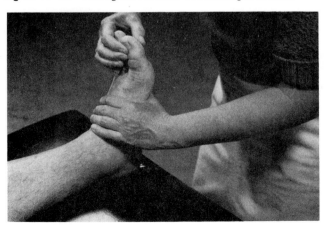

Attachments of Extensor Digitorum Longus and Brevis Muscles

Muscle	Proximal	Distal	Innervation
Extensor digitorum longus	Lateral condyle of tibia, proximal anterior surface of shaft of fibula	One tendon to each lateral four toes, to middle phalanx and extending to distal phalanges	Deep peroneal L5 and S1
Extensor digitorum brevis	Distal, superior surface of calcaneus	Dorsal surface of second through fourth toes, base of proximal phalanx	Deep peroneal S1 and S2

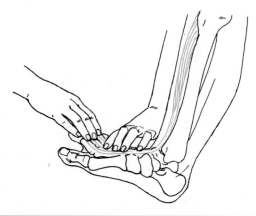

Figure 11–49. Palpating the extensor digitorum longus muscle.

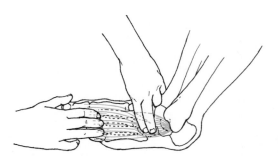

Figure 11–50. Palpating the extensor digitorum brevis muscle.

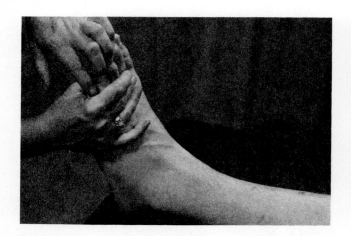

Figure 11–51. Testing the extensor digitorum longus muscle.

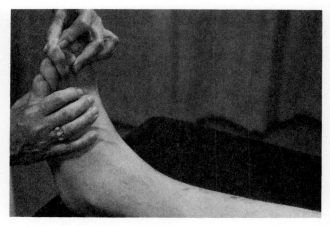

Figure 11–52. Testing the extensor digitorum brevis muscle.

Attachments of Abductor Hallucis Muscle

Muscle	Proximal	Distal	Innervation
Abductor hallucis	Tuberosity of calcaneus and plantar aponeurosis	Base of proximal phalanx, medial side	Medial plantar L5 and S1 (L4)

Attachments of Adductor Hallucis Muscle

Muscle	Proximal	Distal	Innervation
Adductor hallucis	Base of second, third, and fourth metatarsals and deep plantar ligaments	Proximal phalanx of first digit lateral side	Medial and lateral plantar S1 and S2

rum longus; however, the muscle belly is palpated on the dorsolateral surface of the foot. There is no tendon to the fifth digit (Fig. 11–50).

Position. Subject is sitting or supine (Figs. 11–51 and 11–52).

Movement. Extension of the metatarsophalangeal and interphalangeal joints of the lateral four digits.

Resistance. Applied to the dorsal surface of the proximal and distal phalanges.

Stabilization. The ankle and the metatarsals are stabilized.

Substitutions
- The toes deviate laterally as they extend using the extensor digitorum brevis.
- Plantar flexion of the ankle may stretch the extensor tendons and produce extension of the toes by tendon action.
- The subject may quickly flex the toes, then relax.

Intrinsic Muscles of the Foot

The intrinsic muscles of the foot are tested with the patient in either the supine or sitting position. Most subjects are unable to voluntarily contract the intrinsic muscles of the foot individually. The second digit and the second metatarsal are the reference structures for movements of the digits.

Abductor Hallucis Muscle

Palpation. Palpate the medial side of the first metatarsal.

Position. Subject is sitting or supine.

Movement. Abduction at the metatarsophalangeal joint of the first digit.

Resistance. Applied medially to the distal end of the first phalanx.

Stabilization. The metatarsals are stabilized.

Substitutions
- The first digit moves in the sagittal plane by using the flexor hallucis longus and brevis.
- The first digit moves in the sagittal plane by contracting the extensor hallucis longus and brevis.

Adductor Hallucis Muscle

Palpation. The muscle is too deep to palpate accurately.

Position. Subject is sitting or supine.

Movement. Adduction of the proximal phalanx of the first digit toward the second digit.

Resistance. Applied to the lateral side of the proximal phalanx of the first digit.

Stabilization. The metatarsals are stabilized.

Substitutions
- The first digit may flex or extend in the sagittal plane.
- Subject may abduct then relax, giving the appearance of adduction.

Attachments of Lumbrical Muscles

Muscle	Proximal	Distal	Innervation
Lumbricals	Medial and adjacent sides of flexor digitorum longus tendon to each lateral digit	Medial side of proximal phalanx and extensor hood	Medial and lateral plantar L5, S1, and S2 (L4)

Attachments of Plantar Interossei Muscles

Muscle	Proximal	Distal	Innervation
Plantar interossei			
First	Base and medial side of third metatarsal	Base of proximal phalanx and extensor hood of third digit	
Second	Base and medial side of fourth metatarsal	Base of proximal phalanx and extensor hood of fourth digit	Medial and lateral plantar S1 and S2
Third	Base and medial side of fifth metatarsal	Base of proximal phalanx and extensor hood of fifth digit	

Lumbrical Muscles

Palpation. The four muscles are too deep to palpate with accuracy.

Position. Subject is sitting or supine.

Movement. Extension of the interphalangeal joints and assistance in flexion of the metatarsophalangeal joints of the lateral four digits.

Resistance. Applied to the middle and distal phalanges of the lateral four digits.

Stabilization. The lateral four metatarsals are stabilized.

Substitutions
· The dorsal and plantar interossei assist in extension of the interphalangeal joints.

Plantar Interossei Muscles

Palpation. The three muscle bellies are too deep to palpate with accuracy; however, the tendinous expansion onto the medial side of the extensor hood of the lateral three digits is palpable.

Position. Subject is sitting or supine.

Movement. Extension of the interphalangeal joints of the lateral three digits. Adduction of the digits is not practical for most individuals.

Resistance. Applied to the middle and distal phalanges.

Stabilization. Stabilize the lateral three metatarsals.

Substitutions. Extension of the metatarsophalangeal joints of the lateral three digits can substitute by contracting the extensor digitorum longus and brevis.

Dorsal Interossei and Abductor Digiti Minimi Muscles

Palpation
· The muscle bellies of the four dorsal interossei are too deep to palpate with accuracy; however, the tendinous expansion onto the extensor hood of the middle three digits is palpable.
· Palpate the abductor digiti minimi along the lateral side of the fifth metatarsal.

Position. Subject is sitting or supine.

Movement. Extension of the interphalangeal joints and abduction at the metatarsophalangeal joints of the lateral four digits.

Attachments of Dorsal Interossei and Abductor Digiti Minimi Muscles

Muscle	Proximal	Distal	Innervation
Dorsal interossei			
First	First and second metatarsal bones	Proximal phalanx and extensor hood of second digit medially	
Second	Second and third metatarsal bones	Proximal phalanx and extensor hood of second digit laterally	Medial and lateral plantar S1 and S2
Third	Third and fourth metatarsal bones	Proximal phalanx and extensor hood of third digit laterally	
Fourth	Fourth and fifth metatarsal bones	Proximal phalanx and extensor hood of fourth digit laterally	
Abductor digiti minimi	Lateral side of fifth metatarsal bone	Proximal phalanx of fifth digit	Lateral plantar S1 and S2

Resistance

• Dorsal interossei: Applied to the middle and distal phalanges.
• Abductor digiti minimi: Applied to the lateral side of the proximal phalanx of the fifth digit.

Stabilization. The metatarsals are stabilized.

Substitutions. The extensor digitorum longus and brevis muscles extend the metatarsophalangeal joints of the middle digits.

Clinical Tests

Palpation

The structures and landmarks to be observed and/or palpated during assessment of the ankle and foot complex include:

1. Navicular tuberosity.
2. Sustentaculum tali.
3. Heads of the talus.
4. Medial malleolus.
5. Tarsal bones.
6. Base of the fifth metatarsal.
7. Lateral malleolus.

Active and Passive Movements and Contractile Testing

The motions of the ankle and foot that are assessed as part of the evaluation process for active and passive movements and contractile testing include:

1. Ankle dorsiflexion.
2. Ankle plantar flexion.
3. Triplanar inversion.
4. Triplanar eversion.
5. Metatarsophalangeal joint flexion.
6. Metatarsophalangeal joint extension.
7. Interphalangeal joint flexion.
8. Interphalangeal joint extension.

Special Tests

Drawer Test

Indication. The drawer test is performed on subjects who have sustained an ankle sprain or other trauma that could result in ankle instability. The integrity of the structures involved in preventing forward displacement of the tibia on the talus is assessed.

Method. The subject is supine or sitting. The test ankle is relaxed, and slightly in a plantar-flexed position. The examiner stabilizes the distal leg with one hand, while the other hand grips the calcaneus (Fig. 11–53). By pulling the calcaneus forward and causing it to impact the talus, the examiner attempts to displace the talus anteriorly.

Results. Straightforward displacement of the talus on the tibia indicates both medial and lateral ligament instability involving the superficial and deep deltoid ligaments, the anterior talofibular ligament, and the anterolateral capsule. If there is instability and laxity on one side only, then only that side will displace forward. For example, if only the lateral side is involved, the lateral talus will displace forward and internally, resulting in anterolateral rotatory instability of the ankle. The examiner may also feel a clunk as the talus slides from under cover of the ankle mortise.

Varus Stress Test

Indication. The varus stress test is used to assess the integrity of the lateral ligaments of the ankle (anterior and posterior talofibular and calcaneofibular).

Method. The subject is either seated or supine with the ankle in a relaxed slightly plantar-flexed position. The examiner stabilizes the lower leg and grips and inverts the calcaneus maximally (Fig. 11–54). The examiner should palpate all three lateral ligaments with the stabilizing hand as the inversion force is applied.

Results. Lateral gapping and rocking of the talus beneath the mortise indicates instability. All three ligaments must be lax or torn for gross instability to be present.

Valgus Stress Test (Kleiger's Test)

Indication. Valgus stress test assesses instability of the medial side of the ankle, most notably the deltoid ligament.

Method. The subject is positioned as for the varus stress test. The examiner stabilizes the lower leg with one hand and grips the calcaneus with the other (Fig. 11–55). A maximal eversion force is applied to the calcaneus as the lower leg is stabilized. The stabilizing hand should palpate over the deltoid ligament as the eversion force is applied.

Talar Tilt Test

Indication. The talar tilt test assesses the integrity of the calcaneofibular ligament.

Method. The subject is either supine or in a sidelying position with the foot relaxed. Maintaining the foot in an anatomical position brings the calcaneofibular liga-

Figure 11–53. Drawer test.

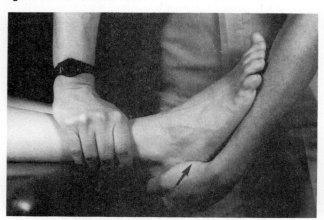

Figure 11–54. Varus stress test.

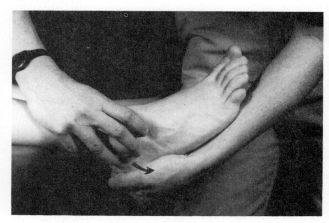

Figure 11–55. Valgus stress test.

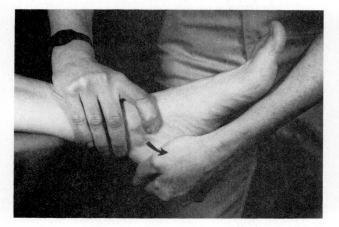

Figure 11–56. Talar tilt test.

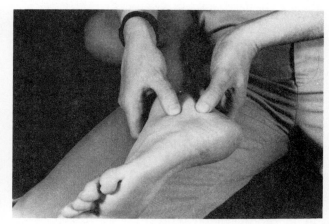

ment perpendicular to the long axis of the talus. The talus is then tilted into abduction and adduction (Fig. 11–56).

Results. Excessive tilting associated with adduction of the talus is associated with laxity or tearing of the calcaneofibular ligament, as it is in this position that the ligament is maximally stressed.

Thompson's Test

Indication. Thompson's test should always be performed when there is suspicion of an Achilles tendon rupture.

Method. The subject is prone, and the knee is flexed to 90 degrees. The examiner squeezes the calf of the leg being tested and observes the response (Fig. 11–57).

Results. Normally, when the calf with an intact gastrocsoleus muscle complex is squeezed, the response is one of passive plantar flexion. In the case of a ruptured Achilles tendon, there will be no associated plantar flexion as the calf is squeezed.

Homans' Sign

Indication. Homans' sign test is indicated in suspected cases of deep vein thrombosis.

Method. The subject may be tested supine, prone, or sitting. The examiner passively extends the knee and then dorsiflexes the ankle. The calf also may be palpated concurrently.

Results. Pain in the calf during ankle dorsiflexion is suggestive of thrombophlebitis, but it is important that other signs of inflammation be present in the calf area before this test is interpreted as positive. The examiner must also be aware that tightness of the gastrocnemius may be responsible for discomfort during this test. For this reason, both legs should be tested, and a distinction made between pain arising from a possible thrombophlebitis or that due to muscle tightness.

Posterior Tibial Reflex

Indication. The posterior tibial reflex is tested to evaluate the integrity of the L5 nerve root level.

Method. The subject lies supine with the test ankle crossed over and resting on the opposite leg. The ankle is placed in a position of mild dorsiflexion by the examiner. The examiner uses the pointed end of the reflex hammer to tap the posterior tibial tendon where it crosses behind the medial malleolus (Fig. 11–58).

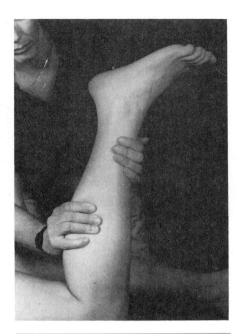

Figure 11–57. Thompson's test.

Results. A response of plantar flexion combined with inversion will be noted. This response should be compared with that in the opposite ankle in order to evaluate the normal response for that subject. A hyperactive reflex may indicate an upper motor neuron problem, whereas a hypoactive response may represent lower motor neuron pathology.

Achilles Tendon Reflex

Indication. The Achilles tendon reflex is assessed to determine the integrity of the S1 nerve root level.

Method. The Achilles tendon reflex can be tested with the subject prone, supine, or seated, although the

Figure 11–58. Posterior tibial reflex.

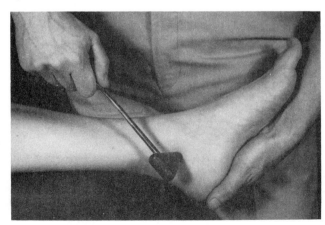

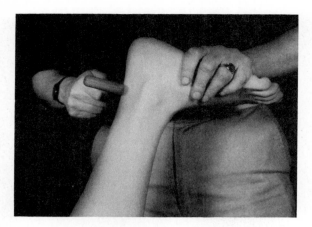

Figure 11–59.   Achilles tendon reflex.

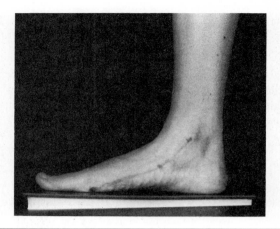

Figure 11–60.   Feiss line.

prone position is preferred. The examiner flexes the subject's knee approximately 90 degrees and applies gentle stretch to the ankle into dorsiflexion. It is important not to forcefully hold the ankle in dorsiflexion as this may mask the reflex response. As the gentle pressure into dorsiflexion is maintained, the examiner taps the Achilles tendon with the broad end of the reflex hammer (Fig. 11–59).

Results.   The normal response should be plantar flexion when the tendon is struck. The response of the involved ankle should be compared to that of the uninvolved ankle. Less response on the involved side represents a hypoactive reflex, whereas an exaggerated response is considered hyperactive.

Functional Tests

Indication.   Functional tests involving the foot and ankle are indicated when there is suspicion of weakness of the L5 or S1 musculature.

Method.   The subject stands for both tests. To assess the functional ability of the L5 musculature, have subject walk on the heels. The S1 musculature is tested by having the subject walk on the toes.

Results.   Inability to walk on the heels represents weakness or paralysis of the L5 musculature that controls dorsiflexion of the ankle. S1 weakness or paralysis of the ankle plantar flexors is manifested by the subject's inability to walk on tiptoe.

Feiss Line

Indication.   The Feiss line serves as a gross means of assessing pronation of the foot, manifested by a flattening of the medial longitudinal arch. The relative position of the navicular tuberosity in the weight-bearing and non–weight-bearing positions is examined.

Method.   The subject is examined both standing and seated, with approximately 3 to 6 inches between the

feet. A line is drawn from the tip of the medial malleolus to the plantar aspect of the first metatarsophalangeal joint (Fig. 11–60).

Results.   Ideally, the navicular tuberosity should lie on or very close to the line drawn. If the navicular falls one third of the distance to the floor, the condition is referred to as first-degree flatfoot. If the navicular falls two thirds of the distance to the floor, the condition represents second-degree flatfoot. If it rests on the floor, the condition is third-degree flatfoot. The Feiss line should be assessed with the patient in both weight-bearing and non–weight-bearing postures, as it is an indication of the rigidity of flatfoot and of whether the subject will be able to wear orthotics.

Joint Play (Accessory Movement)

Talocrural Joint

Distraction (Fig. 11–61)

Restriction.   General hypomobility.

Figure 11–61.   Distraction of the talocrural joint.

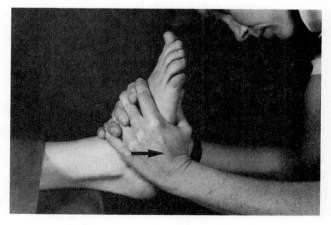

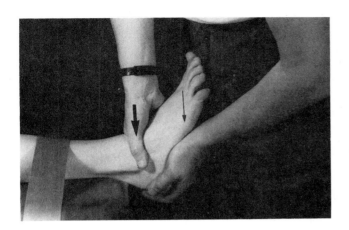

Figure 11–62. Dorsal glide of the talus.

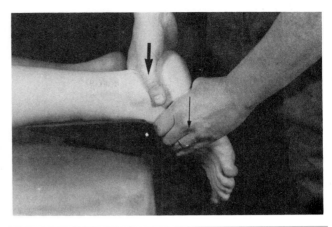

Figure 11–63. Ventral glide of the talus.

Open-Packed Position. 10 degrees of ankle plantar flexion; midway between inversion and eversion.

Positioning. The subject lies supine with the distal leg stabilized by a strap. The examiner stands at the end of the table facing the subject. The examiner clasps the hands together and places them on the dorsum of the foot with the ulnar borders on the talus as close to the joint line as possible.

Movement. The examiner applies a distraction force to the subject's talus. The focus of the application of the force is through the medial aspect of the examiner's hands.

Dorsal Glide (Fig. 11–62)

Restriction. Dorsiflexion.

Positioning. Subject lies supine with the distal leg placed at the edge of the table and stabilized with a strap. The examiner places the mobilizing hand with the web space on the dorsum of the foot over the anterior talus. The other hand cups the calcaneus to provide support and to maintain the open packed position.

Movement. The examiner directs a posterior force through the web space to the subject's anterior talus.

Ventral Glide (Fig. 11–63)

Restriction. Plantar flexion.

Positioning. The subject lies prone with the distal leg at the edge of the table and stabilized by a wedge beneath it. The examiner places the web space of the mobilizing hand on the posterior aspect of the foot over the Achilles tendon, with the thumb and index fingers below the respective malleoli on the talus. The other hand grasps the proximal foot to provide support and to maintain the open packed position.

Movement. The examiner applies a ventral force to the posterior aspect of the talus.

Subtalar Joint

Distraction (Fig. 11–64)

Restriction. General hypomobility.

Open-Packed Position. Midway between inversion and eversion.

Positioning. The subject lies prone with a wedge or small roll beneath the talus for stabilization. The examiner places one hand on the anterior surface of the subject's leg for additional stability. The mobilizing hand is placed so that the heel and palm cup the calcaneus.

Movement. The examiner applies an inferior or distraction force to the patient's calcaneus.

Distal Glide (Fig. 11–65)

Restriction. General hypomobility.

Positioning. Same as for distraction.

Movement. The examiner applies a distal force along the long axis of the foot to the subject's calcaneus.

Figure 11–64. Distraction of the subtalar joint.

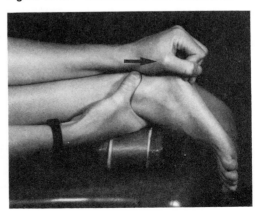

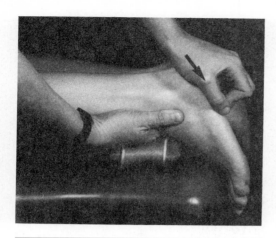

Figure 11–65. Distal glide of the calcaneus.

Midtarsal Joint

Talonavicular Joint

Dorsal and Plantar Glide (Fig. 11–66)

Restriction. General hypomobility.

Open-Packed Position. Anatomical position.

Positioning. The subject may be either supine or long-sitting, with the knee joint flexed. The examiner places the thumb, web space, and index finger of the stabilizing hand over the medial aspect of the talus. The thumb and index finger of the mobilizing hand are placed on the plantar and dorsal surfaces of the navicular.

Movement. The examiner applies a dorsal-plantar force to the navicular in the direction of hypomobility.

Calcaneocuboid Joint

Dorsal and Plantar Glide (Fig. 11–67)

Restriction. General hypomobility.

Open Packed Position. Anatomical position.

Positioning. The subject may be either supine or long sitting, with the knee joint flexed. The examiner grasps the calcaneus with one hand to provide stabilization. The thumb and index finger of the mobilizing hand are placed on the plantar and dorsal surfaces of the cuboid.

Movement. The examiner applies a dorsal-plantar force to the cuboid in the direction of hypomobility.

Tarsometatarsal Joints

Distraction (Fig. 11–68)

Restriction. General hypomobility.

Open-Packed Position. Anatomical position.

Positioning. The subject's foot is placed on a stabilizing wedge, so that the tarsal bone that articulates with the metatarsal being examined is stabilized. The examiner places one hand over the dorsum of the tarsal bone on the wedge to provide additional support. The mobilizing hand is placed with the thumb and fingers gripping the metatarsal on the dorsal and plantar surfaces.

Movement. The examiner applies a distraction force to the metatarsal.

Plantar Glide (Fig. 11–69)

Restriction. General hypomobility.

Positioning. The subject lies supine or sits. The metatarsal adjacent to the one being treated is placed on the stabilizing wedge. The examiner places one hand on the dorsum of the foot over the metatarsal on the wedge to provide additional support. The thenar eminence of the other hand is placed on the dorsal surface of the metatarsal being treated.

Figure 11–66. (A) Dorsal and (B) plantar glide of the navicular.

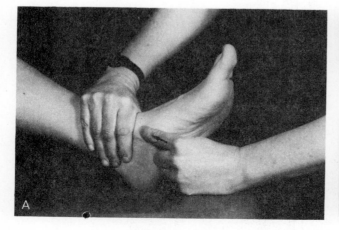
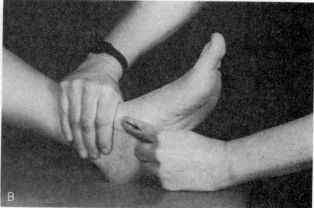

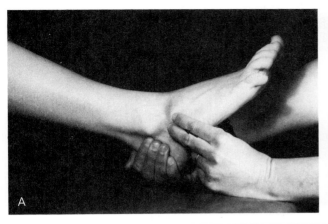 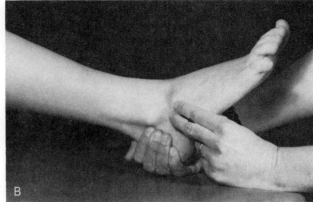

Figure 11–67.   (*A*) Dorsal and (*B*) plantar glide of the cuboid.

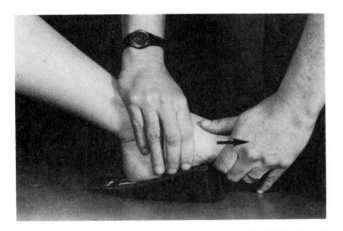

Figure 11–68.   Distraction of the tarsometatarsal joints.

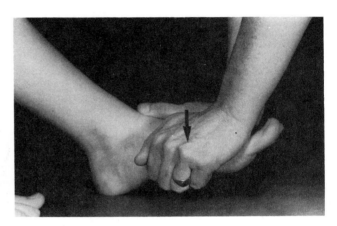

Figure 11–69.   Plantar glide of the tarsal bones.

Movement.   The examiner applies a plantar force through the metatarsal. This mobilization is not only for tarsometatarsal restrictions but is also effective for inter-metatarsal mobility.

First Metatarsophalangeal Joint

Distraction (Fig. 11–70)

Restriction.   General hypomobility.

Open-Packed Position.   5 to 10 degrees of metacarpophalangeal extension.

Positioning.   The subject may be either supine or sitting. The examiner stabilizes the first metatarsal by grasping it between the thenar eminence and the four fingers. The thumb and index finger of the mobilizing hand grip the dorsal and plantar surfaces of the proximal phalanx.

Movement.   The examiner applies a distraction force to the proximal phalanx.

Plantar Glide (Fig. 11–71)

Restriction.   Flexion.

Positioning.   The subject is sitting or supine. A stabilizing wedge is placed beneath the first metatarsal. The examiner puts one hand around the subject's foot on the wedge to provide additional stabilization. The thumb and index finger of the mobilizing hand are placed on the dorsal and plantar surfaces of the proximal phalanx.

Movement.   The examiner applies a force to the proximal phalanx in the plantar direction.

Dorsal Glide (Fig. 11–72)

Restriction.   Extension.

Positioning.   The subject lies prone. A stabilizing wedge is placed beneath the first metatarsal. The examiner puts one hand around the subject's foot on the wedge to provide additional stabilization. The thumb and index finger of the mobilizing hand are placed on the dorsal and plantar surfaces of the proximal phalanx.

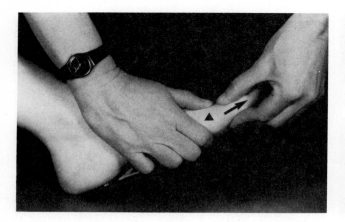

Figure 11–70.   Distraction of the first metatarsophalangeal joint.

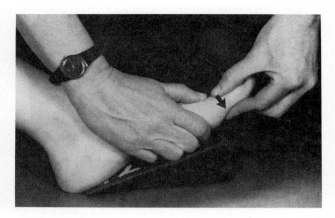

Figure 11–71.   Plantar glide of the proximal phalanx of the great toe.

Movement.   The examiner applies a force to the proximal phalanx in the dorsal direction.

Second to Fifth Metatarsophalangeal Joints and All Interphalangeal Joints

Distraction and Plantar and Dorsal Glide (Fig. 11–73)

Restriction.   General hypomobility, flexion, extension.

Open-Packed Position.   Slight flexion.

Positioning.   The subject lies supine. The examiner stabilizes the proximal articulating bone with one hand. The other mobilizing hand is placed on the distal articulating bone as close to the joint line as possible.

Movement.   The examiner applies a distraction force to the distal articulating bone for general hypomobility. A plantar force is given restrictions in flexion, and a dorsal force for limitations in extension.

Tarsal Bone Mobility Testing

Kaltenborn has described a sequential method of assessing the mobility of the individual carpal bones. The approach to examination of the tarsal area is as follows (Fig. 11–74):

1. Stabilize the second and third cuneiforms and mobilize the third metatarsal.
2. Stabilize the second and third cuneiforms and mobilize the second metatarsal.
3. Stabilize the first cuneiform and mobilize the first metatarsal.
4. Stabilize the navicular and mobilize the first, second, and third cuneiforms.
5. Stabilize the talus and mobilize the navicular.
6. Stabilize the cuboid and mobilize the fourth and fifth metatarsals.

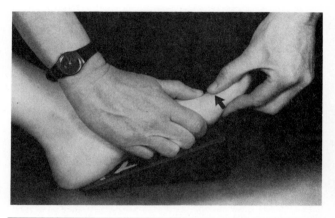

Figure 11–72.   Dorsal glide of the proximal phalanx of the great toe.

7. Stabilize the navicular and cuneiform and mobilize the cuboid.
8. Stabilize the calcaneus and mobilize the cuboid.
9. Stabilize the talus and mobilize the calcaneus.
10. Stabilize the talus and mobilize the tibia and fibula.

Summary of Joint Play of Ankle and Foot

Table 11–1 provides a summary of joint play in the ankle and foot.

Biomechanical Examination of the Foot and Ankle

The examiner's ability to perform an accurate biomechanical examination of the foot and ankle complex is the key to successful management of pathologies involving the lower quarter. Because of the biomechanical in-

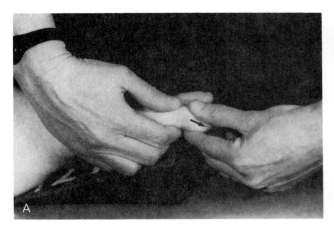
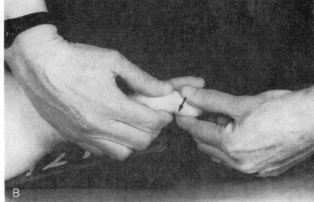
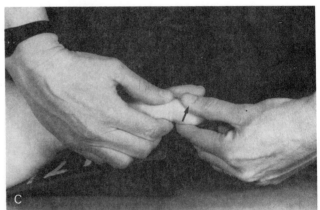

Figure 11–73. (*A*) Distraction of interphalangeal joints. (*B*) Plantar and (*C*) dorsal glide of the distal phalanx.

timacy of the structures that comprise the lower quarter, the examination process involves not only the foot and ankle, but also the pelvis, hip, femur, knee, tibia, and fibula in weight-bearing and non–weight-bearing positions.

The examination of the foot at rest, or in the non–weight-bearing position, is performed in order to determine structural or functional ability and prevent any compensation of the foot. The stance phase or weight-bearing portion of the examination indicates the amount of compensation that occurs for structural abnormalities. The examination process may be organized effectively by grouping the assessment procedures according to the subject's position, as follows:

Supine Examination

1. Hip Rotation. Hip rotation should be tested in various positions of hip and knee flexion to determine whether restriction of motion is due to soft tissue tightness or to a bony deformity. If the available range of motion changes with the alteration of hip and knee position, the limitation is a result of soft tissue tightness. If the amount of hip rotation remains consistent regard-

Figure 11–74. Dorsal view of the anatomical relationships of the tarsal bones.

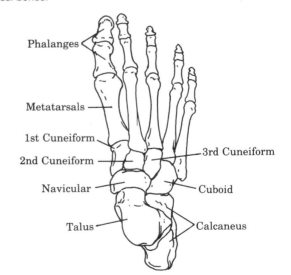

Phalanges

Metatarsals

1st Cuneiform

2nd Cuneiform

3rd Cuneiform

Navicular

Cuboid

Talus

Calcaneus

Table 11–1.   Summary of Joint Play of the Ankle and Foot Complex

GLIDE	RESTRICTION	FIXED BONE	MOVING BONE
Talocrural Joint			
Distraction	General hypomobility	Tibia	Talus
Ventral	Plantar flexion	Tibia	Talus
Dorsal	Dorsiflexion	Tibia	Talus
Subtalar Joint			
Distraction	General hypomobility	Talus	Calcaneus
Distal	General hypomobility	Talus	Calcaneus
Midtarsal Joint: Talonavicular			
Ventral	General hypomobility	Talus	Navicular
Dorsal	General hypomobility	Talus	Navicular
Midtarsal Joint: Calcaneocuboid			
Ventral	General hypomobility	Calcaneus	Cuboid
Dorsal	General hypomobility	Calcaneus	Cuboid
Metatarsophalangeal Joints			
Distraction	General hypomobility	Respective metatarsal	Respective proximal phalanx
Plantar	Flexion	Respective metatarsal	Respective proximal phalanx
Dorsal	Extension	Respective metatarsal	Respective proximal phalanx
Interphalangeal Joints			
Distraction	General hypomobility	Respective proximal phalanx	Respective distal phalanx
Plantar	Flexion	Respective proximal phalanx	Respective distal phalanx
Dorsal	Extension	Respective proximal phalanx	Respective distal phalanx

less of hip and knee position, the limitation is secondary to a bony restriction.

2. Hip and Knee Flexion.   The ranges of hip and knee flexion are assessed and recorded.

3. Flexibility Testing.   Flexibility testing should be performed for the hip flexor musculature (Thomas's test), hamstring musculature (straight leg raise), and the tensor muscle and iliotibial band (Ober's test).

4. Leg-Length Discrepancy.   Measurement of leg length should be performed in weight-bearing and non–weight-bearing positions in order to determine whether a discrepancy exists. Testing should be done for both true and apparent leg-length discrepancy.

5. Torsional Relationships.   Determination of femoral anteversion-retroversion is performed by palpating the greater trochanter and then rotating the hip until the greater trochanter is in its most lateral position. In this position, the femoral condyles are examined and a conclusion is drawn. Normally, with the greater trochanter located in its most lateral position, the femoral condyles should lie completely in the frontal plane. If the lateral femoral condyle lies anterior to the medial femoral condyle, femoral anteversion exists. Femoral retroversion is assessed when the medial condyle lies anterior to the lateral one.

An alternate method of assessment is to place the femoral condyles flat on the examining table in the frontal plane and, with the thigh in this position, to palpate the greater trochanter. Femoral anteversion is present when the greater trochanter is located posterior to its most lateral position. Femoral retroversion is identified when the greater trochanter is palpated anterior to its most lateral position.

Malleolar torsion, a transverse plane measurement, ranges from 13 to 18 degrees of external tibial rotation in normal persons. Measurement of malleolar torsion is

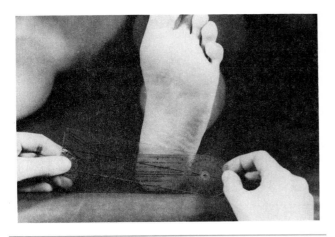

Figure 11–75. Measurement of malleolar torsion.

performed with the subject supine and the femoral condyles in the frontal plane. An angle made by an imaginary line connecting the apices of the malleoli and a line parallel to the floor represents the amount of malleolar torsion (Fig. 11–75). Malleolar torsion greater than 18 degrees results in a toe-out gait, while a value less than 13 degrees produces a toe-in gait. Both of these deformities cause abnormal pronation.

6. Foot Motion. Assess calcaneal inversion-eversion and note the amount of forefoot motion with the calcaneus both inverted and everted.

7. First Ray and Fifth Ray Mobility. The first and fifth metatarsals normally should lie in the same plane as the other metatarsals. If the first or fifth metatarsal lies in a plane superior to the other metatarsals, a dorsiflexed first ray is evident. Conversely, a plantar flexed first or fifth ray is identified when the respective metatarsal lies in a plane inferior to the rest of the metatarsals.

Measurement of the range of motion of the first or fifth ray is considered normal when there is as much movement of the ray into dorsiflexion as there is into plantar flexion from its neutral position. A ray with more dorsiflexion than plantar flexion from the neutral position is termed a dorsiflexed ray, while one with more plantar flexion than dorsiflexion is called a plantar flexed ray.

8. Hallux Dorsiflexion. From 60 to 70 degrees of hallux dorsiflexion is necessary for normal push-off during gait; therefore assessment of the available motion is important. Goniometry should be performed in both non–weight-bearing and weight-bearing positions.

Prone Examination

1. Ankle Dorsiflexion and Plantar Flexion. The range of ankle dorsiflexion and plantar flexion should be assessed with the knee flexed as well as extended. Normal

gait requires 10 degrees of talocrural dorsiflexion with the knee in both flexion and extension. If the available amount of dorsiflexion is less than 10 degrees as measured from the neutral position, the deformity is recognized as ankle equinus and is compensated by pronation at the subtalar joint. The normal range of plantar flexion is 0 to 45 degrees, but this fact is not significant in the biomechanical examination.

2. Measurement of Hindfoot and Forefoot Motion. The examination and assessment of the hindfoot and forefoot should be done with the limb in the frontal plane. The frontal plane position is achieved by having the subject flex, abduct, and externally rotate the opposite hip and by placing the foot on the dorsal surface of the limb being examined (Fig. 11–76).

Before beginning actual examination of the foot, one must identify certain osseous landmarks. These landmarks include the distal third of the leg, the vertical borders of the calcaneus, and the plantar calcaneal border. After these landmarks have been identified, markings are made on the subject with a skin pencil. One line bisecting the distal third of the leg is drawn on the patient. It is important not to use the Achilles tendon as the midline, as this structure usually does not lie centrally. Another line is made representing the bisection of the calcaneus (Fig. 11–77).

3. Subtalar Joint Neutral. The examiner holds the fourth and fifth metatarsal heads with one hand and palpates the talar heads with the other hand. While palpating the talar heads, the examiner gently dorsiflexes the fourth and fifth metatarsal heads to the point of slight resistance. This bending ensures locking of the forefoot

Figure 11–76. Prone position for examining foot biomechanics.

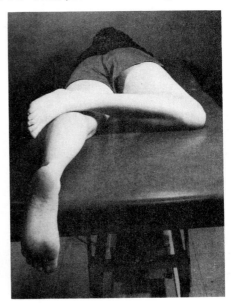

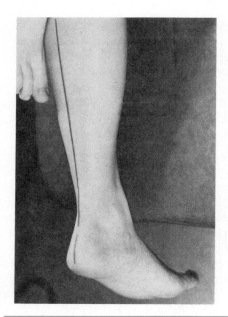

Figure 11–77. Bisection of leg and calcaneus.

when the subtalar joint is in the neutral position. As dorsiflexion of the metatarsal heads is maintained, the foot is moved medially and laterally until congruence of the talar heads is apparent or neither head is prominent (Fig. 11–78). This position is identified as the subtalar joint neutral position of the foot.

Another method of distinguishing subtalar joint neutral position is to observe the concavities superior and inferior to the lateral malleolus. When both concavities appear symmetrical and equal in size, the subtalar joint is in the neutral position. Subtalar neutral is that position where the foot is neither pronated nor supinated and where maximal function can occur.

Goniometry of subtalar neutral is performed with one arm of the goniometer aligned with the bisection of the distal third of the leg and the other arm aligned with the

bisection of the calcaneus. Ideally, there should be a vertical line or a 0-degree relationship. If the calcaneus is inverted relative to the tibia in the subtalar joint neutral position, the condition is defined as hindfoot varus. If the calcaneus is everted relative to the tibia in the subtalar joint neutral position, the condition is termed hindfoot valgus.

Goniometry of maximal hindfoot pronation and supination should also be performed, as measurement will provide an indication of the patient's ability to compensate for hindfoot and forefoot problems. Measuring from the subtalar joint neutral position, the normal subtalar range of motion is twice as much supination or inversion as pronation or eversion.

4. Forefoot to Hindfoot Assessment. While maintaining the hindfoot in subtalar joint neutral position, the examiner compares the forefoot and hindfoot relationship. Normally, the metatarsal heads lie in the same plane as the plantar calcaneal border. Goniometric measurement is performed with one arm of the goniometer parallel to the plane of the metatarsal heads and the other parallel to the plane of the bisected plantar border of the calcaneus (Fig. 11–79). Ideally, the forefoot and hindfoot lie on a straight line. Inversion of the forefoot with respect to the hindfoot is termed forefoot varus; eversion of the forefoot with respect to the hindfoot is called forefoot valgus.

Static Standing Examination

1. Posture. A postural examination should be carried out with the subject standing and the feet maintained in subtalar joint neutral, as well as in the compensated, or relaxed, posture, in order to assess the influence of extrinsic factors causing abnormal foot mechanics (Chapter 3).

2. Tibia Varum. The subject stands with the subtalar joints of the feet maintained in subtalar neutral. One arm

Figure 11–78. Subtalar neutral position.

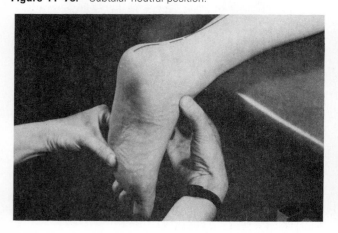

Figure 11–79. Forefoot to rear foot measurement.

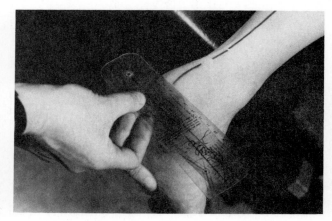

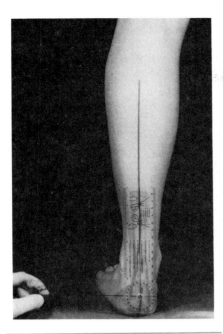

Figure 11–80. Measurement of tibia varum.

of the goniometer is aligned with the bisection of the lower third of the leg. The other arm is parallel to the table or floor (Fig. 11–80). Normal tibia varum falls in the range of 0 to 2 degrees. Tibia varum should also be assessed with the feet in the relaxed, comfortable, compensated posture.

3. Hallux Dorsiflexion. Hallux dorsiflexion is assessed in the standing position by maximally lifting the heel off the table while keeping the first metatarsophalangeal joint and great toe on the table. Normally, 90 or more degrees of hallux dorsiflexion is available in this position as a result of plantar flexion of the first ray.

Dynamic Evaluation. The subject is observed walking, while gait is evaluated. Particular attention should be paid to assessing calcaneal motion, especially at heel strike; foot abduction or adduction; weight transfer between limbs; and tibial position.

Bibliography

Backhouse KM, Hutchings RT: Color Atlas of Surface Anatomy. Baltimore, Williams & Wilkins, 1986

Bateman J, Trott A (eds): The Foot and Ankle. New York, Thieme-Stratton, 1980

Corrigan B, Maitland GD: Practical Orthopedic Medicine. Boston, Butterworth, 1983

Daniels L, Worthingham C: Muscle Testing Techniques of Manual Examination. Philadelphia, WB Saunders, 1986

Gould JA III, Davies GG (eds): Orthopedic and Sports Physical Therapy. St Louis, CV Mosby, 1985

Hollinshead WH, Jenkins DB: Functional Anatomy of the Limbs and Back. Philadelphia, WB Saunders, 1981

Hoppenfeld S: Physical Examination of the Spine and Extremities. New York, Appleton-Century-Crofts, 1976

Jackson DW, Drez D Jr: The Anterior Cruciate Deficient Knee: New Concepts in Ligament Repair. St Louis, CV Mosby, 1987

Kaltenborn M: Mobilization of the Extremity Joints. Oslo, Bygdoy Alle, 1980

Kendall FP, McCreary EK: Muscle Testing and Function. Baltimore, Williams & Wilkins, 1983

Kessler R, Hertling D: Management of Common Musculoskeletal Disorders. Philadelphia, Harper & Row, 1983

Kisner C, Colby LA: Therapeutic Foundations: Foundations and Techniques. Philadelphia, FA Davis, 1985

Losee RE: Diagnosis of chronic injury to the anterior cruciate ligament. Orthoped Clin of North Am 16:1, 1985

Magee DJ: Orthopedic Physical Assessment. Philadelphia, WB Saunders, 1987

Maitland GD: The Peripheral Joints: Examination and Recording Guide. Adelaide, Australia, Virgo Press, 1973

Norkin CC, White DJ: Measurement of Joint Motion: A Guide to Goniometry. Philadelphia, FA Davis, 1985

Saunders DH: Evaluation, Treatment, and Prevention of Musculoskeletal Disorders. Minneapolis, H Duane Saunders, 1985

Schneider RC, Kennedy JC, Plant ML: Sports Injuries: Mechanisms, Prevention, and Treatment. Baltimore, Williams & Wilkins, 1985

Subotnick S: Pediatric Sports Medicine. Mount Kisco, NY, Futura Publishing, 1975

Turek SL: Orthopedics: Principles and Their Application, vol. 2. Philadelphia, JB Lippincott, 1984

Williams P, Warwick R (eds): Gray's Anatomy, 36th British ed. Philadelphia, WB Saunders, 1980

Appendices

Appendix A: Recording Forms for Use in Physical Therapy Assessment Procedures

Range of Motion Record

Upper Limbs

Name: _____

					LEFT							RIGHT			
					EXAMINER										
					DATE										
					SHOULDER										
					Flexion	0–180									
					Extension	180–0									
					Hyperextension	0–45									
					Abduction	0–180									
					Medial rotation	0–65									
					Lateral rotation	0–90									
					Horizontal adduction	0–120									
					Horizontal abduction	0–30									
					SCAPULA										
					Upward rotation										
					Downward rotation										
					Abduction										
					Adduction										
					ELBOW										
					Flexion	0–145									
					Extension	145–0									
					RADIOULNAR										
					Supination	0–90									
					Pronation	0–90									
					WRIST										
					Flexion	0–90									
					Extension	90–0									
					Hyperextension	0–70									
					Abduction	0–25									
					Adduction	0–35									

Range of Motion Record (continued)

Upper Limbs

Name: _____

						LEFT ... RIGHT							

LEFT   RIGHT

						EXAMINER						
						DATE						
						THUMB						
					Flexion MP	0–50						
					Extension MP	50–0						
					Flexion IP	0–80						
					Extension IP	80–0						
					Hyperextension IP	0–90						
					Flexion CMC	30–15						
					Extension CMC	0–70						
					Opposition CMC							
					Abduction CMC	0–60						
					Adduction CMC	60–0						
					Hyperextension MP	0–10						
					SECOND DIGIT						
					Flexion MP	0–90						
					Extension MP	90–0						
					Hyperextension MP	0–30						
					Flexion PIP	0–120						
					Extension PIP	120–0						
					Flexion DIP	0–80						
					Extension DIP	80–120						
					Abduction MCP	0–20						
					Adduction MCP	20–0						
					Hyperextension DIP	0–10						
					THIRD DIGIT						
					Flexion MP	0–90						
					Extension MP	90–0						
					Hyperextension MP	0–30						
					Flexion PIP	0–120						
					Extension PIP	120–0						
					Flexion DIP	0–80						
					Extension DIP	80–0						
					Abduction MCP	0–20						
					Adduction MCP	20–0						
					Hyperextension DIP	0—10						

Range of Motion Record (continued)

Upper Limbs

Name: _____

						LEFT ... RIGHT					
					EXAMINER						
					DATE						
					FOURTH DIGIT						
					Flexion MP	0–90					
					Extension MP	90–0					
					Hyperextension MP	0–30					
					Flexion PIP	0–120					
					Extension PIP	120–0					
					Flexion DIP	0–80					
					Extension DIP	80–0					
					Abduction MCP	0–20					
					Adduction MCP	20–0					
					Hyperextension DIP	0–10					
					FIFTH DIGIT						
					Flexion MP	0–90					
					Extension MP	90–0					
					Hyperextension MP	0–30					
					Flexion PIP	0–120					
					Extension PIP	120–0					
					Flexion DIP	0–80					
					Extension DIP	80–0					
					Abduction MCP	0–20					
					Adduction MCP	20–0					
					Hyperextension DIP	0–10					

REMARKS:

Key: The anatomical position is considered zero and is the starting position for all measurements with the exception of rotation at the shoulder (shoulder is abducted 90 degrees).

Passive motion is recorded unless notation of active motion is made.

Use black pen to record patient's normal range.
Use red pen to record limited range.

Range of Motion Record (continued)

Lower Limbs

Name:												
		LEFT						RIGHT				
					EXAMINER							
					DATE							
					HIP							
					Flexion	0–125						
					Extension	125–0						
					Hyperextension	0–10						
					Abduction	0–45						
					Adduction	0–20						
					Medial rotation	0–45						
					Lateral rotation	0–45						
					KNEE							
					Flexion	0–130						
					Extension	130–0						
					ANKLE							
					Dorsiflexion	0–20						
					Plantar flexion	0–45						
					Inversion	0–30						
					Eversion	0–25						
					FIRST DIGIT							
					Flexion MP	0–45						
					Extension MP	45–0						
					Hyperextension	0–90						
					Flexion IP	0–90						
					Extension IP	90–0						
					LATERAL DIGITS							
					Flexion MP	0–40						
					Extension MP	40–0						
					Hyperextension MP	0–45						
					Flexion PIP	0–35						
					Extension PIP	35–0						
					Flexion DIP	0–60						
					Extension DIP	60–0						

Manual Muscle Testing Record

Upper Limbs

LEFT					RIGHT	
			EXAMINER			
			DATE			
			Upper Limb			
			CN XI—Upper trapezius	Spinal accessory		
			C3–5—Levator scapulae	Dorsal scapular		
			CN XI—Middle trapezius	Spinal accessory		
			CN XI—Lower trapezius	Spinal accessory		
			C4 & 5—Rhomboid major & minor	Dorsal scapular		
			C6 & 7—Serratus anterior	Long thoracic		
			C7—Pectoralis minor	Medial & lateral pectoral		
			C5—Anterior deltoid	Axillary		
			C6—Coracobrachialis	Musculocutaneous		
			C6 & 7—Latissimus dorsi	Thoracodorsal		
			C6—Teres major	Lower subscapular		
			C5—Supraspinatus	Suprascapular		
			C5—Middle deltoid	Axillary		
			C5—Posterior deltoid	Axillary		
			C6—Pectoralis major (clavicular) C7 & 8—(sternal)	Lateral & medial pectoral		
			C5—Infraspinatus & teres minor	Axillary		
			C6—Subscapularis	Upper and lower subscapular		

Manual Muscle Testing Record (continued)

Upper Limbs

Name:								
LEFT						RIGHT		
			EXAMINER					
			DATE					
			Upper Limb					
			C7—Pronator teres		Median			
			C6—Supinator		Radial			
			C6—Biceps brachii		Musculocutaneous			
			C6—Brachialis		Musculocutaneous & radial			
			C6—Brachioradialis		Radial			
			C7 & 8—Triceps		Radial			
			C8—Palmaris longus		Median			
			C8—Flexor carpi ulnaris		Ulnar			
			C7—Flexor carpi radialis		Median			
			C8—1 Flexor digitorum profundus	1	Median			
			2	2	Median			
			3	3	Ulnar			
			4	4	Ulnar			
			C8—1 Flexor digitorum superficialis	1	Median			
			2	2	Median			
			3	3	Median			
			4	4	Median			
			C8—Extensor carpi ulnaris		Radial			
			C6 & 7—Extensor carpi radialis longus (brevis)		Radial			
			C8—Extensor pollicis longus		Radial			
			C8—Extensor pollicis brevis		Radial			
			C8—Abductor pollicis longus		Radial			
			C8—Abductor pollicis brevis		Median			
			C8—Flexor pollicis brevis		Median & ulnar			
			C8—Opponens pollicis		Median			
			C8—Abductor pollicis		Ulnar			
			C8—Flexor pollicis longus		Median			
			C8—Extensor indicis		Radial			
			C7—1 Extensor digitorum	1	Radial			
			2	2	Radial			
			3	3	Radial			
			4	4	Radial			

Manual Muscle Testing Record (continued)

Upper Limbs

Name: _____

							LEFT / RIGHT						
					EXAMINER								
					DATE								
					Upper Limb								
					T1—1 Lumbricals	1	Median						
					2	2	Median						
					T1– 3	3	Ulnar						
					4	4	Ulnar						
					T1—1 Dorsal interossei	1	Ulnar						
					2	2	Ulnar						
					3	3	Ulnar						
					4	4	Ulnar						
					T1—1 Palmar interossei	1	Ulnar						
					2	2	Ulnar						
					3	3	Ulnar						
					T1—Opponens digiti minimi		Ulnar						
					T1—Flexor digiti minimi		Ulnar						
					T1—Abductor digiti minimi		Ulnar						

Manual Muscle Testing Record (continued)

Upper Limbs

Name: _____

LEFT						RIGHT	
			EXAMINER				
			DATE				
			Upper Limb C7—Extensor digiti minimi Radial				

Manual Muscle Testing Record (continued)

Lower Limbs

LEFT					**RIGHT**		
			EXAMINER				
			DATE				
			Lower Limb				
			L1–2—Iliopsoas	Spinal nerve			
			L3–4—Rectus femoris	Femoral			
			L2–3—Sartorius	Femoral			
			S1 & S2—Gluteus maximus	Inferior gluteal			
			L5—Gluteus medius	Superior gluteal			
			L5—Gluteus minimus	Superior gluteal			
			L4–5—Tensor fasciae latae	Superior gluteal			
			L3—Adductor longus	Obturator			
			L3—Adductor brevis	Obturator			
			L3–4—Adductor magnus	Obturator and tibial			
			L2—Gracilis	Obturator			
			L4–S2—Lateral rotators				
			S1—Biceps femoris				
			Long head	Tibial			
			Short head	Peroneal			
			L5–S1—Semitendinosus	Tibial			
			L5–S1—Semimembranosus	Tibial			
			L3 & L4—Quadriceps	Femoral			
			L5–S2—Gastrocnemius	Tibial			
			L5–S2—Soleus	Tibial			
			L5–S2—Gastrocnemius	Tibial			
			L5–S2—Soleus	Tibial			
			L5–S2—Soleus	Tibial			
			L5–S2—Soleus	Tibial			

Name: _____

Manual Muscle Testing Record (continued)

Lower Limbs

Name: _____

LEFT					RIGHT		
			EXAMINER				
			DATE				
			Lower Limb				
			St. L4—Tibialis anterior	Deep peroneal			
			L4 & L5—Tibialis posterior	Tibial			
			L5–S1—Peroneus longus	Superficial peroneal			
			L5–S1—Peroneus brevis	Superficial peroneal			
			S1–2—Lumbricals	Tibial			
			S3—Flexor hallucis brevis	Medial plantar			
			S2—Flexor hallucis longus	Tibial			
			S3—Flexor digitorum brevis	Medial and lateral plantar			
			S2—Flexor digitorum longus	Tibial			
			S1 & S2—Extensor hallucis brevis	Deep peroneal			
			L5–S1—Extensor hallucis longus	Deep peroneal			
			S1 & S2—Extensor digitorum brevis	Deep peroneal			
			L5–S1—Extensor digitorum longus	Deep peroneal			
			L5–S1—Abductor hallucis	Medial plantar			
			L5–S2—1st Lumbrical	Medial plantar			
			L5–S2—2nd, 3rd & 4th lumbricals	Lateral plantar			
			S1–S2—Adductor hallucis	Lateral plantar			
			S1–S2—Abductor digiti minimi	Lateral plantar			
			S1–S2—Dorsal interossei	Lateral plantar			
			S1–S2—Plantar interossei	Lateral plantar			

COMMENTS: _____
_____
_____

Functional Muscle Testing Record

Name: _____

LEFT						RIGHT					
					EXAMINER						
					DATE						
					Shoulder Muscles						
					Flexors						
					Extensors						
					Abductors						
					Adductors						
					Medial rotators						
					Lateral rotators						
					Scapula Muscles						
					Elevators						
					Depressors						
					Abductors						
					Adductors						
					Elbow Muscles						
					Flexors						
					Extensors						
					Radioulnar Muscles						
					Supinators						
					Pronators						
					Wrist Muscles						
					Flexors						
					Extensors						
					Abductors						
					Adductors						
					Thumb Muscles						
					Flexors						
					Extensors						
					Abductors						
					Opponens						

Functional Muscle Testing Record (continued)

Name: _____

		LEFT					RIGHT			
					EXAMINER					
					DATE					
					Finger Muscles					
					Flexors					
					Extensors					
					Abductors					
					Adductors					
					Neck Muscles					
					Flexors					
					Extensors					
					Rotators					
					Lateral flexors					
					Trunk Muscles					
					Flexors					
					Extensors					
					Rotators					
					Lateral flexors					
					Hip Muscles					
					Flexors					
					Extensors					
					Abductors					
					Adductors					
					Medial rotators					
					Lateral rotators					
					Knee Muscles					
					Flexors					
					Extensors					

Functional Muscle Testing Record (continued)

LEFT							RIGHT					
						EXAMINER						
						DATE						
						Ankle Muscles						
						Dorsiflexors						
						Plantar flexors						
						Invertors						
						Evertors						
						Toe Muscles						
						Flexors						
						Extensors						

Comments: _____

_____

_____

_____

_____

Key:
F: Functional—Able to complete maximal number of repetitions
          or distance in a coordinated, timely manner.

FF: Functionally Fair—Able to complete half the repetitions or distance.
               Movements may be slightly uncoordinated or take
               longer to perform than they normally would.

FP: Functionally Poor—Able to complete less than half the number of repetitions
               or distance. The activity may be uncoordinated
               or require extended time.

NF: Nonfunctional—Unable to complete one repetition.

Postural Assessment Record

Standing—Posterior View

NAME _____

AGE _____ HANDEDNESS _____

LEFT   RIGHT

			EXAMINER			
			DATE			
			Head and Neck Head tilt			
			Head rotated			
			Shoulder Dropped			
			Elevated			
			Medially rotated			
			Abduction (valgum)			
			Scapula Adducted			
			Abducted			
			Winged			
			Trunk Scoliosis			
			Pelvis Lateral tilt			
			Rotated			
			Hip Abduction (valgum)			
			Adduction (varum)			
			Knee Genu varum			
			Genu valgum			
			Ankle and Foot Pes planus			
			Pes cavus			

COMMENTS: _____

_____

_____

Check (✔) each box where a postural fault exists.

Postural Assessment Record (continued)

Standing—Anterior View

NAME _____

AGE _____ HANDEDNESS _____

	LEFT				RIGHT		
				EXAMINER			
				DATE			
				Head and Neck Lateral tilt			
				Rotated			
				Mandibular asymmetry			
				Shoulder Dropped			
				Elevated			
				Elbow Cubitus valgus			
				Cubitus varus			
				Hip Laterally rotated			
				Medially rotated			
				Knee External tibial torsion			
				Internal tibial torsion			
				Ankle and Foot Hallux valgus			
				Claw toes			
				Hammer toes			

COMMENTS: _____

_____

_____

_____

Check (✔) each box where a postural fault exists.

Postural Assessment Record (continued)

Standing—Lateral View

LEFT				RIGHT		
			EXAMINER			
			DATE			
			Head and Neck Forward head			
			Flattened lordosis			
			Excessive lordosis			
			Shoulder Forward			
			Tight thoracolumbar fascia			
			Thorax and Chest Kyphosis			
			Pectus excavatum			
			Barrel			
			Pectus cavinatum			
			Lumbar Lordosis			
			Sway back			
			Flat back			
			Pelvis and Hip Anterior tilt			
			Posterior tilt			
			Knee Genu recurvatum			
			Flexed			
			Ankle Forward posture			

NAME _____

AGE _____   HANDEDNESS _____

COMMENTS: _____

_____

_____

_____

Check (✔) each box where a postural fault exists.

Postural Assessment Record (continued)

Sitting on Hands and Knees

NAME _____

AGE _____ HANDEDNESS _____

	LEFT						RIGHT	
				EXAMINER				
				DATE				
				Sitting Posterior pelvic tilt				
				Anterior pelvic tilt				
				Hands and Knees Winged scapula				
				Trunk Lumbar lordosis				
				Thoracic kyphosis				
				Rotated				
				Laterally flexed				
				Hip Decreased flexion				
				Increased flexion				
				Rotated				
				External tibial torsion				
				Ankle and Foot Dorsiflexed				
				Inverted				
				Everted				

COMMENTS: _____

_____

_____

_____

_____

Check (✔) each box where a postural fault exists.

Postural Assessment Record (continued)

Standing on One Foot

LEFT				RIGHT		
			EXAMINER			
			DATE			
			Hip Lateral tilt			
			Trunk Excessive lateral shift			
			Ankle/Foot Pronation/supination			

NAME _____

AGE _____ HANDEDNESS _____

COMMENTS: _____

_____

_____

_____

Check (✔) each box where a postural fault exists.

Gait Assessment Record

NAME _____			AGE _____			
			EXAMINER _____			

EVALUATE WITH SUBJECT WALKING

LEFT				RIGHT		
			DATE			
			Stride Unequal length			
			Slow cadence			
			Short stance			
			Head Forward flexed			
			Deviated laterally			
			Shoulders Nonreciprocal arm swing			
			Unequal arm swing			
			Trunk Forward flexed			
			Deviated laterally			
			Pelvis Excessive rotation			
			Excessive lateral tilt			
			Excessive posterior tilt			
			Excessive anterior tilt			
			Hips Medially rotated			
			Laterally rotated			
			Abducted			
			Adducted			
			Flexed			

Gait Assessment Record (continued)

			Knees Hyperextended			
			Restricted extension			
			Exaggerated flexion			
			Genu valgum			
			Genu varum			
			Ankles Exaggerated preswing			
			Decreased preswing			
			Foot slap			
			Foot drop			
			Excessive dorsiflexion			
			Feet Pes planus			
			Pes cavus			

SUMMARY OF GAIT DEVIATIONS: _____

_____

_____

_____

_____

Check (✔) each box where a gait deviation exists.

Appendix B: Examination Questions

Choose the one best answer to each question.

Chapter 2

1. Three criteria are essential for an accurate muscle test. One of these, validity, requires that "you test what you claim to be testing." How can you best ensure that your muscle test is valid?

   a. Follow the standard procedure for test positions.
   b. Compare the involved side with the normal side.
   c. Repeat the test several times.
   d. Be aware of substitutions and prevent them.

2. Maximal strength of a muscle at a given joint is greater when the muscle contraction is _____.

   a. isometric.
   b. concentric.
   c. eccentric.
   d. isotonic.

3. Resistance applied to a muscle containing predominantly type I muscle fibers is:

   a. greater than that applied to type II muscle.
   b. less than that applied to type II muscle.
   c. the same as that applied to type II muscle.
   d. generally not applied.

4. The force of gravity has the greatest leverage and therefore is able to produce the greatest torque on the body segment when the segment is:

   a. at a 90-degree angle to the joint.
   b. horizontal.
   c. in the anatomical position.
   d. at a 45-degree angle to the joint.

5. Which position of the hip would produce active insufficiency of the hamstrings?

   a. Flexion.
   b. Extension.
   c. Abduction.
   d. Lateral rotation.

6. Muscles that are able to retain a favorable length through a large range allowing the rate of shortening to be less are:

   a. one-joint muscles.
   b. two-joint muscles.
   c. fusiform muscles.
   c. penniform muscles.

7. A person is sitting with the knee flexed 60 degrees. When the knee is extended to 0 degrees, the rotatory component of the force of gravity on the leg _____.

   a. increases.
   b. decreases.
   c. remains the same.

8. A therapist begins testing a subject who is lying supine. The subject can abduct the hip several times without difficulty. What should the therapist do next?

   a. Apply resistance to the distal end of the femur.
   b. Assign a grade of 2 (Poor).
   c. Repeat the test with the patient in the sidelying position.
   d. Apply resistance above the lateral malleolus.

9. When utilizing the break test in muscle testing, resistance should be applied _____.

   a. at the beginning of the range.
   b. at the end of the range.
   c. at the strongest point in the range.
   d. anywhere within the range.

10. Which of the following must be true of a subject before a manual muscle test can be performed?

    a. The subject has voluntary control of the muscles and can understand the therapist's instructions.
    b. The subject has normal range of motion and is free of pain.
    c. The subject has normal strength on one side for comparison with the involved side.
    d. If the subject has partial nerve or muscle trauma, the pattern of injury can be anticipated.

11. Which of the following grades is assigned to a muscle that is able to hold against the resistance of the examiner?

    a. Fair +.
    b. Fair.
    c. Fair −.
    d. Poor +.

12. When is a gross muscle test preferable to a specific muscle test?

    a. When the subject's muscles are too weak to take resistance.
    b. When the subject cannot be positioned correctly for a specific test.
    c. When a surgeon wants to know the strength of a muscle prior to a muscle transfer.
    d. When the therapist does not remember how to perform a specific test.

13. Which of the following statements are true? Goniometric measurements should be taken at the end of the range of motion because _____ .
    1. external landmarks for the axis of motion may change as the joint is moved.
    2. accurate alignment of the goniometer is accomplished with greater ease when the parts are stationary.
    3. accurate alignment of the lever arms with skeletal segments localizes the axis of motion.

    a. 1 only is correct.
    b. 1 and 3 are correct.
    c. 1, 2, and 3 are correct.
    d. 1 and 2 are correct.

14. Which of the following statements are true? In order to measure joint range of motion, the goniometer must be aligned with the _____ .
    1. axis of the joint.
    2. skeletal segments on either side of the joint.
    3. midline of the body part on either side of the joint.

    a. 1 only is correct.
    b. 1 and 3 are correct.
    c. 1, 2 and 3 are correct.
    d. 1 and 2 are correct.

15. The preferred position of the subject when taking goniometric measurements is supine in the anatomical position because _____ .

    a. the end range is assisted by gravity.
    b. a concentric contraction is easily performed.
    c. the joint is in a closed-packed position.
    d. the two joint muscles are relaxed.

16. Functional muscle assessment of the hip extensor muscles when going from a standing to a sitting position would demonstrate what type of contraction?

    a. Isometric.
    b. Concentric.
    c. Eccentric.
    d. Synergistic.

17. What functional muscle assessments would be performed with the subject in the standing position?

    a. Shoulder flexion, scapular downward rotation, ankle dorsiflexion.
    b. Scapular abduction, hip extension, ankle dorsiflexion.
    c. Elbow extension, hip extension, trunk flexion.
    d. Ankle plantar flexion, elbow flexion, wrist flexion.

18. All of the following are inert structures *except* _____ .

    a. nerves.
    b. cartilage.
    c. tendon.
    d. capsule.

19. Passive range of motion testing for assessment of inert structures will be positive for contractile involvement only when _____ .

    a. contractile elements are being shortened passively.
    b. contractile elements are being lengthened passively.
    c. the lesion is located at the periosteal attachment of the tendon.
    d. Passive testing assesses only inert structures.

20. From most to least restricted, the capsular pattern of the shoulder is _____ .

    a. external rotation, abduction, internal rotation.
    b. abduction, internal rotation, external rotation.
    c. abduction, external rotation, internal rotation.
    d. external rotation, internal rotaton, abduction.

Chapter 3

21. Which postural faults are examined from a lateral view with the subject standing?

    a. Forward shoulders, lumbar lordosis, and anterior pelvic tilt.
    b. Lumbar lordosis, dropped shoulder, and coxa vara.
    c. Anterior pelvic tilt, coxa vara, and genu recurvatum.
    d. Genu recurvatum, pes planus, and external tibial torsion.

22. Tightness of the iliotibial band may cause _____.

    a. genu varum.
    b. coxa valga.
    c. external tibial torsion.
    d. lateral pelvic tilt.

23. Excessive pelvic rotation during ambulation may be caused by _____.

    a. tightness in the hamstring muscles.
    b. decrease in ankle dorsiflexion.
    c. tightness of the hip flexor muscles.
    d. weakness of the trunk flexors.

24. Femoral anteversion may lead to _____.

    a. hip lateral rotation.
    b. hip abduction.
    c. limited knee extension.
    d. genu valgum.

Chapter 4

25. When testing the lower trapezius muscle, a grade of 2 (Poor) should be given when a subject _____.

    a. lifts the affected limb through partial range of motion and takes minimal resistance.
    b. lifts the affected limb through full range of motion but is unable to take resistance.
    c. is unable to lift the affected limb, but palpation reveals contraction of the muscle and scapular movement.
    d. raises the affected limb through full range of motion and takes minimal resistance.

26. What shoulder motion is the best to use to test the anterior deltoid muscle?

    a. Medial rotation.
    b. Horizontal abduction.
    c. Shoulder abduction.
    d. Shoulder flexion.

27. All of the following may be tested in a gravity-minimized sitting position *except* the _____.

    a. upper trapezius.
    b. serratus anterior.
    c. rhomboids.
    d. posterior deltoid.

28. Where is the best place to palpate the teres major muscle?

    a. Posterior border of the axilla.
    b. Deep in the axilla.
    c. Immediately inferior to the spine of the scapula.
    d. the midaxillary line on the thorax.

29. Both the rhomboids and the middle trapezius muscles are tested as adductors of the scapula and may easily be confused. When testing the rhomboids how should you position the subject's shoulder to give the rhomboids an advantage over the middle trapezius?

    a. In 90 degrees of abduction.
    b. In adduction.
    c. In 90 degrees of flexion with the elbow flexed.
    d. In medial rotation.

30. Where is resistance applied when testing the rhomboid muscles?

    a. On the vertebral border of the scapula, pushing the scapula into abduction and upward rotation.
    b. On the spine of the scapula, pushing the scapula into abduction and elevation.
    c. On the axillary border of the scapula, pushing the scapula into adducton and downward rotation.
    d. On the flexor surface of the wrist, pushing downward.

31. Which of the following shoulder muscles can be tested against gravity with the subject in the supine position?

 a. Serratus anterior, upper trapezius, anterior deltoid.
 b. Serratus anterior, anterior deltoid, pectoralis major.
 c. Pectoralis major, teres major, middle deltoid.
 d. Anterior deltoid, middle deltoid, serratus anterior.

32. What muscle is being tested when the subject lies prone with the shoulder abducted 135 degrees and raises the upper limb?

 a. Lower trapezius.
 b. Middle trapezius.
 c. Latissimus dorsi.
 d. Posterior deltoid.

33. What muscles are being evaluated when the strength of lateral rotation is tested?

 a. Posterior deltoid and teres major.
 b. Infraspinatus and teres minor.
 c. Subscapularis and supraspinatus.
 d. Latissimus dorsi and pectoralis major.

34. Hawkins test at the shoulder is an impingement test for assessing the _____.

 a. long head of the biceps tendon.
 b. short head of the biceps tendon.
 c. infraspinatus muscle.
 d. supraspinatus muscle.

35. All ot the following are clinical tests for shoulder subluxation *except* _____.

 a. Yergason's test.
 b. the posterior apprehension test.
 c. the anterior apprehension test.

36. Contractile testing of shoulder flexion assesses _____.

 a. the biceps brachii.
 b. the anterior deltoid.
 c. the supraspinatus.
 d. a and b.
 e. All of the above.

Chapter 5

37. To obtain maximal contraction of the brachioradialis muscle as an elbow flexor, the best position for the forearm is _____.

 a. supinated.
 b. pronated.
 c. in mid-position.
 d. in any position.

38. The most common substitution for pronation of the forearm is _____.

 a. lateral flexion of the trunk to the same side.
 b. lateral flexion of the trunk to the opposite side.
 c. abduction and lateral rotation of the shoulder.
 d. adduction and medial rotation of the shoulder.

39. If the subject is capable of 70 degrees of pronation and 85 degrees of supination, the total range of motion is _____.

 a. 15 degrees.
 b. 25 degrees.
 c. 75 degrees.
 d. 155 degrees.

40. Which muscle could flex the elbow if the three elbow flexors were *not* palpable?

 a. The pronator teres.
 b. The flexor pollicis longus.
 c. The supinator.
 d. The pronator quadratus.

41. Tinel's sign at the elbow is a clinical test for assessment of _____.

 a. median nerve involvement.
 b. ulnar nerve involvement.
 c. musculocutaneous nerve involvement.
 d. radial nerve involvement.

42. What tests other than flexion, extension, pronation, and supination should be performed as part of the assessment of inert structures around the elbow?

 a. Tinel's sign.
 b. The valgus stress test.
 c. The varus stress test.
 d. All of the above.

enervation of the musculocutaneous nerve would result in the following contractile finding when assessing elbow flexion:

a. Strong and painful.
b. Weak and painful.
c. Weak and pain-free.
d. Strong and pain-free.

Chapter 6

44. When testing the strength of the wrist extensors, the subject's fingers must be relaxed to prevent _____.

a. active insufficiency of the long finger extensors.
b. substitution by the tenodesis action of the extensor digitorum.
c. passive insufficiency of the flexor digitorum profundus.
d. substitution by the extensor digitorum.

45. A subject who lacks an opponens pollicis and an abductor pollicis brevis muscle is nevertheless able to touch the tip of the thumb to the tip of the little finger. What muscle is substituting for them?

a. Opponens digiti minimi.
b. Abductor pollicis longus.
c. Adductor pollicis.
d. Flexor pollicis brevis.

46. Which of the following is true of goniometry of wrist radial deviation?

a. The axis of the goniometer is placed over the pisiform bone.
b. The stationary arm of the goniometer is placed along the midline of the dorsum of the forearm.
c. The moving arm of the goniometer is placed along the midline of the dorsum of the third finger.
d. Radial deviation at the wrist is also referred to as adduction of the wrist.

47. What is the best way to prevent the flexor digitorum profundus muscle from substituting for the flexor digitorum superficialis muscle?

a. Allow motion to occur only at the distal interphalangeal joint.
b. Stabilize the metacarpophalangeal joint of the finger being tested in extension.
c. Stabilize in full extension the fingers not being tested.
d. Palpate the tendon of the flexor digitorum superficialis on the palmar surface of the proximal phalanx.

48. Which combination of symptoms indicates injury to the median nerve?

a. The middle and index fingers lose the ability to flex and the thumb cannot adduct or extend.
b. The ring and little fingers lose the ability to flex, and the little finger cannot abduct or oppose.
c. The inability of the wrist and fingers to extend interferes with grasp.
d. The middle and index fingers lose their ability to flex, and the thumb cannot oppose.

49. Finkelstein's test is designed to assess involvement of which of the following contractile structures?

a. Extensor pollicis longus and abductor pollicis brevis muscles.
b. Extensor pollicis brevis and abductor pollicis longus muscles.
c. Extensor pollicis longus and abductor pollicis longus muscles.
d. Extensor pollicis brevis and abductor pollicis brevis muscles.

50. All of the following are tests used in the diagnosis of carpal tunnel *except* _____.

a. Tinel's sign.
b. Phalen's test.
c. the three-jaw chuck test.
d. Allen test.

51. The Brunnell–Littler test is a test of _____.

a. all hand intrinsics.
b. the interossei.
c. the lumbricals.
d. the flexor retinaculum.

Chapter 7

52. Which motion can best be measured with a gravity or bubble goniometer?

    a. Neck rotation.
    b. Trunk flexion.
    c. Trunk rotation.
    d. Neck flexion.

53. A normal range of motion for neck flexion measured with a bubble goniometer is approximately _____.

    a. 40 degrees.
    b. 70 degrees.
    c. 100 degrees.
    d. 140 degrees.

54. The alar ligament test assesses stability of the _____.

    a. atlas.
    b. axis.
    c. C3 spinal segment.
    d. occiput on the atlas.

55. What is the position of the head and neck for the vertebral artery test?

    a. Flexion and rotation.
    b. Flexion and sidebend.
    c. Extension and rotation.
    d. Uniplanar extension.

56. The femoral nerve stretch primarily assesses the _____.

    a. L3 nerve.
    b. L5 nerve.
    c. L4 nerve.
    d. L2 nerve.

Chapter 8

57. The facial nerve supplies all of the following muscles *except* the _____.

    a. buccinator.
    b. masseter.
    c. zygomaticus major.
    d. frontalis.

58. An examiner palpating the side of the nose would be feeling for contraction of the _____.

    a. corrugator.
    b. orbicularis oculi.
    c. orbicularis oris.
    d. procerus.

Chapter 9

59. Where do you apply resistance when testing the hip adductor muscles?

    a. Distal to the knee medially.
    b. Proximal to the ankle medially.
    c. Distal to the knee laterally.
    d. Proximal to the knee medially.

60. In what position would you place a subject to evaluate Fair + (3+) strength of the gluteus maximus muscle if there is a 30-degree hip flexion contracture?

    a. Sidelying, hip flexed 90 degrees.
    b. Prone, leaning over the edge of the table with the hips flexed.
    c. Prone, hip extended.
    d. Sitting, hips flexed 90 degrees.

61. Using a full-circle goniometer to measure the hip may produce an inaccurate measurement because _____.

    a. the scale on the full-circle goniometer is smaller and more difficult to read than that on other types.
    b. the scale on a full-circle goniometer requires the subtraction of the measured degrees of motion from 360 to obtain the correct measurement.
    c. the 360-degree goniometer does not allow accurate alignment of the axis because the treatment table is in the way.
    d. None of the above.

62. While you are muscle testing hip flexion in the sagittal plane, the subject moves the hip into abduction and lateral rotation. What muscle is the subject using?

    a. Tensor fasciae latae.
    b. Sartorius.
    c. Gluteus medius.
    d. Gluteus maximus.

63. When testing the rectus femoris muscle as a hip flexor, the best place to palpate is between which two muscles?

    a. Tensor fasciae latae and iliopsoas.
    b. Tensor fasciae latae and sartorius.
    c. Gluteus medius and sartorius.
    d. Sartorius and adductor longus.

64. When muscle testing for hip flexion, the pelvis is in _____.

    a. extension.
    b. anterior tilt.
    c. neutral position.
    d. posterior tilt.

65. The examiner evaluating joint range of motion must be aware that a common substitution for medial rotation of the hip is _____.

    a. inversion of the foot on the test side.
    b. elevation of the buttocks on the "nontest" side.
    c. elevation of the buttocks on the test side.
    d. adduction of the hip on the test side.

66. In goniometry of the hip, for which measurement does the axis of the goniometer *not* fall in the vicinity of the greater trochanter?

    a. Flexion.
    b. Extension.
    c. Medial rotation.
    d. Hyperextension.

67. Thomas' test can be modified to test all the following *except* _____.

    a. rectus femoris muscle.
    b. iliopsoas muscle.
    c. tensor muscle.
    d. gluteus medius muscle.

68. A positive contractile test found in assessment of abduction may implicate all *except* the _____.

    a. tensor muscle.
    b. sartorius muscle.
    c. Iliopsoas muscle.
    d. gluteus medius muscle.

69. Which of these ranges of straight leg raising is considered within normal limits?

    a. Greater than 90 degrees.
    b. Greater than 80 degrees.
    c. Greater than 70 degrees.
    d. 60 to 70 degrees.

Chapter 10

70. Hip flexion may result when resistance is applied to the hamstring muscles during knee flexion because of _____.

    a. passive insufficiency of the hamstrings.
    b. active insufficiency of the hamstrings.
    c. imbalance of strength between hamstrings and quadriceps.
    d. tightness of the hip flexor musculature.

71. In the sitting position, tightness of the hamstrings is evident when the _____.

    a. pelvis remains in anterior tilt.
    b. low back maintains lordosis.
    c. fingers do not touch the toes.
    d. pelvis remains in posterior tilt.

72. The hamstring muscles could substitute for hip adduction if the hip is _____.

    a. medially rotated.
    b. flexed.
    c. laterally rotated.
    d. extended.

73. The starting position for muscle testing knee extension is with the hip _____.

    a. in a neutral position.
    b. flexed 45 degrees.
    c. flexed 90 degrees.
    d. extended.

74. Normal range of the **Q** angle in males is _____.

    a. 10 to 15 degrees.
    b. 15 to 20 degrees.
    c. 0 to 5 degrees.
    d. 5 to 10 degrees.

75. A finding of intense pain during contractile testing of knee extension may indicate _____.

    a. rupture of the quadriceps muscle.
    b. femoral nerve injury.
    c. patellar tendinitis.
    d. iliotibial band syndrome.

76. The most reliable test for anterior cruciate insufficiency is _____.

    a. Lachman's test.
    b. the anterior drawer test.
    c. the Slocum's test.
    d. the pivot shift.

Chapter 11

77. A substitution in muscle testing for ankle dorsiflexion and inversion is _____.

    a. action of the extensor digitorum longus and peroneus tertius muscles.
    b. quick dorsiflexion then relaxation.
    c. active contraction of the tibialis posterior muscle.
    d. active contraction of the tibialis posterior and extensor hallucis longus muscles.

78. Where would you palpate the tibialis posterior muscle?

    a. Anterior to the lateral malleolus.
    b. Anterior to the navicular.
    c. Posterior to the medial malleolus.
    d. Distal to the cuboid bone.

79. What would you evaluate to substantiate a deep peroneal nerve lesion if ankle dorsiflexion was not evident?

    a. Weakness of the peroneal muscles.
    b. Contraction of the extensor digitorum brevis.
    c. Sensory deficit medially on the leg.
    d. Decreased Achilles tendon reflex.

80. The most common substitution for ankle plantar flexion during goniometric measurement is _____.

    a. forefoot flexion.
    b. inversion.
    c. eversion.
    d. supination.

81. In measuring ankle dorsiflexion, the moving arm of the goniometer is placed parallel to the _____.

    a. midline of the first metatarsal.
    b. bottom of the heel on the plantar side.
    c. dorsal midline of the second metatarsal.
    d. lateral midline of the fifth metatarsal.

82. The varus stress test of the ankle assesses the integrity of all of the following ligaments *except* the _____.

    a. tibiofibular ligament.
    b. calcaneofibular ligament.
    c. anterior talofibular ligament.
    d. posterior talofibular ligament.

83. Feiss line uses the following bone as a reference to assess pronation grossly:

    a. cuboid.
    b. calcaneus.
    c. navicular.
    d. talus.

84. Thompson's test is designed to detect which of the following dysfunctions?

    a. Laxity of the talocrural joint.
    b. Rupture of the Achilles tendon.
    c. Hindfoot pronation.
    d. Active insufficiency of the gastrocsoleus complex.

Answers to Examination Questions

Chapter 2

1. d
2. c
3. a
4. b
5. b
6. b
7. a
8. c
9. b
10. a
11. a
12. b
13. c
14. d
15. a
16. c
17. c
18. c
19. b
20. a

Chapter 3

21. a
22. b
23. c
24. d

Chapter 4

25. c
26. d
27. a
28. a
29. d
30. a
31. b
32. a
33. b
34. a
35. a
36. d

Chapter 5

37. b
38. b
39. d
40. a
41. b
42. d
43. c

Chapter 6

44. d
45. d
46. b
47. d
48. d
49. b
50. d
51. c

Chapter 7

52. d
53. b
54. b
55. c
56. a

Chapter 8

57. b
58. d

Chapter 9

59. d
60. b
61. c
62. b
63. b
64. d
65. c
66. d
67. d
68. c
69. b

Chapter 10

70. b
71. d
72. c
73. b
74. a
75. c
76. a

Chapter 11

77. d
78. c
79. d
80. a
81. d
82. a
83. c
84. b

Index

Page numbers followed by an *f* indicate figures; *t* following a page number indicates tabular material.

367